Third Edition

Appraisal and Diagnosis of Speech and Language Disorders

HAROLD A. PETERSON, Ph.D.
University of Tennessee

THOMAS P. MARQUARDT, Ph.D.
University of Texas

 Prentice Hall, Englewood Cliffs, New Jersey 07632

Library of Congress Cataloging-in-Publication Data

Peterson, Harold A., (date)
  Appraisal and diagnosis of speech and language disorders / Harold
A. Peterson, Thomas P. Marquardt.—3rd ed.
    p.   cm.
  Includes bibliographical references and indexes.
  ISBN 0-13-200149-7
  1. Speech disorders—Diagnosis.   2. Language disorders—Diagnosis.
I. Marquardt, Thomas P.   II. Title.
  [DNLM: 1. Language Disorders—diagnosis.   2. Speech Disorders—
diagnosis.   3. Speech Articulation Tests.   4. Language tests.   WM
475 P485a   1994]
RC423.P47   1994
616.85′5075—dc20
DNLM/DLC
for Library of Congress   93-33657
                                                              CIP

Acquisitions editor: Charlyce Jones Owen
Editorial assistant: Caffie Risher
Editorial/production supervision and
    interior design: Linda B. Pawelchak
Cover design: Amigo Design
Production coordinator: Mary Ann Gloriande

 © 1994, 1990, 1981 by Prentice-Hall, Inc.
A Paramount Communications Company
Englewood Cliffs, New Jersey 07632

Printed in the United States of America
10 9 8 7 6 5 4 3 2 1

ISBN 0-13-200149-7

Prentice-Hall International (UK) Limited, *London*
Prentice-Hall of Australia Pty. Limited, *Sydney*
Prentice-Hall Canada Inc., *Toronto*
Prentice-Hall Hispanoamericana, S.A., *Mexico*
Prentice-Hall of India Private Limited, *New Delhi*
Prentice-Hall of Japan, Inc., *Tokyo*
Simon & Schuster Asia Pte. Ltd., *Singapore*
Editora Prentice-Hall do Brasil, Ltda., *Rio de Janeiro*

This edition is dedicated to the memory of

Sol Adler

a friend, a colleague, and an advocate of children's use of the language of their culture

Contents

5   Language Testing   111

6   Evaluation of Uncertainty: Developmental Skills, Motor Skills, and Nonverbal Intelligence   161

Part Three

Preface

*Our ignorance is never so clearly shown up by our inability to explain exist-
ing facts, as it is by specious explanations of imaginary phenomena. In other
words, not only do we lack principles for arriving at the truth, but we hold
others that enable us to commit errors.*

Fontanelle
Histoire des Oracles

The scope of practice in speech-language pathology has changed dramatically
since the authors of this text began their professional careers. Work settings that
include contact with populations of infants and preschoolers, hospital nurseries for
at-risk infants and well-baby clinics, hospital operating rooms and trauma centers,
rehabilitation centers, nursing homes and home health care, and school settings and
speech and hearing clinics often require highly specialized equipment and expertise. Electronically assisted measurement devices, viewing and imaging equipment
that were exotic only a generation ago, may now be accepted as standard.

Even with this diversity of clinical settings, what has remained constant is the
task of the speech-language diagnostician—the obligation to observe and describe

speech and language behavior, the anatomic (physical/neurological) capabilities and/or limitations, and to make judgments as to what can/should be done about the presenting behaviors. We won't always be sure—we won't always know the variables behind a problem and the most efficient intervention. Occasionally what we "know" may be wrong. We must be prepared to learn from the patients as well as from our mentors.

Our task with this text is to present the philosophy of appraisal and diagnosis, which is that you must know what it is you want to know before selecting a test protocol. That is the first requirement, the *sine qua non*. The next step is to decide whether the available devices provide valid measurements and if they are sufficiently reliable for your descriptive purposes.

HAP
TPM

1

The Philosophy of Diagnosis

It is the customary fate of new truths to begin as heresies and end as superstitions.

T. H. Huxley

The appraisal and diagnosis of speech and language disorders are primarily descriptive tasks. An adequate description should define the speech and language skills observed, judge the communication ability, determine the relevant variables in the speaker, and make obvious a plan of action for remediation if warranted. Consequently, before discussing the specifics of speech and language description, it is appropriate that we first concern ourselves with the philosophical basis for testing, test construction, and the concept of "normal." Those three variables are inexorably bound. Your philosophical basis for testing will flavor your test selection, and your definition of normal will be some function of the test content and format you choose. We will comment on the need for nonformalized as well as formalized assessment procedures and briefly discuss ethics and responsibilities involved with the diagnostician's task.

APPRAISAL AND DIAGNOSIS

Before we continue, we need to define two terms—*appraisal* and *diagnosis*—and the way in which we will use them. *Appraisal* implies calibrated observation and measurement. Measurement requires obtaining direct quantitative data. Some of these data can be compared with published "norms"—some cannot. Diagnosis requires placing measurements and other observational data into context and perspective in order to decide whether a problem exists and to differentiate one problem from others that may have similar performance aspects. The diagnosis is then a function of the descriptions that we have collected, and not all of these descriptions will have been easily quantifiable.

Some of the tests we discuss in the ensuing chapters are identified as "diagnostic" and others as "screening." The term "diagnostic" used in this way is a misnomer. No single test, apart from the case history and other significant observational descriptions, can be diagnostic by itself. The term is intended to denote those instruments that provide more detailed observations.

THE NEED TO BE DESCRIPTIVE

Test constructions change over time, just as theories change. A new theory is proposed when, in the mind of the theorist, the previous explanation was incomplete. Tests are constructed to fit theoretical biases and to calibrate specific types of observations. More important than the specific tests we select to use as observational tools is our clear understanding of the behavior we set out to describe. The assignment of terms, such as "stuttering" or "aphasia," or "learning disability," is not a description but an abbreviation for a constellation of behaviors. Terms or categories such as these may be helpful for filing purposes, but they do not describe what the person does or does not do. Call this the first law of diagnostics: *Describe the behavior.* If you cannot describe it, you do not understand it; or, you cannot expect to understand the behavior if you cannot describe it. Description does not guarantee understanding, but description makes understanding possible.

This emphasis on description is important whether or not we can use "standardized" tests to aid our observation. It becomes increasingly important when, as speech-language clinicians,[1] we are called upon to evaluate "special" populations such as nonverbal or language-delayed children or those who are referred to us as learning disabled. With a great number of these children, test results may be inaccurate or even misleading. Muma (1973) has stressed the point that standardized assessment procedures by themselves will not usually yield an adequate description of language function. In his *Language Handbook* (1978), he makes a stronger statement:

> Behavior is relative, conditional, complex, and dynamic. Accordingly, clinical assessment must be relative, contextual, process oriented, and dynamic. Contrary to some views, it should not be categorical, quantitative, or normative. These three traditional

[1]The word "clinician" as used here is not in contrast to "therapist" or "pathologist" or similar terms but is a generic term to denote one who works in a clinical setting or is involved in clinical activity.

notions need to be challenged. Clinical assessment should be about an *individual* as he functions in natural contexts (Bronfenbrenner 1977) or deals with systems and processes directly relevant to natural behavior. (p. 211)

Siegel (1975) provided similar advice to clinicians:

In my mind, the best "instrument" available is a clinician who has some knowledge of research and theory in language, some experience in describing and dealing with important communication behaviors, and some reservoir of confidence in his or her own abilities to observe behavior, develop hypotheses, and change ideas and approaches when necessary. (p. 213)

Neither of these quotes denies the applicability of standardized testing—of formalized measures. They *do* remind the clinician of the importance of going beyond restricted, structured assessment techniques. Leonard and others (1978) extended Siegel's philosophy in an article about nonstandardized approaches to assessment, which they considered

. . . a necessary supplement to the use of standardized tests for the assessment of language behavior. We adopt the position that the use of nonstandardized measures is essential in gaining sufficient information about the child's linguistic system in order to devise effective intervention strategies. (p. 371)

In other words, we do need observations in addition to the standardized quantitative, normative comparisons. Normative comparisons are a function of controlled circumstances and can help us make a judgment of speech and language deviance. That is, we can compare how the patient at hand performed in relation to other patients of the same age with the same or comparable stimuli. They do not necessarily describe the communicative function of this person in his "natural" environment. The behavior we observe, in either a controlled or nonrestrictive circumstance, is only a sample from which inferences are made. It is never a complete description of all behavior under all conditions.

The formalized and nonformalized assessments we make are subject to interpretation, and that includes a judgment of communicative effectiveness within a situation. A determination of functional effectiveness requires at least the circumstance, or variety of circumstances, in which the child is attempting to communicate (Menyuk 1963, 1964; Sroufe 1970). What a child does, in other than imitative performance, may be taken as some evidence of linguistic competence, but lack of performance should not routinely be accepted as evidence of lack of competence (Cazden 1967).

Bloom and Lahey (1978) described three dimensions of language: content, form, and function. The bulk of the normative data that are available bear on language form. Form is described in terms of the acoustic-phonetic shape of segments of the utterance. In other words, quantitative comparisons are available for phonology, morphology, and syntax, but very few comparisons are available for content and function. Content refers to topics or concepts and the interaction between content and information processing. Language function judgments are concerned with the context or circumstances in which the utterances occur and may be methodically analyzed as in Searle's (1969) Speech Acts theory.

Searle separates the "speech act" intention and understanding into separate aspects to explain events: "The speaker means something; the sounds he emits mean something; the hearer understands what is meant; the speaker makes a statement, asks a question, or gives an order" (p. 3). To Searle these are the utterance act (the words produced); the propositional act (referring or predicating—basically the intent); the illocutionary act (stating, questioning); and the perlocutionary act (the effect on the actions and beliefs of the listener—a request is granted, an answer is given, etc.). These definitions bear on the "relative, conditional, complex and dynamic" behavior referred to by Muma and are part of the "knowledge of research and theory" required by Siegel.

We need to describe our subject's skill in speech and language in terms of overall communicative skill. Part of the task then is to decide if the behavior presented is normal. In order to make a judgment of normalcy, we need information on expected levels of performance or guidelines for comparison.

Test scores are not descriptions of behavior. A well-constructed set of test items is intended to provide information on what the subject can do. On the other hand, failure on a set of items may more accurately be a statement what she *did not* do rather than what she *cannot* do. The purpose of the normed test result is to allow a comparison of our client's test performance with the performance of similar individuals in similar circumstances.

Beyond the question of the test score, according to Salvia and Ysseldyke (1988), is what to do about it in terms of recommendation. Olswang and Bain (1991) posit two questions that they believe are crucial in attempting to identify when a child is likely to benefit from intervention. The first has to do with whether the child's language skills are commensurate with other aspects of development, and the second is whether the child demonstrates an immediate potential for change. The questions are concerned both with how the child compares with other children and how the child's speech-language skills compare with his other developmental skills. In other words, at times a chronological age (CA) comparison may be appropriate; and at other times, if we assume a cognitive variable, a mental age (MA) comparison may be appropriate. In order to put that caveat in perspective, we must first describe the concept of "normal."

THE CONCEPT OF NORMALCY

Our clinical task is to define a set of procedures that will help to separate "normal" from "abnormal" performance and to gather sufficient description to suggest what can be done about the problems we identify. A number or test score by itself is never an adequate description for our diagnostic task, but quantification is at least part of the requirement for making comparisons. Normal and abnormal are reciprocal terms and need clarification. For example, in a statistical or probability sense, normal means average. One such average that most of us are familiar with is the measurement of intelligence and the expected or average intelligence quotient (I.Q.) of 100. A "quotient" (proportional score) of 100 implies that the person tested performed no better and no worse than is expected for his age.

Two points should be made relative to an average score. One is that the practical interpretation of intelligence and similar scores considers average to be a range rather than a single point on the scale. The normal range on most intelligence tests, for example, the *Wechsler Intelligence Scale for Children–Revised* (1974) and the *Stanford-Binet Tests of Intelligence* (1960), is from 90 to 110, or one standard deviation on either side of the mean. The Wechsler and the Stanford-Binet tests have been constructed with one standard deviation equivalent to 10 points, and both consider a score between plus and minus two standard deviations (a score of 80 to 120) to be within gross normal limits. In other words, a score of 90 on one of these tests would be considered "average," and a score as low as 80 would be interpreted as "low average." A receptive vocabulary test, which we discuss in a later chapter, the *Peabody Picture Vocabulary Test–Revised* (Dunn and Dunn 1981), uses a standard deviation of 12 to 13 points with a standard mean score of 100. Consequently, gross normal limits of performance according to the Peabody test are from 75 to 125 for the plus or minus two standard deviation range.

The second point to be made concerning average scores is that the individuals who are measured should belong to the population with which they are compared. Again, using intelligence scores as an example, the mean or average I.Q. in a university class of undergraduate seniors would probably be between 115 and 120; the mean I.Q. in a grammar school in a low socioeconomic area may be between 90 and 95, and so forth. In general, a range of scores rather than a single score should be considered normal, and normal or average depends on the population used for comparison.

It is important to remember that statistical description based on quantified data does not carry with it a value judgment. Performance above or below some average value is not necessarily good, bad, or otherwise. This is true whether the statistical comparison we are using is concerned with height, weight, shoe size, words in a vocabulary, speech sounds correctly produced, or any other of the variety of behaviors, talents, or attributes available for measurement. A numerical value may be helpful information as part of our total description, but by itself, it only serves as an exemplar of a person's one-time measurement and comparison to a specific population on a described task. It has no intrinsic evaluation or judgmental connotation.

It is also important to point out that the intrinsic nature of the test has an important bearing on our interpretation of an individual's performance. Some measures, such as tests of achievement and intelligence, are designed to obtain a maximum performance. Results from these tests are determined by innate ability, learned ability, and motivation (Lyman 1986). Typical performance tests, in contrast, are used to obtain information on what the person tested typically does, rather than what she is capable of doing. Obviously, the distinction between what an individual *does do* in comparison to what she is *capable of doing* is an important one to remember when measuring performance.

At this point, we need to consider some statistical concepts. Our primary focus will be on central tendency and dispersion attributes of a "bell-shaped curve," or normal distribution (DuBois 1965). A distribution of this type is not found in test manuals because it is based on an infinite number of observations that vary randomly. However, given a large enough number of subjects, we might expect behavioral attributes to approximate this type of distribution. The normal distribution is central to our discussion because it has a number of important features.

Figure 1–1 illustrates the normal distribution of an attribute such as intelli-

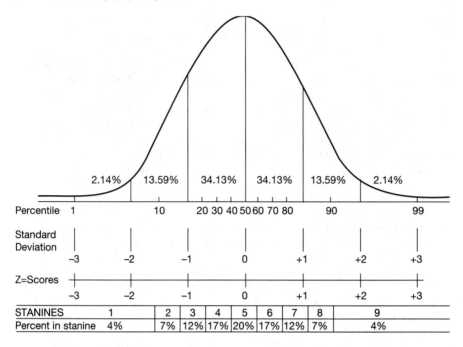

2.14%	13.59%	34.13%	34.13%	13.59%	2.14%		

Percentile	1	10	20 30 40 50 60 70 80	90	99

Standard Deviation	−3	−2	−1	0	+1	+2	+3

Z=Scores	−3	−2	−1	0	+1	+2	+3

STANINES	1	2	3	4	5	6	7	8	9
Percent in stanine	4%	7%	12%	17%	20%	17%	12%	7%	4%

FIGURE 1–1   Normal distribution curve showing expected proportion of the population within each area of the curve. Also shown with the standard scale divisions are approximate percentile rankings.

gence in a population. The highest point on the distribution is the mean (average score) and also the median (score at which 50 percent of the cases fall below and 50 percent fall above) and the mode (most frequent score). On other types of distributions, we might expect the measures of central tendency (mean, median, and mode) to be different values. In addition to the range of scores (difference between the highest and lowest scores), an important measure of variability is the standard deviation. The standard deviation is equal to the square root of the squared deviations from the mean of the distribution. This mathematical description may seem complex but is actually quite simple. If we determined the difference between each score and the mean, some would be positive and an equal number would be negative; adding them together would yield zero. To solve this problem, each difference between scores is squared to make all the numbers positive. The total difference between each score and the mean is divided by the total number of scores to find an average. The square root is then derived to neutralize the effect of having squared each number. The standard deviation is particularly important to our discussion because it is more stable than other estimates of variability and serves as the basis for standard scores.

Areas of the normal distribution curve in Figure 1–1 are sectioned off at equidistant intervals along the horizontal axis to indicate standard deviations. The relative fatness of the curve is intended to show the approximate proportion of the population in each of these sections. Approximate percentile rankings are also shown on the horizontal axis. For example, slightly more than 34 percent of the population is expected to score between the mean and the minus one standard deviation point. The midpoint on the horizontal axis is where 50 percent of the population should score higher and 50 percent should score lower. It is, therefore, the 50th percentile. Since 34.13 percent of the population is expected to fall within this range, the minus one standard deviation score is approximately at the 16th percentile. Similarly, the minus two standard deviation score is between the 2nd and 3rd percentile.

A percentile score is a relative ranking. If the child's score is at the 3rd percentile, then 97 children out of 100 are expected to do better. Don't confuse percentage and percentile because they are not the same thing. If a child responds correctly to 10 out of 20 items on a test, he has successfully completed 50 percent of the items. But if 90 out of 100 children his age respond correctly to more than 10 items, he is at the 10th percentile.

The bell-shaped curve is a random or probability distribution. If we were to measure some randomly distributed attribute in a large population of normal children, two-thirds of their scores would be within one standard deviation on either side of the mean, and approximately 95 in 100 would be within two standard deviations of the mean. If our criterion for "non-normal" performance was any score more than two standard deviations from the mean, we would expect to be correct in this assignment 95 times in 100 (or 19 times in 20), but we also have a statistical probability of being wrong in our determination one time in 20.

Z-scale. The z-scale is used to determine the difference between any score and the mean of the group and is computed by dividing the difference between a score and the group mean by the standard deviation. The scale has a mean of zero and a standard deviation of one with approximately one-half of the values positive and one-half negative. The practical value of the z-scale is that if you have several test scores for a child where the mean and standard deviation are known, the test scores can be converted to a common base for your comparison. That is, the z-scale scores, deviations from a standard base, would make for an easier interpretation than the raw scores.

Stanine. The stanine is similar to the standard deviation and is shown as marked intervals along the horizontal axis in Figure 1–1. "Stanine" is a term generated by Air Force psychologists during World War II (stanine = standard nine) and was used to represent bands of values. With the exception of the extreme stanines of 1 and 9, which are open-ended, each stanine is exactly one-half of a standard deviation in width. The mean of the stanine scale is 5, and the standard deviation is 2. Note that the 5th stanine straddles the 50th percentile point—or the mean of the normal distribution. The 5th stanine includes approximately 20 percent of the population (one-fourth standard deviation with approximately 10 percent of the population on each side of the midpoint on the standard distribution scale). The range of normal (2 standard deviations) on the stanine scale is from the limits of the third through the seventh stanines. If we add the proportions (20 percent for the fifth stanine, 17 percent each for the fourth and sixth, and 12 percent each for the third and seventh, for a total of 78 percent) of the population, then the range for "normal" is from approximately the 10th to the 90th percentile.

Standard Error of Measurement (SEM).   If a child completed the same test an infinite number of times and if we assumed no learning, we would expect that her scores would be normally distributed with the mean of this distribution equal to her *true* score and with a standard deviation estimated by the standard error of measurement. The SEM is related to the reliability of the test and is similar in size to the standard deviation of scores for the subjects used to standardize the measure. In general, the larger the population tested, the smaller the SEM. The reason for including the SEM is to provide an estimate of the range of scores that will include the true score of the child tested. Earlier, we mentioned the probability of a child's obtaining a score at one point on the scale, by chance, when she really should be at a different point on the scale. The true score range, or confidence band by this reasoning, is equal to the obtained score plus or minus the standard error of measurement.

An example may help to clarify this concept. The manual for the *Peabody Picture Vocabulary Test–Revised* (PPVT–R) (Dunn and Dunn 1981) lists specific SEM values according to age level ranges for both raw scores and standard scores for the two versions of the test. For standard score equivalents, the median value provided for the SEM for all ages is 7 points. This means that if the child we tested on the PPVT–R received a standard score equivalent of 95 on the first administration of the test, her true score is plus or minus 7 points from this number and is between 87 and 102.

Centering Tendency.   In the discussion of the normal distribution, the relative fatness in the middle of the bell-shaped curve implied that proportionally more of the population belonged near the midpoint than at the extremes of the scale. The idea of statistical centering suggests that if a child scored near the low end of the scale, on retest he may score relatively higher. If he scored at the high end of the scale, the probability is that he will score lower the next time we test him. The SEM values of different age groups for the PPVT–R are skewed to reflect this fact. The score sheet indicates that if the child's obtained score was 75, his true score is probably between 71 and 85—from 4 points lower to 10 points higher than the obtained score. (Remember that the 7-point SEM for the PPVT–R was symmetrical and based on results of subjects from all age groups.) This discussion on the range of expected score shift becomes more than academic when we interpret the significance of the child's score. Our best estimate of the child's performance is the score we obtained—equivalent to a standard score of 75 (5th percentile). This is a moderately low level of performance, but statistically his score could be as high as 85— approximately at the 15th percentile and nearer to the minus one standard deviation than to the minus two standard deviation point. Knowledge of the SEM obviously makes a difference in the judgment concerning intervention.

The important point we wish to stress is that caution must be used in interpreting a test score. As McCauley and Swisher (1984) point out, the use of a norm-referenced test for judgment of progress in therapy is risky because the test score may be interpreted as progress, or lack of progress, when it may instead reflect an error of measurement. The obtained score is the best estimate of the true score, but the probabilities are that the true score is in a range around the obtained value. Unfortunately, relatively few tests provide standard error information. Where possible, tests should be used that are constructed and normed to allow this interpretation. We can then treat the test score with a concern for the range of normal scores and the probable error of measurement.

Fey (1990) suggests that especially if you plan to use a test to measure the effectiveness of your intervention, your speech-language measurement device must have a reliability coefficient of at least 0.90. Correlation is not a measure of cause and effect but of relationship. The square of the correlation, called the "coefficient of determination," reports the common variance of the instruments being used. In other words, if the two measures have an $r = 0.90$, then approximately 80 percent ($.9 \times .9 = .81$) of the variability is captured in common by the measures—but 20 percent of the reason for variances is still not identified.

Age scores are particularly difficult to treat as comparative measures. They may have been determined as the average performance or where 80 percent of children of a given age performed on that particular test, but we do not know the range of normal scores on those measures. In that way, the relevance of age-referenced scores is difficult to interpret. Lawrence (1992) cautions that even "age-equivalent" derivations from standard tests are often misleading—and are certainly not appropriate for making clinical decisions or measuring clinical progress.

Some of the tests we discuss in later chapters specify a normal range of scores in terms of means and standard deviations, some in terms of percentile rankings and stanines, and some in neither. These comments on distribution scores will be of no particular value for the tests that use age scores and similar interpretative indices, except possibly as a reminder that they also should have a normal range (albeit unknown). For a large number of tests that use statistical interpretations, however, it is pertinent to note that at least part of the determination of normality or abnormality is based on a statistical or probability judgment, which also includes an estimate of probable error. From our earlier probability discussion, it is obvious that if we use the minus two standard deviation point (approximately 3rd percentile) as our criterion for abnormal we will be safer in our judgment (greater confidence level) than if our cutoff for normal is the 16th percentile (minus one standard deviation). The underlying assumption is that the test is well standardized, valid, and appropriate for the child tested. If the child tested speaks primarily Spanish and the test is in English, the deviation of the score has not occurred by chance.

A number of the tests that we review use percentile scores to separate normal from abnormal performance. At least some of the articulation tests we consider use the 16th percentile (one standard deviation below the mean) as the cutoff between "adequate" and "inadequate" articulation skill. Some of the language tests recommend the 10th percentile (two stanines or one and one-fourth standard deviations below the mean) to represent an important deviation that warrants further evaluation.

There are also criterion-referenced tests, for example, that may place a behavior at an age score at which 80 percent of the norming population was successful. This means that a child who did not adequately perform on the tested task could be at approximately the 20th percentile—a point within one standard deviation of the expected mean and therefore within normal limits.

The point we have been attempting to make in this discussion of statistical concepts is that "normal" is a range of scores on a probability curve. As clinicians, we should be aware of the relative value of the scores we use in making our normal and abnormal judgments. In terms of the probability of error in our scoring judgments, it would follow that "deviations" may be additive. That is, if the child scores below expected levels of performance on only one measure and related measures place him in the normal range, then two immediate choices are available. It may be that our first test result was spurious and we need an alternative and more detailed measure before making a judgment. It is, of course, also possible that there is a deficiency restricted to one aspect of behavior, which will need to be explored with additional testing.

Up to this point, we have discussed making judgments of normal or abnormal as if the next patient who walks through the doors of our clinic is a randomly selected individual from a normally distributed population and as if the probability of his performing within the normal range on a test we administer is high (approximately 95 out of 100 if we use the two standard deviation range or 80 out of 100 if we use the two stanine range). This is hardly the case. Quite obviously, patients come to clinics because they have a problem, and they come to speech, language, and hearing clinics because they have a communication problem. When tests of communicative functioning are administered, we expect that the patient will frequently perform outside the normal range if the tests selected are appropriate to the disorder demonstrated. This observation in no way diminishes the applicability of using statistical concepts to aid in making our decision, but it is noteworthy because communicatively impaired patients typically represent the lower end of the score distribution when speech and language skills are assessed. Finally, it should be pointed out that some tests use the performance of a sample from a communicatively impaired population to serve as the standardization group for the test. For example, tests for aphasia frequently provide norms based on a sample of aphasic subjects. It should be kept in mind then that our interpretation will be based on the reference group to which the patient is compared, a point to which we will soon return.

TESTS: STANDARDIZATION, VALIDITY, AND RELIABILITY

As you no doubt have gathered by now, tests are systematic procedures that yield a score. Two parts of this description are important. The procedures are *systematic* or *standardized* in terms of administration and scoring, and they yield a *score* that allows interpretation of the performance of the individual tested. Tests are important because they aid in making decisions, and if they do not aid in making decisions, then they are not worth the time and effort they require to administer and score (Nunnally 1972). On the other hand, many tests are objective and, therefore, may be of more value than our subjective impressions.

Standardization is the process by which the test or measurement device is administered to a sample from a population with specified physical (age, sex, etc.) and nonphysical (language exposure, socioeconomic status, etc.) characteristics according to specified explicit procedures. Data from the test administration can then be analyzed to determine the mean, standard deviation, and other statistical attributes of the obtained scores. In order to interpret the performance of a new subject by reference to these data, we must assume that the person in question is representative of the population, or at least very similar to the population from which the original sample was drawn and on which the test was standardized. In other words, the subjects within the sampled population must be similar in important respects to the average person in the standardization population. As we have noted, the characteristics of the sampled population utilized to standardize tests that purport to measure a variable may differ considerably. Whether or not you choose to use a particular test because of, or in spite of, the standardization population, it is important that you have a defensible rationale for your decision.

Other important considerations in choosing a measurement tool are the validity and reliability of the instrument. *Validity* is typically described as how well the test does what it purports to do. This is a circular definition analogous to defining a hammer as "something you hammer with" and a horse as "something you horse around with." It is a sufficient definition insofar as it utilizes function to make the meaning known. No test is ever completely valid, and tests are only valid to the extent that they serve their function. The primary functions of tests and the basis on which their validity is determined are prediction, assessment, and trait measurement (Nunnally 1972). These three functions are termed criterion-related validity, content validity, and construct validity.

Criterion-related or "predictive" validity concerns the effectiveness of the test in predicting the individual's behavior in specified situations external to the test (Anastasi 1968). For this purpose, performance on the test is correlated with the behavior to be predicted. One example of a test based on this type of validity is the *Predictive Screening Test of Articulation*, which uses articulatory performance at the first grade to predict whether the child will need therapeutic intervention or whether she will acquire articulatory proficiency without treatment by the third grade. Here performance on a test is used to make a decision regarding treatment. A second example relates to the use of tests to predict improved performance for the patient over time. The *Porch Index of Communicative Ability* uses the results of testing at one month to predict the performance of the patient at six months post onset of brain damage and, therefore, performs a prognostic function.

Content validity relates to the assessment function. It involves the careful inspection of the test items to determine if the test covers the behaviors that are to be measured. Rather than being predictive, it involves a sampling of the behaviors that reflect poor or good performance in a particular situation at a particular time (Nunnally 1972). It is not important that all possible content be integrated into the test items, only that the important behaviors are examined. For example, in an articulation test, various phonemes are tested but only in a limited number of contexts. The important behaviors evaluated are the phonemes. The contexts need not all be evaluated, only a representative number. Content validity is sometimes confused with "face" validity. Face validity is the superficial examination of items to assess whether the test items actually cover the behaviors that are to be measured. As such, face validity serves the important function of weeding out items that appear inappropriate, but it is not identical to content validity.

The *construct validity* of a test is the degree to which the test measures psychological traits (constructs). It requires the gradual accumulation of information from many sources. It is broader in scope than the other types of validity we have discussed. Nunnally (1972) has succinctly defined the process of establishing construct validity:

In essence, construct validation consists of weaving a network of meaningful relations between a new measure and other supposed measures of the same trait. If such relations hold, the new measure then can be trusted in subsequent use. If such relations do not hold, subsequent use of the instrument should be held suspect. (p. 33)

Two primary means used to establish construct validity are factor analysis (major factors and their weightings are used to account for the obtained test scores) and correlations with other tests (concurrent validity). An example of this process might be your development of a new test of aphasia. You select items that appear to measure behaviors typically associated with the disorder, administer the test to a sample of aphasic patients, and analyze the resultant test scores to determine the major factors (traits, constructs) that appear to account for the scores. A second procedure would be to correlate the scores with the scores from a second test of aphasia that is generally agreed to be valid. A high correlation would be indicative of good construct validity for your new test.

The validity of a test then depends upon its purpose; it may be highly valid for one purpose but not for another. This statement points out the fact that many tests serve more than a single function and may need to be validated for each of the purposes.

Reliability means repeatability and focuses on the issues of consistency of test scores and the precision of the test. The consistency of test results may be a function of the person being tested, of the test instrument, or of the tester. A test may be reliable without being valid, but a test cannot be valid unless it is reliable. For example, let us say that we want to determine the volume of liquid in a beaker that has been bent out of shape. If we had only a rubber ruler that stretched whenever we made a measurement, it would be neither reliable nor valid. If the ruler were stable, we could determine the height of the beaker in a reliable fashion, but we could not determine the volume of liquid in the beaker. If we now selected a cup, poured the liquid into the cup until filled, and repeated this process until all the liquid had been poured, we would have reliable and valid measures of the volume. This is so because the cup is a valid measure of volume, and the process of measurement could be repeated to demonstrate that we would come out with approximately the same number of cups of liquid every time we did so.

Several procedures are used to establish the reliability of a test, and they all involve correlation. One method is to examine the relationship of scores from two alternate forms of the same test administered to the same subjects. This *alternate-form reliability* is ideal because it examines all the sources of variability that can have an effect on test scores. A second procedure is the *test-retest reliability* method which involves administering the test to the same subjects at two different times. A third method, *split-half reliability*, involves, for example, the correlating of scores on the odd-numbered items from a test with the scores from the even-numbered items. This method generally overestimates the reliability of the test because there is no instability of the scores over time that would be entailed within alternate-form and test-retest reliability procedures. Consequently, measures of internal consistency, like the Kuder-Richardson formulas, are used. The Kuder-Richardson formulas estimate the reliabilities that would be obtained from all possible subdivisions of the test and examine the overlap or correlations between items of the test (Nunnally 1972).

In summary, the results obtained from the variety of tests and observations must be placed in context to interpret their relative importance. Each of the test scores is only a single index and is, therefore, not the whole picture of the patient. Moreover, the interpretation of results of each of the indices used is dependent on the appropriateness and the quality of the measuring instrument (and the skill of the test administrator). The second law of diagnostics might well be to *interpret each of the quantification numbers with caution.* Or, with data in hand, stand firmly with both feet about three inches off the ground. It is harder to jump to conclusions from that pose.

TESTING NONSTANDARD OR "SPECIAL" POPULATIONS

Earlier, in the section on reliability and validity, we discussed test selection in terms of whether the person to be tested should logically be compared with the population on which the test was standardized. A discrepancy would amount to a test bias. If the discrepancy between test subject and comparative population were not recognized, it could also be termed an examiner bias.

Our biases or our expectations can be a variable in test interpretation. For example, if our task is to screen the speech and language skills of the third grade of the local school, or the entire class of incoming freshman at a college or university, we may well expect to find 95 percent of the subject population to be normal as previously defined. When we, as speech-language clinicians, screen those children and adults who are referred to us because someone has been concerned about their speech, the statistics are more likely to be reversed. Our clinical biases tend to be more operative in one situation than in the other. This example is meant to imply a difference between clinical and statistical significance. Where the testing is done, with whom it is done, and the purpose for which it is done may affect our clinical judgment.

Our clinical expectations become an important variable when the population to be tested is culturally different from that which we usually see. Our intent in the speech and language screening is to make a judgment of the efficiency of the communication patterns displayed. Our implicit assumption is that we and the person we are judging share the same communication patterns—the same vocabulary and the same communicative intent. This is a markedly difficult assumption to make when the tester and the testee represent different cultures.

Because of obstacles that cultural barriers may raise, there is an expanding array of literature that questions the reliability and validity of test results obtained with culturally different children (for example, Adler 1971, 1973; Cazden 1970; Grimshaw 1969; Severson and Guest 1970). Most of the speech and language measures available have been standardized on middle-class children. Most have used restricted geographic samples. Weiner and Hoock (1973) have discussed the difficulty of standardization assumptions on some frequently used tests when used with the "standard" culture populations. Consider how much more confounded our "standardized" assumptions become with a population which has different culturally generated speech and language patterns.

Adler (1973) has listed some of the linguistic and nonlinguistic factors that may generate a bias against the culturally different child's performance, such as the tested items being outside the cultural experience of the child, the verbal style being culture-specific, or just the fact that the poor or rural or ethnic-culture child may be intimidated by the test situation. He reduced the array of specific impediments to two basic problems: motivation and communication. Adler stated that the safest assumption the examiner can make when testing a culturally different child is that it will be difficult to get the child to perform at her potential. Motivation implies a tangible reward but may also include an apparent interest and appreciation on the part of the examiner. Communication barriers may be obvious or may be more subtle. The examiner may not always know which words or syntactic structures used are culture-specific. Because of this uncertainty, Adler urges the examiner to be redundant in the presentation of test instructions and, whenever possible, to utilize a sufficient number of practice items to illustrate to the child what is expected. Put another way, a posttest performance of a child may reflect her better understanding of the task she is to perform as much as it represents her improved performance on the task itself.

Our basic purpose in an evaluation procedure is to measure the tools of communication and the subject's efficiency in using them. If we have not obtained the person's "best effort," our judgment of capability may be faulty. If the tasks or items we have used for evaluating her are not similar to what is used in her linguistic environment, we may not be measuring her "real" communicative efficiency. And, if the speech and language measures we are using are not appropriate to the population she represents, our judgment of what is expected behavior may be biased. In other words, what we perceive as "language deficiency" may instead be a "language difference." It may be assumed (Burling 1973; Wolfram and Fasold 1974; and others) that the "nonstandard dialect" is an equally well-formed and complex linguistic system. However, unless we understand the phonological structure, the grammar, and the function of the language we are listening to, we cannot judge the efficiency of the speaker's use of it.

There is a philosophy, expressed by some, that suggests that when testing minority children (culturally different, in the way we have used the term), we should measure them against a separate yardstick. For example, the *Denver Articulation Screening Exam* (Drumwright 1971) was constructed with norms for use with "culturally disadvantaged" rather than with the general population of children. Musselwhite (1983) reported "SES [socioeconomic status] related norms" for use with Carrow's (1973) *Test for Auditory Comprehension of Language*. With 299 Head Start children, 95 percent of whom were black, just over half (56 percent) scored more than one standard deviation below the middle SES mean, and 15 percent scored more than one standard deviation below the low SES mean.

De Avila and Havassy (1974), however, list three cautions relative to the development of "local" norms in the testing of these children. They believe that there is a risk for (1) developing lower expectations for certain ethnic-racial groups; (2) reducing children's aspirations to succeed, possibly as a result of lowered expectations; and (3) reinforcing the genetic-inferiority argument especially with regard to intelligence testing.

Both "local norms" and "general norms" would appear to have their place in the description of the child's performance. It may be useful to compare the child with a peer group for some purposes and to maintain the larger population comparison for other purposes.

Related to the cultural difference notion, there is some expressed concern that materials used in testing may be racially biased or that a disparity of race between examiner and child may be a variable. This position seems to be primarily supported by implication—for example, Adler (1971). Seymour, Ashton, and Wheeler (1986), however, reported that this was not true for a population of randomly selected African-American and European-American children in grades one through four:

> Neither race of the examiner nor the race of the child depicted in the stimulus materials affected the language performance of randomly selected black and white children when language performance was measured in terms of response length and response latency. (p. 146)

This obviously does not mean that the examiner should not be conscious of dissonances that may occur as a function of race or culture. Such differences are not inherent, but the examiner should be conscious of the potential for dissonance and the effect it may have on performance in the test situation.

STANDARDS, NORMS, DIVERSITY: DIFFERENCES VERSUS DISORDERS

When we talk about standards or norms against which to make comparisons of a subject's performance, we imply (or state) a normal and representational group for that standard. That implication may have been easier to accept some years ago than it is today with the changing demographics of the population. A summary of the social and economic data from the 1990 census in *USA Today*, May 29, 1992, reported that nearly 20 million (7.9 percent) of the approximately 249 million people in the United States are foreign born. The decade of the 1980s showed the largest influx of immigrants in 50 years. One in four people in the United States is black (12.1 percent), Hispanic (8.5 percent), Asian (2.9 percent) or Native American (0.8 percent). Relative growth in the decade of the eighties showed an increase of 6.0 percent white, 13.2 percent black, 107.8 percent Asian, 53.0 percent Hispanic, and 37.8 percent Native American. Approximately one in seven, or 13.8 percent of the population speaks a language other than English at home.

The ASHA School Services Division (Peters-Johnson 1992) reported that the number of limited English proficient speakers four years and under increased from 1.8 million in 1976 to 2.6 million in 1990.

If the normative sample for determining standards of performance for the speech and language tests we give was representative of the population as a whole (e.g., based on age, sex, socioeconomic status, ethnic groups), then statistically the comparisons should still be valid insofar as the target items are the same. On the other hand, when the target phonemes, morphemes, syntactic elements, contents, and so on are different, then the statistical validity base for interpretation of normal is suspect (Seymour 1992). That point by Seymour may represent the difference between "difference" and "disorder."

The importance of this demographic variation for the speech-language clinician would be the recognition of the cultural and linguistic bases and biases that may be influencing the speaker's language patterns. Identifying a speaker's language production as "disordered" or "delayed" may be considered a pejorative judgment, while "different" has no such negative connotation. One theoretical choice, therefore, is to construct speech and language tests that reflect the speech and language units, sequences, and contents of the various populations for comparison with what is expected of a child or adult of that age or in that circumstance, in order to prevent a linguistic or cultural bias in interpretation. For example, "Hispanic" in the percentages given earlier does not separate among Spanish dialects spoken in Cuba, Mexico, Spain, or Puerto Rico. As Seymour (1992, p. 640) puts it:

> Unless a test can capture the commonalties among language and cultural groups, so that the behaviors being tested are culturally and linguistically free of bias, test scores will reflect considerable group differences and large standard errors of measurement. Consequently, the test would have serious problems of validity.

Lahey (1990) has reminded us that the first goal of an assessment procedure is identification. An interested parent, teacher, doctor, or other observer, has had a concern that the child may be having difficulty learning the language or using language in a particular environment. As a diagnostician, your first task is the assessment that allows you to answer "yes" or "no" to the question of whether or not there is a problem.

The scores you get from the measures used should indicate whether the language behavior observed is different from the expected (standard) target items. Your knowledge of the cultural and linguistic background of the child would help you decide if the deviation reflects a "difference" (apart from the mainstream) or a "disorder" (different from the rule system of his language). It is difficult to assume, however, that every clinician faced with this task will have sufficient exposure and expertise in the various dialects to make the required judgments. Adler (1991) has proposed a checklist and set of rating scales relative to speech and language form and function to be completed by an assessment team. The scales include, in addition to the speech-language person, a native speaker of the dialect and a standard English speaker who also has knowledge of the nonstandard dialect. The result would be less of a quantitative score than a qualitative judgment of the degree to which the presented language patterns interfere with communication.

As part of an American Speech-Language-Hearing Association Clinical Forum on treatment efficiency, Olswang and Bain (1991) argue for a data-based rationale for deciding when intervention is recommended. Since language is not only multifaceted, as we discuss in later chapters, it is "influenced by at least four factors (biological, cognitive, psychosocial and environmental)" (Committee on Language Learning Disorders, 1989). Again, which deviations are disordered and which are different?

Our task in this discussion is not to argue the political and cultural nuances of when to intervene, what type of intervention may be appropriate, and what it will be called, but to describe testing procedures and to caution the diagnostician to be aware of a variety of influences on both the test maker and the test user.

TESTING THE COMMUNICATIVE FUNCTION—NONSTANDARDIZED TESTING

Tests for communicative function are less common than tests of form. Most of the available tests are designed to measure grammatical forms such as phonemes, morphemes, syntax, and semantics; function (pragmatics) is implied by the child's command of the forms or is measured (judged) as efficiency of communication. Our first task, therefore, is to attempt to establish some communicative interchange with the child to be evaluated.

In a previous section, we cited Adler's assumption that it may be difficult to get the language-different child to perform to her potential. It would be wise for the prudent clinician to approach all children in this way. It is a reasonable assumption to make concerning all children, especially pre–school-aged children. In the next chapter, we define rapport as mutual trust, the ingredient necessary to obtain the kind of personal information requested in the case history interview. We are also asking for a great deal of trust on the part of the child. Even if she is not afraid of the unknowns in your office, the child—and many adults—will at least be shy or uncertain of what is expected of them. The three-, four-, or five-year-old child who is "completely cooperative" may well be the exception rather than the rule. With this in mind, it may also be logical to expect something less than a full array of completed test results.

ETHICS AND RESPONSIBILITIES

We have been discussing some of the difficulties of testing and test interpretation. There are also some other general comments to be made concerning our responsibilities in an evaluational endeavor. At some time or other, we have all heard the exhortation to "treat the whole child." A more realistic statement might be a reminder that "there is a whole child to be treated." Inherent in this paraphrase is the assumption that none of us is adequate to the task of being all things to all people. The Code of Ethics of the American Speech-Language-Hearing Association (1992) reminds all speech and hearing professionals that they must ". . . possess appropriate qualifications" and that they must ". . . use every resource available, including referral to other specialists as needed, to effect as great improvement as possible in the persons served."

Fortunately, that means we are not required to know everything about all problems for all persons. We are neither ethically nor legally required to be right at all times—only to use our best professional judgment and to recognize what we do not know. That means we are allowed to change our minds about the type of treatment and about what we can do to ameliorate problems we have identified—and to seek referral for help when we cannot handle a problem. We are ethically bound to be qualified, certified, capable, and available—but we are not required to "cure" all problems presented.

Dr. Karl Menninger (1958) stated it rather succinctly:

> The physician announces (and implies) that he is qualified (trained), authorized (certified), prepared (in equipment and time) and willing to render services to one who

needs them. . . . The physician gives the patient his attention and having heard what the patient complains of, makes a decision as to whether or not he—the doctor—can justifiably accept the responsibility of attempting to help this person as a patient. . . . He promises to seek the best way to help this patient . . . what the patient pays for is not relief of symptoms but the professional services of the physician. (pp. 19–20)

Two points are to be noted from the ASHA Code of Ethics and Menninger's quote. First, the clinician must be trained, qualified, and available to do the best he can for the patient or to find someone better qualified to handle those aspects of the patient's behavior that are not within his (the clinician's) realm of competence. Second, Menninger's "nonguarantee" stipulates that the clinician has no ethical or professional responsibility to be right at all times. Clearly, this means that our best judgment of cause-and-effect relationships and remediation predictions may not be correct. We should always accept our own as well as others' judgments as being tentative rather than absolute. The judgment we make will be the best and most reasonable we can make according to how we interpret the total problem, but it is changeable. It may be inscribed on parchment, but it should not be treated as if it were chiseled in stone. Don't *expect* to be wrong, but don't commit to a judgment at the expense of the patient.

The third diagnostic law may be stated as follows: *It is ethically acceptable to be wrong—fallability is forgivable—it is legal to change your mind.*

One More Caution

Darley (1964) quoted Beck (1959) in a statement of the basic formulations of science. Briefly stated (and paraphrased), they were

1. behavior is understandable—deviant as well as normal behavior
2. cause-and-effect relationships are expected to maintain some consistency under similar circumstances
3. the simplest consistent explanation is probably correct
4. behavioral causes are measurable

Darley was stressing the need for a scientific approach in speech and language diagnosis. Scientific problem solving is based on the asking of answerable questions. He cautioned the clinician to put more credence in a fact than in a guess or an intuition. "If a fact and a guess are in conflict, the clinician uses the fact. He comes to depend more upon what he can hear, see, feel, and verify than upon his intuition. He concentrates upon behavior that can be observed, measured, classified and manipulated" (p. 4).

In agreement with Darley, our emphasis is on measurement and direct observation, wherever possible. At the present state of the art—or science—we cannot determine and measure all the cause-and-effect relationships in speech and language disorders. It is still pertinent to assume that behavior is quantifiable. Further, it is imperative that we separate our inferences from our quantifications. We can measure performance. Competence, or capability, are inferences we make from performance or lack of it.

SUMMARY

This chapter has been concerned with the philosophy of testing. We have included comments on what "normal" means; some definitions of terms such as standardization, reliability, and validity; and a caution that not all children and adults are from the same cultural background or speak the same dialect as we do—nor do they have the same interest in test performance as we may like. We must recognize the purposes we have in testing, the appropriateness of the measurement devices we are using, and the applicability of the norms of behavior that those tests imply. Further, we must recognize the ramifications of our descriptions and judgments. We must know what value to assign to the obtained scores.

We stated, somewhat facetiously, three diagnostic laws: to describe rather than to categorize; not to be too sure of each of the numbers we generate; and to make it possible to change our minds about interpretation or significance of the "facts" we generate. They may have been stated facetiously, but the intent is for the clinician to take them seriously.

We commented about a "whole communication system to be treated"—or tested. An efficient communicative system includes appropriate rules and performance in phonology, morphology, syntax, and semantics. Language is "all of a piece." When we make formal or informal value judgments of a child's communication skill, we must also keep in mind the content of what she says (the concepts discussed) and her goals or functions—the reason to speak.

Weiner (1969) formulated one of the strictly linguistic assumptions for decoding a speech sample as "in the problem of decoding, the most important information which we can possess is the knowledge that the message we are reading is not gibberish." In other words, our first assumption must be that the child knows what she is talking about and what she is expressing is at least consistent with her understanding of the rules of her language.

In terms of culture-fair testing, Wechsler (1958) has expressed the opinion that "no test is or can be entirely culture-free." Communication skill, however, should not be considered purely an accident of geography or completely conditioned by local mores. Obviously these factors may intrude to a greater or lesser degree, but our task is to make an evaluation of communication skill and efficiency in the communicative functions presented. As clinicians, we are being asked to express a professional opinion as to the nature of the problem, if there is one, the prognosis or probable outcome, and the manner of therapeutic intervention.

REFERENCES

ADLER, S., Dialectal differences: Professional and clinical implications. *J. Speech Hearing Dis.*, 36, 90–100 (1971).

ADLER, S., Data gathering: The reliability and validity of test data obtained from culturally different children. *J. Learning Dis.*, 6, 429–434 (1973).

ADLER, S., Assessment of language proficiency of limited English proficient speakers: Implications for the speech-language specialist. *Lang. Speech Hearing Serv. Schools*, 22, 12–18 (1991).

ANASTASI, A., *Psychological Testing*, 3rd ed. New York: Macmillan (1968).

BECK, S. D., *The Simplicity of Science*, New York: Doubleday (1959).

BLOOM, L., AND M. LAHEY, *Language Development and Language Disorders*. New York: John Wiley (1978).

BRONFENBRENNER, U., Toward an experimental ecology of human development. *Ameri. Psychol.*, 32, 513–531 (1977).

BURLING, R., *English in Black and White*. New York: Holt, Rinehart and Winston (1973).

CARROW, E., *Test for Auditory Comprehension of Language*. Lamar, Tex.: Learning Concepts (1973).

CAZDEN, C., On individual differences in language competence and performance. *J. Spec. Educ.*, 1, 135–150 (1967).

CAZDEN, C., The neglected situation in child language research and education. In *Language and Poverty*, ed. F. Williams. Chicago: Markham Press (1970).

CODE OF ETHICS. *American Speech-Language-Hearing Association 1992 Directory*. Rockville, Md.: American Speech-Language-Hearing Association (1992).

COMMITTEE ON LANGUAGE LEARNING DISORDERS, Issues in determining eligibility for language learning. *Asha*, 31, 113–118 (1989).

DARLEY, F. L., *Diagnosis and Appraisal of Communication Disorders*. Englewood Cliffs, N.J.: Prentice Hall (1964).

DE AVILA, E., AND B. HAVASSY. The testing of minority children—A neo-Piagetian approach. *Todays Education*, 63, 72–77 (1974).

DRUMWRIGHT, A., *Denver Articulation Screening Exam*. Denver: University of Colorado Medical Ctr. (1971).

DuBOIS, P. H., *An Introduction to Psychological Statistics*. New York: Harper & Row (1965).

DUNN, L. M., AND L. M. DUNN, *Manual for The Peabody Picture Vocabulary Test revised*. Circle Pines, Minn.: American Guidance Service, Inc. (1981).

FEY, M. C., Understanding and narrowing the gap between treatment research and clinical practice with language impaired children. In *The "Future of Science and Services" Seminar*, ed. C. M. Shewan. *Asha Reports, No. 20* (1990).

GRIMSHAW, W., Language as an obstacle and as data in sociologic research. *Items, Soc. Sci. Res. Council*, June (1969).

LAHEY, M., Who shall be called language disordered? Some reflections and one perspective. *J. Speech Hearing Dis.*, 55, 612–620 (1990).

LAWRENCE, C. W., Assessing the use of age-equivalent scores in clinical management. *Lang. Speech Hearing Serv. Schools*, 23, 6–8 (1992).

LEONARD, L. B. AND OTHERS, Nonstandardized approaches to the assessment of language behaviors. *Asha*, 20, 371–379 (1978).

LYMAN, H., *Test Scores and What They Mean*, 4th ed. Englewood Cliffs, N.J.: Prentice Hall (1986).

MENNINGER, K., *Theory of Psychoanalytic Technique*. New York: Basic Books (1958).

MENYUK, P., Syntactic structures in the language of children. *Child Develop.*, 34, 407–422 (1963).

MENYUK, P., Syntactic rules used by children from preschool through first grade. *Child Develop.*, 35, 533–546 (1964).

MCCAULEY, R. J., AND L. SWISHER, Use and misuse of norm-referenced tests in clinical assessment: A hypothetical case. *J. Speech Hearing Dis.*, 49, 338–348 (1984).

MUMA, J. R. Language assessment: Some underlying assumptions. *Asha*, 15, 331–338 (1973).

MUMA, J. R., *Language Handbook: Concepts, Assessment, Intervention*. Englewood Cliffs, N.J.: Prentice Hall (1978).

MUSSELWHITE, C. R., Pluralistic assessment in speech-language pathology: Use of dual norms in the placement process. *Lang. Speech Hearing Serv. Schools*, 14, 29–37 (1983).

NUNNALLY, J., *Educational Measurement and Evaluation*. New York: McGraw-Hill (1972).

OLSWANG, L. B., AND BAIN, B. A., Clinical forum: Treatment efficacy—when to recommend intervention. *Lang. Speech Hearing Serv. Schools*, 22, 255–263 (1991).

PETERS-JOHNSON, C., Professional practices perspective on . . . multicultural issues. Report of School Services Division, *Asha*, 34, 14 (1992).

SALVIA, J., AND YSSELDYKE, J. K. *Assessment in special and remedial education*, 4th ed. Boston: Houghton Mifflin (1988).

SEARLE, J. R., *Speech Acts Theory*. New York: Cambridge University Press (1969).

SEVERSON, R., AND K. GUEST, Toward the standardized assessment of the language of disadvantaged children. In *Language and Poverty*, ed. F. Williams, Chicago: Markham Press (1970).

SEYMOUR, H. N., The invisible children: A reply to Lahey's perspective. *J. Speech Hearing Res.*, 35, 640–641 (1992).

SEYMOUR, H. N., N. ASHTON, AND L. WHEELER, The effect of race on language elicitation. *Lang. Speech Hearing Serv. Schools*, 17, 146–151 (1986).

SIEGEL, G., The use of language tests. *Lang. Speech Hearing Serv. Schools*, 4, 211–217 (1975).

SROUFE, L., A methodological and philosophical critique of intervention-oriented research, *Develop. Psych.*, 2, 150–155 (1970).

WECHSLER, D., *Manual for the Wechsler Adult Intelligence Scale*. New York: Psychological Corporation (1955).

WECHSLER, D., *The Measurement and Appraisal of Adult Intelligence*. Baltimore: Williams and Wilkins (1958).

WECHSLER, D., *Wechsler Intelligence Scale for Children—Revised*. San Antonio, Tex.: Psychological Corp. (1974).

WEINER, N., The human use of human beings, as quoted in R. Jakobson, C. G. M. Fant, and M. Halle, *Preliminaries to Speech Analysis*. Cambridge: M.I.T. Press (1969).

WEINER, P. S., AND W. C. HOOCK. The standardization of tests: Criteria and criticisms. *J. Speech Hearing Res.*, 16, 616–626 (1973).

WOLFRAM, W., AND R. W. FASOLD, *The Study of Social Dialects in American English*. Englewood Cliffs, N.J.: Prentice Hall (1974).

2

Information Gathering

*Although it may seem rather obvious, it is worth restating that as clinicians
we must listen before we speak.*

L. L. Emerick and J. T. Hatten

The first part of this chapter is concerned with the nature and purpose of information gathering, including some of the barriers between the interviewer and the information. In that respect, it is an extension of the previous chapter. We then discuss some of the mechanics of interviewing—how one goes about setting up and accomplishing the interview. Next we consider some sample questions that may be on a case history form. Last, we present some examples of social and early developmental measures that are usually completed by interview.

THE PHILOSOPHY OF INFORMATION GATHERING

Much of the context or background information we need in order to interpret the significance of the behaviors we observe is gathered by interview, and all interview information is subject to bias. The informant's biases are an intervening and often unmeasurable variable between us and the information we are seeking. Some of the available instruments of child development, such as the *Vineland Adaptive Behavior Scales*, are categorized as "interview" rather than "measurement" devices in this chapter because the descriptions available to us are secondhand rather than direct— the data are interpretive rather than observed. The purpose of our information gathering by either direct or indirect means is to determine the current status of the patient and to determine what (and if) changes are to be desired, the direction of these desired changes, and impedance to change. The amount of distortion in our data that can be attributable to the intervening informant bias will, at least initially, be difficult to calibrate. For this reason, it may well be appropriate to take all such indirect information with a grain of salt.

THE TASK AND THE TOOLS

As diagnosticians, we have two main tasks. The first is to analyze and describe the presenting speech, language, voice, fluency, hearing, or other problems. The second is to distinguish the relevant variables in order to understand the dimensions of the problem. The two tasks can be reduced to questions of *what* and *why*. *What* is the nature of the problem, and *why* did it come to be?

The first task is what we have labeled *appraisal*, or the measurement of the various abilities, and it occupies the bulk of the ensuing pages. The second task, *diagnosis*, is accomplished by putting the measurement results and observations in context. Determining the context of the problem is the concern of this chapter. The information we gather is to be collated with information supplied by other professional workers from their observations. With the integration of the many aspects of the client's behavior, it may be possible to arrive at some tentative cause-and-effect relationships. This task is termed a differential diagnosis and entails distinguishing the problem from similar problems with which it may be confused. From a tentative understanding of cause and effect, decisions can be made concerning prognosis and treatment.

Basically, the diagnostician has two types of tools: measurements or tests and interview or background information. A test allows the examiner to make measurable judgments without an intervening reporter to distort the picture. A test allows reasonably exact observations, and, if quantification is not possible, the clinician can at least reduce her observations to objective, understandable, agreed-upon statements. When she can measure what she is observing and can reduce observations to a numerical value, it is possible to chart improvement or lack of improvement and to determine if the therapeutic intervention is appropriately directed. If the improvement cannot be quantified, it is difficult to defend the judgment of improvement. Quantification is especially important in this age of accountability. For example, later in this text we mention a device called an oral manometer. With an oral manometer, oral air pressure produced with the nares open and with the nares occluded is compared to determine the ratio of the two measurements. This ratio helps determine the efficiency of the velopharyngeal valving mechanism—the closer the ratio is to 1.00, the more capable the speaker is in his ability to close off the nasal port to generate oral air pressure. An alternative to the ratio of nares open to nares closed is a report that the speaker has "some nasal emission." Obviously, the latter term expresses an important observation, but the oral manometer ratio yields a quantification of nonverbal velopharyngeal functioning.

The second major tool of the diagnostician is the history-type interview. The examiner wants to obtain information about antecedent and continuing conditions related to the communication difficulty and whatever predisposing, precipitating, and maintaining factors may be present. The determination of these kinds of variables will help delineate the nature of the problem and what can be done about it. An effective interviewer has to be more than a pleasant "asker of questions." The late Wendell Johnson characterized a good interviewer as a "professional eavesdropper." "Professional" in the sense that he has an ethical obligation to maintain the confidentiality of the information gathered and "eavesdropper" in the sense that he should not influence or intrude upon the information supplied. This is an important concept because it can seriously affect the amount and nature of the information made available. If we ask a question, or slant a question, in such a way that the client (parent) is aware we expect a particular answer, then it is highly probable that we will get the answer—whether it is true or not. If you think an answer could be embarrassing, ask the question in a straightforward manner, and it is less likely to cause embarrassment. To do this, a special relationship must exist between the interviewer and the one being interviewed—a relationship called rapport. Rapport is not something that one establishes before beginning the interview. It is a process or quality that is necessarily maintained throughout the interview to reduce the impedance to communication and sharing. Rapport means mutual respect. In practical terms, that means the informant becomes willing to divulge personal information because she can respect the professional purpose of the interview and because the interviewer has shown respect for the informant. In order to fulfill our ethical and professional responsibility to adequately describe the patient, we need as much unfiltered information as possible.

The Purpose and the Pitfalls

The professional purpose of the interview is clear when it is apparent to the one being interviewed that the questions being asked have a point and that the point is both valid and obvious. The questions must not be ambiguous or random. The nature of the information desired by the interviewer should be apparent. Questions should require a factual answer and not just opinion. They should not require merely agreement or denial. The interviewer may have to supply definitions or examples of the kind of information desired, but be aware that such prompts may also influence the answers received. Do not be afraid to ask for further explanation when answers are contradictory or when the tone of the response does not appear consistent with the words.

The Apostolic Function, or Giving Advice

Balint (1957) wrote a fascinating book entitled *The Doctor, His Patient, and the Illness.* The book was concerned primarily with the practice of psychotherapy by professionals not specifically trained in psychotherapy. When discussing interviewing, he stated that if you ask a question, all you may get is an answer. He stressed the importance of listening to the tone of the responses as well as to the words. Filling in answer blanks on the case history form is easy, but listening for information relevant to an understanding of the problem is much more difficult.

By virtue of the role played by the interviewer, the implied role of authority, it is frequently expected that the interviewer will be asked for advice. And what is more natural (although possibly dangerous to the best interests of the client) than giving advice? Balint devotes two chapters to what he terms "The Apostolic Function," which means going out and making the world over in our own image. What we say we would do is not necessarily most appropriate for the patient. Professional advice concerning treatment of communicative disorders is appropriate and expected. When the advice requested or offered is less obviously part of our professional jurisdiction, it may still be accepted as from an authoritarian base. The pharmacology of "therapist" has not been determined. We are frequently not aware of how much of ourselves we prescribe and the effect of that dosage. The philosophy we espouse and the words we use in asking questions or supplying information may be interpreted differently from what we intend.

Guiding Principles in Diagnosis

Darley (1964, pp. 9–14) lists six guiding principles in diagnosis and appraisal:

1. *Beware of a priori conceptions.* Each of us is prone to see what we expect to see and to rationalize behavior in terms of a notion we are fond of. It is an occupational hazard for all of us as clinicians to let our biases and preconceptions do our thinking for us. The scientific method demands that we observe the behavior and translate or define it as carefully as possible, without letting our biases interfere with what we observe.

2. *Stick to first-order facts.* Use as few inferences as possible; describe rather than speculate. A break in fluency in a child's speech should be reported as a revision, a part-word repetition, or whatever else it was without labeling it as "stuttering."

3. *Choose the simplest explanation consistent with the facts.* For example, a child may display a tongue-thrust swallow and distorted sibilant sound productions. This does not necessarily mean the distorted sibilants are caused by the tongue thrust.

4. *Keep your conclusions tentative rather than absolute.* Do not be afraid to change your mind. Remember that your ethical and professional obligation is to seek the best possible solution to the communicative problem presented. You are not ethically bound to be correct. Your conclusions and recommendations are professional opinions; they are not pronouncements. Based on your tentative results, you can chart a tentative course of treatment that will include further sampling of behavior. With new data, the picture may become more clear and complete. Diagnosis is not necessarily completed before therapy begins.

5. *Respect the relevance of norms.* Understanding what is deviant depends upon understanding what is normal. For example, only approximately one-third of the population has completely normal dental structure. In this case, "normal" is not necessarily average.

6. *Seek the counsel of other professionals.* Other professional workers may be in a better position to supply the necessary information than we are from our vantage point. Do

not play at being neurologist, psychologist, social worker, educator, or other specialist that you have not been trained to be. The code of ethics of the American Speech-Language-Hearing Association, for example, states that the patient's welfare is of paramount importance. Among other mandates, the clinician is to ". . . establish harmonious relations with colleagues and members of other professions." She must refer the patient when her limitations to provide the best available treatment are clear.

The Scientific Method.   A similar way of looking at Darley's statements is with the assumption that we are engaged in a scientific endeavor. The method of science, as commonly described, consists of asking answerable questions. The organization of a research project follows an outline such as the following:

1. definition of the problem
2. development of hypotheses to be tested
3. development of a procedure for testing the hypotheses
4. collection of data
5. analysis of data
6. support or rejection of hypotheses

Let us assume that our "research project" is a child referred because someone was concerned about the intelligibility of her speech. The six steps just mentioned are then translated in the following way:

1. *Definition of the problem.* Statements to the effect that the child is hard to understand or that she has an articulation problem are not sufficiently descriptive for us to pose hypotheses to be tested. We must at least give an articulation test or otherwise methodically determine error sounds. We need information on the consonant contexts of the errors. We need to know whether or not the errors are consistent and whether or not the incorrect sounds can be produced correctly in imitation (stimulability). We need to know the place and manner of error productions in contrast to the expected place and manner of articulation. In other words, we need to know whether there is consistency in the pattern of error. We need to know if there are mechanical reasons that could cause or contribute to the speech pattern we hear. In essence, we need whatever information we can get to help us narrow or define the problem.
2. *Development of hypotheses to be tested.* Depending partly on the types of information gathered in our definition, possible hypotheses could be related to hearing loss, dental malocclusion, language patterns related to familial or cultural ethnicity, speech and language patterns as a function of unique linguistic rules, inadequate motor control, or velopharyngeal insufficiency. There may also be other possibilities.
3. *Development of a procedure for testing the hypotheses.* Essentially, this statement means that we must test in such a way that we may believe our results. An important factor may be the willingness or the ability of the child to cooperate in the testing endeavor. Does she understand what is being asked of her? Are the directions clear? Is she sufficiently interested or motivated to perform? Have we established sufficient rapport? Not the least of the variables is whether we can accept the test as a valid measure.
4. *Collection of data.* Simply stated, this means testing for the possible alternatives we listed as hypotheses. For example, in addition to our articulation testing, we would

expect to administer at least a test of hearing acuity, appropriate language tests of morphology and syntax, and a complete evaluation of structure and function of the oral-peripheral mechanism. Case history or early developmental information may alert us to areas of more specific interest.

5. *Analysis of data.* In some cases, we can now make relatively clear positive or negative statements. Additional judgments may be reserved for a later time. A summary of our data collection is intended to rule out probable causes of the articulation problem we had earlier described, rather than to determine a single cause. In most cases, it is more realistic to look for interrelationships or coexisting factors than to expect a single cause-and-effect relationship.

6. *Support or rejection of hypotheses.* As indicated earlier, some of our hypotheses will be rejected at this point, and some will remain as possibilities that cannot yet be rejected. We will, at least, have some tentative conclusions. For example, our first decision is whether or not the speech and language behavior we have measured is importantly different from what is expected.

The Content of Science: Resolution of Uncertainty.   Schultz (1973) has compared the clinical evaluation procedure to information theory (Shannon and Weaver 1964). According to the formulations of Shannon and Weaver, the amount of information conveyed by a message is equivalent to the amount of uncertainty resolved by receipt of the message. By the Schultz comparison, clinical evaluation is a process of generating hypotheses or tentatively predicting judgments with their relative probabilities, for example the probability of hearing loss in a school-aged population. The examination procedures are then tests of the hypotheses. When the hypotheses are reduced to one by virtue of the observations made, the clinician's uncertainty has been resolved, and the examination is concluded. Schultz (p. 153) posed a variety of possible hypotheses, such as "designation of current status, diagnostic categorization, (re)habilitative requirements." The type of hypotheses entertained would determine the type of observations made and the discriminant ability of the tests selected. The magnitude of the uncertainty determines the value of the test procedure. If there is no resolution of the clinician's uncertainty, new hypotheses must be raised. We only get answers by asking questions, and a good answer requires asking a good question.

Schultz (1973) stated the final advantage of the evaluation model as follows:

> The early establishment of a set of hypotheses enhances data gathering and data retention efficiencies. Alternatively, the later in the process the hypotheses are first delineated, the more likely it is that the set will include the "true" hypothesis. The examiner must contend with these antagonistic decision pressures; but she knows that, in the event of an unsuccessful outcome (irresolution), she can reformulate any or all of her hypotheses, reconsider the available data, and attempt economically to secure the increment necessary to her evaluative decision. (p. 153)

Darley's six guiding principles in appraisal and diagnosis, the six-step outline of the method of science, and the resolution-of-uncertainty evaluation model described by Schultz all speak to the same point.

To be effective, our procedures of appraisal must be organized around the specific questions that will be most productive for our diagnostic-descriptive purposes.

WHAT IS THE PROBLEM—
AND WHOSE PROBLEM IS IT?

When we are talking about the "case history"—the history of the client across the desk from us—we should remember that none of us live in isolation. We are not in a world of our own choosing and only to a limited degree can we control our own destiny. If this philosophical statement is true for the more talented among us, consider how much more true it may be for the more dependent among us, including those who are communicatively handicapped.

A nine-year-old young man came to our clinic with his mother, referred because of a problem with fluency. During our conversation, he reported that he had stuttered, as far as he could remember, since he began to talk. But, he said, he did not stutter when he was in the second grade. He was now in the third grade and stuttered once more. When asked why, he reported that his father had died when he was very young and that an uncle who lived down the street from him acted as his father. The uncle, who was his authority figure, told the boy that all males in the family stuttered. In the previous year when he was in the second grade, the uncle repeatedly asked him why he did not stutter. The boy reported that he felt it was easier to stutter than to argue with his uncle. The "problem" in this case was not the relative fluency of the boy but his perception of what choices were available to him.

Obviously, the uncle was not necessarily the cause of the stuttering, and the boy may or may not have stuttered in the second grade; we have only his report on which to base our judgment. Possible etiologies of stuttering and differences between "disfluency" and "stuttering" will be explored in a later chapter. The point to be made here is that an initial cause of a problem and a maintaining cause may or may not be the same thing. Similarly, a judgment that a problem exists (in someone's mind) and a description of behaviors characteristic of the problem may have little resemblance. The direction of therapy intervention must be based on what is changeable (be it perception or behavior) and behavior that is changeable now—not what may have been changeable at an earlier time.

A quality control engineer in an electronics plant suffered a stroke and was left with a residual aphasia. Following a period of therapy, he was functioning well at a social conversation level. He had also regained the use of his right arm and hand and was spending the majority of his time in his backyard shop restoring and making furniture. He did not have the speed and dexterity necessary to return to his former employment, but he appeared happy with his life and the one-time furniture-making hobby that now produced income as well as enjoyment. It was not yet a "successful rehabilitation" story, however, because his wife was not willing to accept his woodworking as an occupation or her new role as the wife of an artisan. Acceptance was gained in time, but the point of this anecdote is that the definition of the problem may not be restricted to the one with the communication handicap.

These two stories are a reminder that a description that includes only the speech, language, and/or hearing skills of the client before us may not be adequate for successful intervention. We earlier agreed with Beck (1959) that behavior is understandable, but we must also attempt to learn upon what logic the behavior is based. The client interview is where the diagnostic information gathering begins—a process that includes not only behavioral description but also perceptions about the circumstances, beliefs, habits, and pressures that mitigate both for and against remediation.

Our diagnostic endeavors are an attempt to develop as complete a description as possible in order to determine where significant deviations lie, what changes are desired and/or expected, and what circumstances or restrictions may interfere with or limit the desired changes. These efforts are also importantly tied to prognostic decisions since we need to know where the remediation process is to lead in order to locate the most efficient means of getting there.

OBSERVING, TESTING, MEASURING

The gathering of information does not begin with testing or with the formal interview of the client or "important others." The gathering of observational data begins when we first see the client, which may very well be before the formal diagnostic process is begun. For example, observations related to physical mobility and responsiveness to questions and greetings may be made when we meet the client in the waiting room.

Later we discuss the choice of structured versus unstructured testing in the assessment of language. The observations of behavior in response to controlled circumstances should be supplemented, augmented, and corroborated by as many unstructured situational observations as are available and necessary. It is entirely possible that our client may demonstrate different social, developmental, and language behaviors in different situations—the classroom versus the therapy room, the waiting room or hallway versus the diagnostic room, his home versus your clinic.

We would like to observe the client's functional communicative efficiency and also his best effort. No one, child or adult, wants to be in a situation where he feels inadequate or foolish and expects to fail. At the same time, your task as diagnostician is to determine what the client can do and what he cannot do. You should expect to find inadequacies by virtue of your role in the situation. As an evaluator, demonstrate your interest in the client as a person, not as a subject. Praise participation and attempted performance and not just success. Be alert for changes in performance that may indicate a lack of attention and may require a break in activity. Especially with young children, begin with tasks that require less verbal participation so that they will have a chance to succeed early and you will have the opportunity to praise their participation. The development of trust and confidence is critical to your task of describing behaviors and not simply obtaining test results.

THE MECHANICS—HOW TO GO
ABOUT THE INTERVIEW

As stated earlier, to be a good interviewer, you cannot be a completely dispassionate "asker of questions." You must be interested, and you must listen. The roles of interviewer and interviewee are not equal. The person being interviewed is assumed to be the one who has come for help, and the interviewer is the professional being asked to supply that help. It is expected that you as the interviewer will ask most of the questions and guide the direction of the interview while most of the information will come from the informant. In your role of authority, however, you must not be authoritarian, aloof, critical, or judgmental. As an interviewer, you cannot afford to act superior and still maintain the trust required to obtain the personal information you seek.

The admonition to listen is to keep you from asking for information that has already been supplied in response to a previous question. Nothing will turn off an informant faster than being asked the same question two or three or more times. That would indicate a lack of interest on your part, and the informant would then likely revert to "answers" instead of providing information.

Tell the Informant What Information You Want and Why

It is not safe to assume that the informant understands the purpose of the interview or the nature of the information requested. Explain the purpose of the interview, the type of information being sought, and the use to which the information will be put. It may be helpful to remind the informant that you may not ask all the appropriate questions but that you are asking for her cooperation in obtaining as much information as possible to better understand the nature of the problem being presented.

Informed Consent

Tell the informant who you are. If you are a student in a training program, say so. If there are observers, say so. Everyone has the right to be fully informed, and informed consent requires that you be honest and that you be explicit and clear in your explanations. Tell the informant with whom the information will or will not be shared. Anonymity cannot be maintained, but the information will be kept confidential. If a report is to be sent, obtain the patient's (or parent's) agreement on a signed release-of-information form.

Be Economical with Time—Make Your Questions Clear

The informant should not get the impression that you are in a rush to complete the interview to go on to more important matters, but don't waste time. Give the patient time to answer the questions you pose, but don't encourage "best" answers. The general atmosphere you establish will go a long way toward expediting the information-gathering process. Your questions will be more efficient sources of information if you ask them straightforwardly and primarily in words of one syllable.

"How old was Johnny when he was toilet trained? When could he stay dry during the day and during the night?" might be more efficient questions than having to sort through clarifications and restatements of something like, "Was it difficult to get Johnny used to bathroom habits, you know, like . . . did he take a long time to be toilet trained? How old was he?"

Don't ask yes or no questions that must be followed immediately by other questions required to get the rest of the answer. "Has Johnny been sick much?" may be less efficient than questions like "What illnesses has Johnny had?" "How severe were they?"

Take Notes, but Be Brief

The economical use of time requires that the interviewer be thoroughly familiar with the interview outline, with the types of information to be gathered, and with the essence of what is expected. That way the interviewer can move rapidly through the interview without leaving too much time for the informant to frame "best" answers. This also requires that the interviewer take notes as briefly and as expeditiously as possible. Try not to leave long silences while you record everything word by word. Very seldom would you need an exact quote for an answer. Routine, long silences for transcribing answers will tend to inhibit the information to be gathered, and excessive note taking will interfere with eye contact. The note taking should not be surreptitious. Many informants seem to find it reassuring that you are taking notes, which at least implies that their answers are important, but it is preferable to use a clipboard or pad so the informant cannot read what you have written.

Listen

Listen not only to answers given so that you may keep from asking for information already supplied, but also listen for apparent contradictions. If you think there is a contradiction in the answers you have received, ask about it, but avoid forcing the informant into being defensive. When you complete the interview, you will have to summarize the information you have gathered, so it is appropriate that you clarify possible points of confusion. Listen to what the words say—and to the tone of the responses. Listen for the concern that may show between the words. Listen for cues that may tell you whether the answers you have been given are real. Have you been given information as well as answers? Listen for questions that the informant asks or wants to ask.

When the Interview Is Over, Close It Gracefully

When the interview is completed, thank the informant for her cooperation and explain again why you have been asking the questions. It is probably not a good idea to volunteer a summary of your impressions of the informant's concern at this point. It may, however, be appropriate to ask if there is anything else that the informant thinks you should know to better understand the problem being presented. This sort of invitation may frequently yield a summary on the part of the informant—what she thinks is of primary importance.

Tell the informant that the information you have gathered will be assembled with the speech, language, and other data by you, or whoever is in charge of the case disposition, and that a summary of the findings and recommendations will be discussed with her. Thank her for her cooperation and say goodbye.

CASE HISTORY INTERVIEW

A case history, or case study data, must satisfy four criteria: relevancy, sufficiency, representativeness, and reliability (Wallin 1963). There are many versions of case history forms in use, but there are no standardized forms. Theoretically, a complete case history may be gained by simply asking the patient (or parent or knowledge-able adult) to "tell me all about it"—or it may be many pages in length with every conceivable question written in advance, and still it may not adequately discover all the pertinent answers. The appropriate question is not how long a case history *should* be, but rather how long *must* it be. A case history interview must be as long as a piece of string—long enough to do the job.

In addition to the information necessary for filing and retrieval, such as name, address, birth date, file number, referral source, and similar information of a book-keeping nature, case history interviews should cover such topics as family history, physiological data, early developmental history, speech history, educational history, personal behavioral characteristics, socioeconomic data, and the interviewer's state-ment of general impressions.

It is obvious that communication problems in an adult may elicit different areas of concern than communication problems in children. For example, if the patient is a recently laryngectomized adult, we would not logically be concerned about early developmental history or speech history or areas that were not of con-cern before the removal of the larynx. On the other hand, one of the authors of this text was once at a loss to explain an inability to read by an aphasic patient he was evaluating. The lack of reading skill in the patient did not fit with the rest of his abilities/disabilities—the subject was the owner/operator of a local restaurant. The mystery was solved when this examiner thought to ask if the man could read Eng-lish (he was a recent émigré to the United States) prior to the cerebral insult—and he could not. The pertinent history of the case should be complete enough to dis-cover the value of the important variables. When new information becomes avail-able, it can be added as an aid to interpretation.

Some clinical settings may use a preassessment questionnaire as a means of setting the stage for the parental interview. This could serve as a means of giving the parent time to describe in more detail her concern with the child's communica-tion problem, consult a baby book or other diary materials, or in general terms rule out areas of unlikely concern. Such a preassessment questionnaire may serve the purpose of alerting the parent or guardian to the types of information sought in the case history interview, as well as alerting the interviewer to other areas that may be of concern.

There probably are nearly as many variations for this aspect of information gathering as there are clinics. What they have in common is the need for identifying information for filing purposes and health and general developmental background of the child, and because it may be pertinent, they frequently include educational background of the family—for example, language other than English spoken in the home. Figure 2–1 is a case history form that illustrates the type of background information to be sampled.

Family History

Information concerning age, education, occupation, and prior or current speech and language disorders in parents or relatives may provide clues to other questions that need to be asked. A parent may be concerned about what she per-ceives as early signs of stuttering in her child because someone in her family had "stuttering problems." On the other hand, she may have a lower level of concern

```
                        CASE HISTORY (CHILD)


NAME_____AGE_____SEX _____
ADDRESS_____BIRTH DATE _____
_____ZIP _____
COMPLETED BY_____PHONE NO. _____
DATE_____


                        FAMILY HISTORY


Father:
  1. Full Name_____Age _____
     If dead, state cause and age at death _____
  2. Living at home, divorced, remarried, etc. _____
  3. Education _____
  4. Present occupation _____
  5. Did he ever have a speech defect?_____Voice defect? _____
     At what age did the defect clear up? _____
     Speech defects among relatives _____


Mother:
  1. Full Name_____Age _____
     If dead, state cause and age at death _____
  2. Living at home, divorced, remarried, etc. _____
  3. Education _____
  4. Present occupation _____
  5. Did she ever have a speech defect?_____Voice defect? _____
     At what age did the defect clear up? _____
     Speech defects among relatives _____


Brothers and Sisters:
                                      Speech   School Grade &
Name                    Age    Sex    Defect   Performance
_____  _____  _____  _____    _____

_____  _____  _____  _____    _____

_____  _____  _____  _____    _____

_____  _____  _____  _____    _____

How many living at home?_____
```

FIGURE 2–1   Sample case history form

PHYSIOLOGICAL DATA

Height_____Weight_____Current Health (good, poor) _____
Physical deformities _____
Date of last physical examination _____Physician_____

Diseases:	Age	Sever-ity	Change in Speech		Age	Sever-ity	Change in Speech
Chicken Pox	____	____	____	Diptheria	____	____	____
Measles	____	____	____	Encephalitis	____	____	____
Scarlet Fever	____	____	____	Mumps	____	____	____
Rheumatic Fever	____	____	____	Meningitis	____	____	____
Pneumonia	____	____	____	Whooping	____	____	____
Influenza	____	____	____	Cough	____	____	____
Asthma	____	____	____	Allergy	____	____	____
Hay Fever	____	____	____	High Fevers			
Other respiratory				(104°)	____	____	____
illnesses	____	____	____	Earaches	____	____	____
Others	____	____	____	Convulsions	____	____	____

Surgery: _____
_____

Injuries: _____
_____

Injuries or illnesses relatable to speech problems: _____
Current or past medications: _____
Hearing:
   Parent's evaluation of child's hearing _____
   Ear infections_____Otological care or surgery _____
Comments: _____

SPEECH HISTORY

1. a. Age first words spoken: _____
   b. Age 2-3 word combinations spoken: _____
   c. Age first sentences spoken: _____

2. a. Rate of speech development:
      Fast_____Average_____Slow_____
   Clearness of child's speech before age 6:
   below average_____average _____above average_____

3. Verbal output—Evaluation:

	More than average	Average	Less than average
a. Amount of babbling	_____	_____	_____
b. Amount of talking when first began	_____	_____	_____
c. Amount of talking at present			
d. Present rate or speed of talking (fast, slow)	_____	_____	_____

FIGURE 2–1   Sample case history form (continued)

4. Description of child's conversation at home: none_____
   brief responses_____ speaks easily_____ gestures
   with words_____

   Child's speech with peers: none_____ brief responses_____
   speaks easily_____ gestures with words_____

   Child's speech with strangers: none_____ brief
   responses_____ speaks easily_____ gestures with
   words_____

5. Intelligibility of child's speech: easily understood_____
   understood if listener knows the topic_____ words
   understood now and then_____ completely
   unintelligible_____ gestures understood_____

6. Language(s) other than English spoken at home:_____
   understands second language_____ speaks second
   language_____

7. Describe how your child gets along with other
   children/adults _____

   _____

8. Parents' description of speech problem (now) _____

9. When was the problem first noted?_____ Description of speech
   at that time? _____
   Who was first concerned (parent, teacher, relative,
   etc.)? _____
   Has any change occurred in speech? _____
   To what do you attribute this change? _____

10. Previous speech evaluation? _____ Agency_____ Date _____
    Comments _____

    _____

SCHOOL HISTORY

1. Present grade_____ School _____
2. Age and date of first school attendance _____
3. Other schools attended (year and dates) _____
4. Grades failed_____ grades skipped _____
5. Easy subjects _____
6. Difficult subjects _____
7. Problems in school _____
8. Recreational interests and hobbies _____

DEVELOPMENTAL HISTORY

Pregnancy:
  Mother's health (illnesses, medicines, accidents) _____

  _____
  Previous pregnancies _____
  Rh factor_____ Toxemias _____
Birth:
  Home_____ Hospital _____
  Physician_____City/State _____

FIGURE 2–1   Sample case history form (continued)

Delivery:
  Normal_____Instrument_____Breech_____Caesarian _____
  Condition at birth:
  jaundiced_____blue_____breathing_____crying _____
  red_____purple_____other _____
  Length of labor_____ Anaesthetic_____ Birth weight _____
  Term_____ Physical deformities _____
Feeding:
  Breast-fed_____ Bottle-fed_____ Nutritional disturbances _____
  _____
Age of
  First tooth_____ Sitting_____ Creeping_____ Crawling _____
  Walking_____ Self-feeding_____ Dressing _____
  Toilet training_____ Comparison with other children _____

PERSONAL CHARACTERISTICS

Please indicate how often these behaviors occur in the child
by circling the letter that most often describes it.indicates
that it occurs often; S indicates seldom; N indicates never

Nervousness	O S N	Tongue sucking	O S N
Sleeplessness	O S N	Hurting pets	O S N
Nightmares	O S N	Setting fires	O S N
Bedwetting	O S N	Constipation	O S N
Playing with sex organ	O S N	Thumb sucking	O S N
Walking in sleep	O S N	Face twitching	O S N
Shyness	O S N	Fainting	O S N
Showing off	O S N	Strong fears	O S N
Refusal to obey	O S N	Strong hates	O S N
Rudeness	O S N	Queer food habits	O S N
Fighting	O S N	Temper tantrums	O S N
Jealousy	O S N	Whining	O S N
Selfishness	O S N	Stealing	O S N
Lying	O S N	Running away	O S N
Excitability	O S N	Destructiveness	O S N
Easily discouraged	O S N	Preference for	
Convulsive attacks	O S N	older children	O S N
		Preference for	
		younger children	O S N

Your comments:

SOCIOECONOMIC DATA

1. Type of community (city, town, country, etc.) _____
2. Home (owned, rented, bedrooms shared, etc.) _____
3. Economic condition of family (poor, very poor,
   comfortable, well-to-do) _____

INTERVIEWER'S IMPRESSIONS

                    Interviewer _____
                    Supervisor _____

FIGURE 2–1   Sample case history form (continued)

because "Uncle Charlie stuttered as a child, but he got over it." Similarly, information about siblings, their ages and school performance, may or may not be pertinent to the child in question. How many siblings are there, and what are their ages? Is there a sibling rivalry? To what extent might parental aspirations or levels of expectations for the child be a factor? Our task as "professional eavesdroppers" requires that we not make moral judgments or offer unsolicited advice on child rearing. We must remain nonjudgmental so that we can maintain the interviewee's trust while asking for very personal information. From the parent we are seeking an outline of the child's semantic environment. The child's evaluative reactions will have to come from him. A statement that a child is "a good student" is a value judgment on the part of someone. A statement that a child receives "As and Bs in English and history and arithmetic" is a factual report. When you pool all your information for a diagnostic description, you can interpret the significance of facts. You cannot interpret the significance of value judgments.

Physiological Data

Height, weight, current health, childhood diseases, injuries, hospitalizations, surgery, and current or past medications may all be examples of the kinds of data collected in this section. A probable question that arises is whether reported injuries or illnesses are relatable to the speech problem. From our previous discussion of the "scientific method" and the "resolution of uncertainty," it may be assumed that we are not looking for *the* cause of a speech and language difficulty but for a number of possible factors that could contribute to the problem. A child may be reported to have begun to stutter just after he had his tonsils removed or just after the family was involved in an automobile accident. This reported coincidence in time does not necessarily imply a cause-and-effect relationship. Accept the statement, but record it as a value judgment. We also need to know the parent's definition of stuttering. What did the child do? What was the speech like before and after the incident in question? Is it possible that the perceived problem began earlier or later?

An arrest in the development of speech and language skills following prolonged high fevers or encephalitis, for example, may be a more acceptable cause-and-effect relationship, but it is not the end of the search. These may be significant factors but are not of themselves sufficient.

Early Developmental History

Our concern with development begins very early. Questions we raise would have to do with mother's health during the pregnancy (prenatal) and go on to perinatal and postnatal, as well as early developmental milestones. Concerning the mother's physical and emotional health, were any complications reported, such as severe nausea or vomiting, toxemias, viral infections, anemia, bleeding, X-ray treatments, nutritional or metabolic disturbances? If so, when during the pregnancy did they occur? Is there any history of miscarriages? Is there a blood incompatibility, such as Rh factor? What was the term of pregnancy? What was the birth weight of the child? How does that compare with other children of the family? Was labor induced? Was the baby in a breech position? Were forceps required for delivery? Was the mother under anaesthesia or analgesia during delivery? Concerning the baby, was there a report of discoloration, of blueness or jaundice at birth? Was there any delay in respiration? Did the infant require incubation? For how long? If there are complications that could be of a genetic nature, is there a birth-defects facility in your area that could provide genetic study and counseling?

In terms of early development, was there any indication of hypo- or hyper-tonicity? Did the infant have any difficulty nursing? Was she breast-fed or bottle-fed? Was there ever a feeding problem? Was she a "colicky" baby? How old was she when she could sit up, crawl, stand alone, walk, and feed herself? When was she toilet trained during the day and during the night? How do these developmental ages compare with other children in the family? How do these ages compare with published norms, for example, age norms provided by Aldrich and Norval (1946) who cite sitting up at approximately six months; crawling or creeping at seven months; standing alone at ten to eleven months; walking at approximately twelve months. In a later chapter of this text, motor developmental measures are discussed more fully.

Speech History

Questions concerning the early speech history of the child may serve a sort of double-barreled purpose. It is usual to ask for approximate ages of babbling and cooing, of early attending behavior to speech, age of first word, age when two- and three-word utterances were assembled, and similar questions on amount and intelligibility of the verbal output. There have been a number of early studies that reported on the age of first word and similar milestones, but they reflect differences in definition of first word by the experimenters. "First-word" data for normal children range from ten to approximately eighteen months. With this range for first word, two-word utterances are to be expected by twenty-four months of age.

We said there was a double purpose in these questions. In addition to ages that can be compared to general ages of expectancy, the second purpose is to get a judgment by the parent as to whether these ages are earlier or later than they expected. If an older child said his first words at ten months, a later age for the child in question may be considered late although still within the normal range. Part of the information we are asking for with these questions is whether the parents are concerned about the child's speed of development.

In *The Onset of Stuttering* studies (Johnson and others 1959), there was a consistent lack of agreement between judgments of "late" and the child being later than the usual age in reaching developmental milestones. In this series of studies, 246 children who were judged by their parents to be stutterers and their parents were compared with 246 children who were judged by their parents as nonstutterers and their parents. More experimental (stuttering) mothers than control group mothers rated their children as being much slower than average, but a comparison of the ages when the two groups of children said their first words and when they said their first sentences did not differ. In other words, ages in the speech history may give us data for comparison with children in general, as well as with other siblings in the family. Judgments of early, average, or late may yield information concerning the *parents'* norms, aspirations, and expectations.

In this section, we would also ask for a description of the child's functional communication. How easily does he speak with children his own age or with strangers? Is his speech easy to understand? Is it understood only if the topic is known? Is it not understood? Does he rely on gestures with or without accompanying words? Are other languages spoken in the home? Does the child use more than one language? Who was first concerned about the child's speech? How would the parent describe the speech at that time? How would it be described now? Have any changes occurred in the child's speech? To what does the parent attribute the change?

Educational History

As with many of the other sections of our case history interview, the educational history may or may not be significant to the understanding of every child studied. With children of school age, it is sometimes helpful to know what their educational history has been. Have any grades been failed? Have any grades been skipped? What are the easiest subjects; what are the most difficult? What kinds of marks does he usually obtain? Have there been any drastic changes? Are there any other reported problems in school?

Here again, we are not dictating questions to be asked but reminding the interviewer to construct as complete a picture as possible to determine if there are areas of potential significance that need to be explored. For example, questions concerning social interaction or academic performance in school may allow us to determine if the child's performance is consistent with other performance predictions we may have in terms of intellectual potential, social maturity, and other related indices. Is academic performance consistent with parental expectation?

Personal Characteristics

Under this general heading may be a list of behaviors such as nervousness, sleeplessness, nightmares, shyness, showing off, jealousy, excitability, tantrums, strong fears, strong hates, whining, destructiveness, and the like. The kinds of behavioral characteristics questioned may be normal behaviors to some degree in all children. The behaviors you list may occur often, seldom, or never in the child in question. This section may be considered an attempt to "flesh out" our description of the child's nonverbal behavior and to add one more dimension to the total picture. Are any of the behaviors described relatable to the "cause" of the speech problem? Are any of them likely to have been caused or aggravated by the child's lack of communication skill?

Socioeconomic Data

Socioeconomic classification systems may have a number of variables in their formulae, but most commonly they include source (rather than amount) of income, occupation, and education of the parents. Of these three, one study (Helton 1974) found mother's education to be the factor that best predicted the child's language skill. The purpose in gathering the social, cultural, and economic information is to help you determine cultural influences or opportunities available to the child. Social-cultural exposure may be important in terms of language form and possibly language function. Do not, however, assume that socioeconomic status tells you everything. Only Aristotelian logic assumes that class determines behavior. Non-Aristotelian logic assumes that behavior determines class. The distinction is important for your remedial intervention. In the extreme, if class determines behavior, language intervention would logically include increasing family income and moving the family across town. While that is not necessarily a poor idea in itself, it may be much more productive to the child's language skills to recommend the kind of language stimulation and interaction commonly found in a more "culturally advantaged" environment.

Interviewer's Impressions

The premise on which we began this chapter is that we wish to gather as much information as possible that is pertinent to our understanding of the child and the problem presented. Our understanding can be no more complete than our data—and the data no better than our interpretation. This section, therefore, is an invitation to put into words those on-the-spot thoughts and impressions that may not be available when we look back over the answers at a later date. For example, statements concerning the mood of the interview and the quality of the interaction may be obvious at the time but may not be equally obvious later.

OBSERVATION AND INDIRECT TESTING

Different clinical settings have functioned with different procedures. It is difficult to assume that there is only one best way to operate. Some clinicians do an interview first and then test the child, on the assumption that they will have more understanding of the behavior they see. Others do the testing first and then the interview because they feel they can better channel interview questions to areas of prime concern. Clinics with more personnel available may split the task with one clinician taking the case history while another tests the child. If the patient concerned is a child, most clinicians agree that, when possible, it is helpful to observe the child apart from the parent and interacting with another clinician and also to observe interactions of child and parent. Sometimes these observations can add considerable information.

The following case is not necessarily unique, but consider it as an example. A four-year-old boy was brought to the Hearing and Speech Center because of the parents' concern with the child's fluency. The subject displayed normal fluency when he was interacting with a clinician. The descriptions of speech given by his mother did not coincide with our observations of his speech. The boy's mother had also brought a five-year-old son with her to the center, and when the mother was asked to go into the diagnostic room to continue the activities the clinician had initiated, the other son went along. When the two boys communicated with each other, the speech fluency of both sounded normal, but when the two were competing for their mother's attention, the disfluency in the four-year-old that the mother had described was very evident.

This anecdote only points out that our observations or our test results are not complete in themselves and frequently require "outside" information that is not always available to us. Many children, due to their age or the way in which they view the test situation, may not be willing to separate themselves from their parent or may not be willing to perform for us, whether or not the parent is present. Especially for these children, and as supplemental information for "performing" youngsters, the social and early developmental scales that are discussed later in this chapter may be looked on as extensions of the case history or interview information. While they are, by our earlier definition, "secondhand" information, one or more of the measures discussed may be useful.

Also, consider the fact that the parent or interviewee probably knows the child considerably better than you do. If the parent is listening/watching while you go through your "formal" testing procedure, she may well comment that "He does that at home frequently," although your subject failed to supply the targeted forms in the test environment. That comment should be considered to have value and you should be alert for examples in the child's speech that would indeed indicate that he may have the targeted forms in his repertoire. For that matter, some otherwise "direct" tests, such as the *Sequenced Inventory of Child Development*, which we discuss in a later chapter, do include some parental report items as primary data. One of the common tools in the evaluation of an adult stroke victim is the *Functional Communication Profile* (also described in a later chapter), which utilizes some reported (not observed) as well as observed behaviors.

"ENABLE ME, ARMOR ME, EMPOWER ME"— THE EMPOWERMENT REHABILITATION MODEL

The case history and background information help us determine the parameters of the problem and what limitations may exist and thereby acquire some clues as to what the potential outcome may be.

What has been missing in the previous discussion is the role of the patient in providing background information, in putting the direct and indirect observations in perspective, and in setting rehabilitation goals. Especially when that patient is an adult, she should be part of the rehabilitation team (O'Hara and Harrell 1991). O'Hara and Harrell have constructed an "empowerment model" for use primarily with traumatic brain injury (TBI) clients that does just that. When the adult patient first suffers a head injury she is a victim and

> may lose control not only over cognitive, physical, and emotional function, but over autonomous decision making about many aspects of [her] life. This victimization includes the loss of an internal locus of control, and the quest for a gradual resumption of self-control. Thus, the victim's path of rehabilitation is one toward the goal of self-redefinition as survivor. (p. 14)

Empowerment of the patient/family is an emerging issue in the treatment of brain damage. At admission to some hospitals, the staff meets with the patient and family to explore in detail what they want the rehabilitation program to accomplish. The "survivor" and family may well be limited to regaining their functioning prior to the incident. But if they are to be survivors—that is, allowed to return to social and economic self-control, they must be part of the goal-setting, information-gathering, and measurement processes. The survivor has needs and feelings that must be allowed objective expression. The restrictions and opportunities of the social and economic environments to which the survivor will return also need definition.

One of the authors once worked with a geologist who had a stroke while inspecting a coal mine. The man was fortunate to receive immediate medical attention. He reported that while in a vigilant coma, he overheard the physicians surrounding his hospital bed (who were not aware that he could hear) express the opinion that "poor George" was not expected to last the night. "Poor George" not only lasted the night but reported that he was so motivated by the remark that to prove them wrong he was sitting on the edge of the bed in the morning waiting for his breakfast. Within a very short period of time, "George" was back at work. He had not lost his ability to function as a geologist. He could still tell you where in the state to go and how far down to dig to find whatever minerals you sought, but prior to the cerebral insult he could read a 400 page text in four hours and it now took him three times that long. His complaint was not that he was "handicapped" but that his boss no longer trusted him as a reliable source of information.

"George" is probably an exception in the speed and extent of his recovery but, by his report, he "chose" (was motivated) to be a survivor and not a victim. The survivor with his motivations, needs, feelings, and skills is an important part of the empowerment rehabilitation model. O'Hara and Harrell also suggest that treatment providers need to develop better means of assessing motivation on the part of the victim/survivor, as well as assessing themselves as providers—and motivators. This assessment task not only requires gathering of information from and about the patient, but the supplying of information *to* the patient.

This text is concerned with the gathering of information to describe communication problems that may exist and is not about the intervention to remediate those problems. But successful intervention requires adequate description and the sharing of information: in the appraisal mode—what information do we want and why; in the intervention mode—what are we doing in therapy and why. Whether your client is a child or an adult, each must be adequately informed in order to be part of the process.

SOCIAL AND EARLY DEVELOPMENTAL SCALES

The Vineland Adaptive Behavior Scales

An important distinction between tools of measurement and the case history as information-gathering methods is that there is an intervening variable between the examiner and the behavior to be described in the interview. Since we cannot be certain of the accuracy of the responses obtained in the interview or the biases of the reporter, we must be cautious in our information gathering and interpretation of responses. The *Vineland Adaptive Behavior Scales* (Sparrow, Balla, and Cicchetti 1984) have attempted to control this potential source of variance by utilizing a large number of questions related to discrete behaviors.

The forerunner to the *Vineland Adaptive Behavior Scales*, the *Vineland Social Maturity Scale*, was developed by Doll a half century ago (published in 1935; reprinted in 1947 and 1965). The original purpose of this scale was to determine social placement of retarded individuals in a residential school. It included a series of items used to explore six aspects of behavior: self-help, locomotion, occupation, communication, self-direction, and socialization.

Most intelligence tests provide information on mathematical and language skills that can be used to determine academic placement. Doll, however, wanted to develop a measure of social intelligence that evaluated the ability to deal with people rather than symbols. A parent or caregiver who knew the child well served as the informant, and judgments of credit or noncredit for performance on the items of the scale were made by the examiner.

The *Vineland Adaptive Behavior Scales* are more than just an update of the earlier measure with new norms. They are a complete revision, vastly expanded and changed in internal format. The measure remains a secondhand source in that a parent or caregiver provides the information and the purpose of determining an individual's daily social functioning is the same. However, the measure has been expanded from one to three scales that differ in length and method of administration. The Survey Form (297 items) usually takes 20 to 60 minutes to administer; the Expanded Form (577 items) typically takes 60 to 90 minutes to complete; and the Classroom Edition (244 items), administered as a questionnaire by a teacher, takes about 20 minutes. The Survey and Expanded forms cover an age range from birth to 18 years and 11 months, and norms are based on a representative national sample of 4,800 handicapped and nonhandicapped subjects. The Classroom Edition has an age range from birth to 12 years and 11 months, and norms are based on a representative national sample of 3,000 children.

The *Vineland Adaptive Behavior Scales* retain the same areas of testing as the original scale, but the six areas of behavior assessed are defined as four "domains," which are further divided into subdomains. *Communication* includes receptive, expressive, and written language; *Daily Living Skills* include personal, domestic, and community aspects; *Socialization* encompasses interpersonal relationships, play and leisure time, and coping skills; and *Motor Skills* is divided into gross motor and fine motor. An optional *Maladaptive Behavior* domain is included for "behavior problem" individuals five years and older.

While the original Vineland scoring system included full credit, half credit, and "no opportunity" options, the Vineland Adaptive simplifies this system. Two points are credited for what was once full credit (always or usually performed); one point is used as a replacement for half credit (sometimes or partially performed); and zero is equivalent to no credit. "No opportunity" and "don't know" item responses are scored according to the surrounding scores, as in the original version of the test. These items, of course, must be viewed with more caution. A child could be credited for "no opportunity" when the question is whether he can provide his telephone number on request (Communication domain) when there is no telephone in his residence or whether he can peddle a tricycle (Motor Skills) when he has no tricycle. Specific items within the various domains are identified as allowing or not allowing partial or no opportunity credit. Each subdomain includes basal levels (below which all items are given two points or full credit) and ceiling levels (above which all items are scored as zero). Most of the items retained from the original version of the test have been reworded to make them less ambiguous. This improved specificity of the items has the effect of requiring less "judgment" on the part of the examiner and improves the level of agreement between examiners.

Raw scores from each subdomain and the sum of the raw scores for each domain can be converted to standard scores (mean = 100, SD = 15) and percentile ranks as well as an "adaptive level" and age-equivalent scores.

Reliability and Validity.   Split-half reliability or internal consistency coefficients across the domains and across age groups of the *Vineland Adaptive Behavior Scales*, with few exceptions, exceed 0.80. Split-half coefficients for subdomains by age show more variability, but the means for all age groups within each subdomain show acceptable internal consistency. Test-retest reliability coefficients for domain scores across age groups are in the high 0.80s and 0.90s, and interrater reliability is reported to be in the mid to upper 0.90s.

Construct validity is subject to an interpretation of what a measurement of "socialization" in the matter of self-help, self-direction, communication, and so on, is expected to include. The items on the scales (content validity) appear to reflect the realm of behaviors described. Correlations reported between the Vineland Adaptive and the original Vineland are low (*r* = 0.55), which is not surprising given the expanded content of the revised scale.

The intent of the original Vineland was to provide a "social intelligence" estimate for residential placement of children. The correlations reported for the agreement on the *Vineland Adaptive Behavior Scales* and the *Vineland Picture Vocabulary Test–Revised* (Dunn and Dunn 1981) were low but positive, and correlations with the Wechsler intelligence tests (WISC and WAIS) were slightly higher but still low. However, the measures are different in intent and content, and so it is logical to expect that agreement would be positive but not high.

Considering its intended use, the *Vineland Adaptive Behavior Scales* are more useful than the original *Vineland Social Maturity Scale* by virtue of the expanded description of profiles, the standardization sample, and the standard score conversions. For general clinical purposes, it is probably most useful for establishing a profile of "domains" of adaptive behavior development. But, like other tests of this type, the Communication domain is used to describe general communicative function rather than the precision of language form and content and does not provide sufficient information for planning clinical intervention.

Birth-to-Three Development Scale

The *Birth-to-Three Development Scale* (Bangs and Dodson 1986) is one more of those "old" version instruments that has been republished with a slightly new face and some additional data. There are now three parts to the scale: the Screening Test of Learning and Language Development (Bangs and Dodson), an Intervention Manual (Bangs), and a Checklist of Learning and Language Behavior (Bangs). The earlier (1979) version of the Birth-to-Three was criterion referenced to identify behaviors above and below age level in six-month age groups. Five maturational areas were included: Language Comprehension, Language Expression, Problem Solving, Social-Personal, and Motor Behavior. The 1986 version includes the same five areas, but "Problem Solving" is now called "Avenues to Learning." The new edition is norm referenced with standard scores, percentile ranks, and stanines for each of the five areas. The standard score conversion is a T score with a mean of 50 and a standard deviation of 10. A range of one and one-half standard deviations is considered normal, a score from 35 to 65. The Screening Test has 16 to 18 items in each of the 5 subtests. Each of the items was successfully completed by a minimum of 80 percent of the norming population.

There is some potential for confusion in the score conversion. For example, the conversion table for a thirty-month-old child who was credited with 14 (of 17) points on the Language Comprehension subtest could be credited with a standard score from 42 to 47 and a percentile rank from the 15th to the 40th percentile because the raw scores include decimal numbers. That is, a score of 14 points = 15.9 percentile, 14.3 = 22.7, 14.6 = 30.8, 14.9 = 40.1. These scores range from the third to the fifth stanine. How can a child receive a fractional score on one adminis-- tration of the scale if the scoring options are pass (+1) or fail (0)? A raw score of 14 is at the mean for twenty-six months and within the normal range (conversion T score 35) for thirty-five months. With the new standard score norm-referenced edition, the examiner now has a suggested range of normal variation. However, the value of a conversion score from a fractional raw score must be questioned.

The Checklist of Learning and Language Behavior is criterion referenced with 8 items for each six-month division in contrast to the 16 to 18 items for each six-month division on the Screening Test. The normative base for the Checklist consisted of 20 children each from Texas, Tennessee, and Utah, all judged to be normal in development and near the top of the age range in each of the six-month divisions. That is, four-to-six-month-old children were included in the zero-to-six-month range, and so on. With 8 items at each of the six-month age divisions, each item is credited with 0.75 months.

Receptive-Expressive Emergent Language Scale (REEL)

The *Receptive-Expressive Emergent Language Scale* (REEL) (Bzoch and League 1986, 1991) was also developed for measurement of language skills in infancy and purports to measure language emergence in age periods from zero to 36 months. Age-level separations for the first year are by one-month divisions (0–1, 1–2, 2–3, etc.), for the second year by two-month divisions, and for the third year by three-month divisions. At each age period, there are three receptive and three expressive language statements. If the informant's description convinces the examiner that two of the three items are satisfied, the child is given credit for that age level performance. An expressive language age (ELA), a receptive language age (RLA), and a combined language age (ELA + RLA/2 = CLA) can be determined, or the age scores can be divided by chronological age and multiplied by 100 to yield a set of language-age quotients.

The REEL is not a normed test, and as such there is no reported range of normal performance. The "two-of-three" criterion, however, would seem to add some flexibility to the measurement. In the most recent printing of the test (1991), Bzoch and League reported three studies of infants—a longitudinal study of 50 "normal" children who were tested monthly over a two-to-three year period and 77 infants in two cross-sectional studies that supported the validity of the age-referenced scores.

Language Development Survey

The *Language Development Survey* (LDS) (Rescorla 1989) fits the "second-hand information" category in the way we have been discussing developmental measures. The LDS is designed to test children from 24 to 30 months of age. It is a collection of 309 words in 14 semantic categories—such as food, toys, outdoors, animals, places, body parts, actions, and so on. The parent is asked to "check off words which your child says"—spontaneously not imitatively. The parent is also asked to list other words the child uses and whether the child combines two or more words in phrases and to give examples of three of the child's longest and best sentences or phrases. In other words, a checklist of understandable vocabulary is produced. The task can be accomplished in about 10 minutes. The intent of the instrument, however, is not size of vocabulary per se, but the determination of whether or not the child meets what would be considered a criterion level for normal early language growth. Three "delay levels" are offered for interpretation of results:

> Delay level 1: fewer than 30 words AND no combinations
> Delay level 2: fewer than 30 words OR no combinations
> Delay level 3: fewer than 50 words OR no combinations.

Nelson (1973) has pointed out, for example, that the age at which children's vocabulary reaches 10 words (about 15 months) is a more stable measure of language development than when first words are spoken. Also, rather than predicting in normal language development two-word combinations would occur at 18 to 24 months, a better indicator is that two-word combinations are likely to occur when the child has fifty words in her vocabulary (Nelson 1973).

Rescorla's delay level 1 criterion had the smallest number of "false alarms" (identified as delayed when normal) and delay level 3 was most sensitive (86 percent correct identification in her interpretation).

> In summary, the criterion of fewer than 50 words OR no word combinations on the LDS enabled us to identify the majority of both language-delayed and normal children, with very low rates of both false positives ("false alarms") and false negatives ("misses"). (p. 593)

The LDS was patterned after the *Early Language Inventory* (ELI) developed by Bates and her colleagues (1988) (Dale, Bates, Reznick, and Morisset, 1989). The ELI was designed as a parent-report instrument for information to pediatricians concerning development of children 18 to 36 months old. Included in its profile are judgments on the child's gestural development, receptive language, expressive vocabulary, and grammatical development.

The original sample for the LDS was obtained from just over 400 children receiving medical care in one public and four private clinics serving a wide range of socioeconomic levels. Validation studies (on eighty-one children) were accomplished primarily by comparison of LDS scores with items from the *Bayley Scales of Infant Development* (Bayley 1969) concerned with pointing to pictures and objects. Correlations were $r = 0.80$ to 0.85, which would appear to be quite good agreements for the tasks and the age of the populations.

Summary—Validity and Reliability of Developmental Scales

The social and early developmental scales we have discussed,[1] and others we have not discussed, have been assembled more from empirical than from statistical bases. The exception is the *Vineland Adaptive Behavior Scales*. The REEL and the Birth-to-Three have reported attempts to demonstrate construct validity on small samples of children, but they are screening tests and subject to interpretive bias—or variability, especially due to their short length. By its "two-of-three" format for age designation, the REEL has some more protection from bias than does the Birth-to-Three. The LDS is not intended to provide an age-scale result but rather is essentially a criterion-referenced screen. If the two-year-old child has not surpassed the selected delay level, it may be appropriate to refer the child for more elaborate observation and evaluation.

The measures we discussed were included because they are characterized by an intervening variable—the informant—between the examiner and the subject's behavior. If the examiner observes a behavior, the child can obviously be credited. If the behavior is reported by another, as examiners we do not have the same assurance that it would be credited by our own definition of the behavior. If the child fails to perform for us as examiners, however, we cannot say that the child would not have performed in more familiar surroundings. For this reason we have use for these scales in our evaluations, even though the variability of reporter and hence the variability of the test result are inherent weaknesses.

One other note of caution! Do not be fascinated by an age score even if it is reported as a developmental quotient. Our earlier discussion of age-referenced versus norm-referenced tests made the point of unknown variability. An age score is only a year–month conversion of a raw score. A quotient is no more and no less than the comparison of that age score with the child's chronological age multiplied by 100. The value of the standard score, the age-score, or the quotient is only as good as the instrument used to determine it.

TABLE 2–1   Social and early developmental scales

Name	Age Range	Areas Examined
Vineland Adaptive Behavior Scales	0–19 yrs	Communication, Daily Living Skills, Socialization, Motor Skills, plus Maladaptive Behavior
Birth-to-Three Developmental Scales	0–3 yrs	Language Comprehension and Expression, Avenues of Learning, Social-Personal, and Motor Behavior
Receptive-Expressive Emergent Language Scale	0–3 yrs	Receptive and expressive language
Language Development Scales	24–30 mos	Minimum vocabulary usage

[1]A summary of the scales appears at the end of this section as Table 2–1 with age ranges and areas examined.

REFERENCES

ALDRICH, C. A., AND M. NORVAL, A developmental graph for the first year of life. *J. Pediatrics*, 29, 304–308 (1946).

BALINT, M., *The Doctor, His Patient, and the Illness*. New York: International Universities Press (1957).

BANGS, T., AND S. DODSON, *Birth to Three Developmental Scale*. Allen, Tex.: DLM Teaching Resources (1986).

BATES, E., I. BRETHERTON, AND L. SNYDER, *From First Words to Grammar: Individual Differences and Dissociable Mechanisms*. New York: Cambridge University Press (1988).

BAYLEY, N., *Bayley Scales of Infant Development*. New York: The Psychological Corporation (1969).

BECK, S. D., *The Simplicity of Science*. New York: Doubleday (1959).

BZOCH, K. R., AND R. LEAGUE, *Receptive-Expressive Emergent Language Scale*. Gainesville, Fla.: Computer Management Resources (1986, 1991).

CODE OF ETHICS, *American Speech-Language-Hearing Association 1986 Directory*. Rockville, Md.: American Speech-Language-Hearing Association (1986).

COPLAN, J., J. R. GLEASON, R. RYAN, M. G. BURKE, AND M. L. WILLIAMS, Validation of an early language milestone scale in a high-risk population. *J. Pediatrics*, 70, 677–683 (1982).

DALE, P. S., E. BATES, J. S. REZNICK, AND C. MORISSET, The validity of a parent report instrument of child language at 20 months. *J. Child Language*, 16, 239–249 (1989).

DARLEY, F., *Diagnosis and Appraisal of Communication Disorders*. Englewood Cliffs, N.J.: Prentice Hall (1964).

DOLL, E. A., *Vineland Social Maturity Scale*. Circle Pines, Minn.: American Guidance Service, Inc. (1947, 1965).

DUNN, L. M., AND L. M. DUNN, *The Peabody Picture Vocabulary Test–Revised*. Circle Pines, Minn.: American Guidance Service, Inc. (1981).

EMERICK, L. L., AND J. T. HATTEN, *Diagnosis and Evaluation in Speech Pathology*. Englewood Cliffs, N.J.: Prentice Hall (1974).

HELTON, J., The value of occupation, education, and income in predicting PPVT scores of preschool-aged children: Some comments on criteria commonly utilized for social-class stratification. Unpublished master's thesis, University of Tennessee, Knoxville (1974).

JOHNSON, W., AND OTHERS, *The Onset of Stuttering*. Minneapolis: University of Minnesota Press (1959).

JOHNSON, W., F. L. DARLEY, AND D. C. SPRIESTERSBACH, *Diagnostic Methods in Speech Pathology*. New York: Harper & Row (1963).

NELSON, K., Structure and strategy in learning to talk. *Monogr. Soc. Res. Child Develop.*, 38 (1–2, Serial No. 149) (1973).

O'HARA, C. C., AND M. HARRELL, The empowerment rehabilitation model: Meeting the unmet needs of survivors, families, and treatment providers. *Cog. Rehabil.*, pp. 14–21 (1991, January/February).

RESCORLA, L., The language development survey: A screening tool for delayed language in toddlers. *J. Speech Hearing Dis.*, 54, 587–599 (1989).

SCHULTZ, M. C., The bases of speech pathology and audiology: Evaluation as the resolution of uncertainty. *J. Speech Hearing Dis.*, 38, 147–155 (1973).

SHANNON, E. E., AND W. WEAVER, *The Mathematical Theory of Communication*. Urbana: University of Illinois Press (1964).

SPARROW, S. S., D. A. BALLA, AND D. V. CICCHETTI, *Vineland Adaptive Behavior Scales*. Circle Pines, Minn.: American Guidance Service, Inc. (1984).

WALLIN, P., The predicting of individual behavior from case studies. Cited in W. Johnson, F. L. Darley, and D. C. Spriestersbach, *Diagnostic Methods in Speech Pathology*. New York: Harper & Row (1963).

3

Articulation
Testing

There is no point in giving a test except for a definite purpose.

Wendell Johnson
People in Quandries

INTRODUCTION

The testing of articulation, the premises underlying testing, and the interpretation of test results have, appropriately, gone through a number of changes as a reflection of the dominant theories of the time. In the fifties (e.g., Templin 1957), phonemes were treated as minimal elements that were mastered sequentially as a function of age and motor skill. Age-of-acquisition norms were a reflection of this sequential learning of phonemes as the child matured. Coarticulation, the concept that speech sounds are affected by the production of other sounds in a sequence, was not seriously considered in the context of articulation testing until the sixties (e.g., McDonald 1968). The significance of coarticulation to the understanding of speech production and perception is that a description of articulatory behavior must entail more than the attachment of an invariant label to a variant signal. Also in the sixties (e.g., Chomsky and Halle 1968), attention was drawn to distinctive features of speech sounds. In distinctive-feature theory, phonemes are viewed as clusters of dichotomous elements (voicing, friction, etc.). Phonological development from this theoretical vantage point was seen as a series of distinctive features to be mastered in the course of maturation.

Articulation tests in the "age-of-acquisition" era were of the "sun, bicycle, bus" variety, in which emphasis was placed on the effects of initial, medial, and final word positions, but little consideration was given to the effects of context or consonant clusters. With the advent of distinctive-feature theory, the description of errors changed but not necessarily the stimuli used to elicit responses.

Feature descriptions should predict phoneme confusions, and marking should predict the direction of the confusion. For example, /t/ and /k/ are similar in feature composition with the exception of "front" versus "back" place of articulation. Marking is defined as a productive and/or perceptual order of difficulty—if the feature is marked, it is assumed to be more difficult. In the example, /t/ is unmarked for place, and /k/ is marked. Therefore, /t/ is a maturationally logical substitution for /k/, but /k/ is not a likely substitution for /t/. The importance of the concept of features is that it assumes a rule-governed and generative ordering of a set of hierarchical relationships. For example, front tongue sounds should be mastered before back tongue sounds, and continuancy should be mastered before stridency.

It follows that the next generation of speech-sound error interpretations would maintain the phonological deep structure (rule-generated productions) with errors described in terms of processes. We examine this concept in more detail later in this chapter, but essentially the distinction between a feature analysis and a process analysis is that the "phonological processes" are descriptions of production rather than descriptions based on a combination of production and perception.

Given the diversity of theories related to speech-sound development, it is not surprising that there are probably more tests of articulation than of any other aspect of language. However, articulation tests, like children, are not all created equal. Unlike children, they were created from different theoretical bases; but like children, they do not all perform equally well in the tasks they are designed to perform. We will not review all available articulation tests, but a sufficient variety will be presented to capture test variations and the diversity of rationales from which they were constructed. Your choice of tests to use in the clinical enterprise will be based on your purposes in testing and on your biases.

SCREENING VERSUS DIAGNOSTIC TESTS

One logical division of articulation tests is into screening and diagnostic categories. Screening tests are used to make decisions about whether articulatory development is adequate or inadequate. Diagnostic tests are used to provide a more detailed description of the child's ability to produce a wide range of speech sounds in a variety of syllable positions and phonetic contexts. Diagnostic tests might also be viewed as a means of describing the problem in a manner that will provide a basis for intervention, such as a description of the sound features in error or the phonological processes that characterize the sound productions. Your choice based on these categorizations will depend on your purposes in testing.

Many of the tests we discuss are not easily categorized as screening or diagnostic. Therefore, the first operational division we make is between articulation tests that are primarily single phoneme compared to those that provide more phonetic detail. It will be evident in this categorization that some tests treat the phoneme as a minimal unit; for other tests, the minimal unit is a sound feature described either in articulatory and perceptual terms or in articulatory terms only. A major variable in test selection is the importance assigned to the effects of context. In some tests, consonant sounds are tested in initial, medial, and final word positions; in other tests, the medial position is eliminated either because of relatively little information contributed by a medial position production or because the syllable is considered the basic unit of articulation and consonants do not occur in the middle of a syllable. If the syllable is considered the basic unit of production, then the description will be of the releasing or arresting function of the consonant. Your choice of test based on contextual effects and theoretical orientation will depend, at least in part, on your biases.

Finally, if you agree that speech sounds may represent morphological as well as phonological functions, you will assign a different interpretation to, for example, an omission of an /s/ to represent plurality from an /s/ expected to represent possession or an /s/ as the last phoneme of a root word. We will reserve our discussion of morphology for a later chapter. At this point, we consider testing articulation skills and description of phonological processes.

Articulation tests vary considerably in their procedures and interpretations. Key issues related to the administration and analysis of the results of any of the tests are the method of eliciting responses, scoring procedures, the effects of stimulation, and interpretation of test results based on age of acquisition.

SPONTANEOUS AND IMITATIVE RESPONSES

In the administration of a test with picture stimuli, the examiner has a choice of showing the subject the picture and asking him to name it or providing the word and asking him to repeat it. The first method is called spontaneous, and the second is imitative. There is some difference of opinion expressed in the literature as to whether the two methods of administration yield comparable results.

The earliest reported study concerned with this issue was done by Morrison (1914), who concluded that the two methods yielded similar results. Her subjects were kindergarten and primary school children with "marked" articulatory inaccuracies. Templin (1947a) reported a slight, but not statistically significant, increment from spontaneous to imitative test method with a group of preschool and kindergarten children. Snow and Milisen (1954) used both an imitative and a spontaneous method to test first-, second-, seventh-, and eighth-grade children. Their results showed a consistently higher level of performance for the imitative method, especially among the older children.

Anthony and others (1971) tested three- to five-year-old children and reported no statistically significant difference in the results from the two methods. They indicated, however, that the children probably concentrated more on the pronunciation than the recognition of the picture and, therefore, gave a less self-conscious articulation example in the spontaneous method. Paynter and Bumpas (1977) found no significant difference between scores for the two methods with 3–0 (years–months) to 3–6 children. Siegel and others (1963) reported a statistically significant difference between the imitative and spontaneous testing methods for 8 of the 40 sounds tested with 100 kindergarten children. The differences found were significantly in favor of the imitative method although they were small in magnitude. From inspection of their tabulated data, some of the difference in production may have been related to the familiarity of the words and the ease with which the words could be pictured. In view of these diverse findings, an equitable compromise on test procedures may be that the spontaneous method is preferable as a means of eliciting a representative sample from older children, but equivalent results may be expected from the two methods with younger children—probably through kindergarten and first grade.

These findings also indicate the importance of the picture stimuli utilized to elicit responses. For example, it is difficult to draw a picture that has a high probability of eliciting the words "there" or "smooth" to test the production of a voiced /ð/ sound. In general, and in the interest of saving time, it is probably more efficient to ask young children to repeat the words after the examiner. With older children and adults, a sentence test is more likely to yield valid results. If the person being tested does not read fluently enough to provide "spontaneous-sounding" speech, a picture "word" test may be used to elicit spontaneous responses.

STIMULABILITY

Our discussion of methods for eliciting responses suggested that articulation-test procedures attempt to sample the subject's typical performance. A second procedure as part of the testing is to determine if the subject can correct error sounds following the presentation of the correct sounds at several levels of complexity, for example, in isolation, in syllables, and in words. This procedure is called stimulability testing and involves asking the subject to "watch and listen carefully" as the clinician produces the stimulus sound two or three times and then to repeat the stimulus that was presented. The errors observed during the articulation-test procedure and stimulability testing are recorded the same way; the examiner notes correct production, a substitution, a distortion, or an omitted phoneme. The results of the stimulability testing are recorded with the level of complexity at which the stimulation was attempted. Stimulation of the error sound, and then testing to determine correct production, would usually be carried out for the sound in isolation, syllables, words, and phrases or sentences.

Stimulability data are obtained because of their prognostic value. On the basis of data obtained from 100 kindergarten-aged children—50 classified as having mild articulation problems and 50 with severe articulation problems—Farquhar (1961) concluded that children with mild articulation problems are more likely to make the error sound correctly following stimulation. Furthermore, she found that when the subjects were retested seven months later, there was greater spontaneous improvement in articulation for the mild group than for the severe group of children. When the results of this study are applied to the spontaneous versus imitative method of administration of articulation testing, it can be concluded that an imitative method is apparently less likely to affect the test results if the child has a "severe" articulation problem.

Milisen (1957) suggested that the error phonemes and the stimulability data be listed in adjacent columns. The first column would list error phonemes in order of distractability, so that those errors most distracting to an audience would be at the top of the list. The same sounds in the second column would be listed with the most stimulable at the top. The sounds that are near the top on both lists would be worked with first in therapy to effect a rapid and noticeable change.

SCORING

If your interpretation of an articulation test score were number of correct productions, then, logically, marking the targeted items as correct or incorrect would derive the important information. Recording an incorrectly produced item as a substitution, distortion, or omission has a slightly different purpose. Jordan (1960), as discussed later, reported that the total number of tested items in error was relatively more important than the omission of some number of targeted items. The number of target items that were distorted or substituted was further down the list in determining the judged severity of the problems. For the sake of description of the nature of the articulation problems, recording the specific phoneme that was substituted for the intended phoneme is a useful device. Noting that the intended production was "distorted" is not very descriptive. Beyond the adequate/inadequate judgment, your purpose in testing the subject's articulation—to provide a description of the speech pattern—is better served by fine phonetic notation or by a phonological process description. More will be said of phonological processes later; but for now assume that the more descriptive your scoring, the more information you will have to plan a therapy intervention if there is a problem.

NUMBER AND TYPE OF ERRORS

There is no universal interpretation among articulation test makers regarding the importance of total number of errors on their tests. This lack of consistency is based on the fact that some articulation tests are interpreted on the basis of age of acquisition of speech sounds, some on the frequency of their occurrence, and so on. Consequently, for some tests, the specific speech sounds in error are more important than the total number of errors. For other tests, total number of errors of the sounds tested is more important. Rarely would type of error be important. We discuss age of acquisition of speech sounds in the following section, but for the moment, let us review several studies related to the total number and types of articulation errors and their relationship to judgments of defectiveness.

Historically, the total number of speech-sound errors has been considered the primary factor in judgments of defectiveness. However, there have been few studies that have explored this relationship. Perrin (1954) correlated judgments of trained and untrained listeners with the number of defective sounds, and Barker

(1960) derived a numerical value for defectiveness of articulation, but both of these studies used small samples. The Perrin study used only 7 subjects while Barker included 45 children. A more complete attempt at determining which factors of misarticulation contribute to defectiveness judgments was completed by Jordan (1960). His study included 150 children who evidenced mild to severe articulation deviations. The correlations within this study were made between judgments of defectiveness of tape-recorded samples of conversational speech and results from the *Templin-Darley Tests of Articulation*. He found a statistically significant correlation of 0.72 between number of defective items on the Templin-Darley test and judged severity. It would seem a generally safe assumption that total number of articulation errors is related to the defectiveness of articulation.

There is a frequently stated assumption (e.g., McDonald 1965a) that children develop correct articulation by progression through several stages of production. In general, as language skills develop, speech sounds first are omitted, substituted, distorted, and then produced correctly. Support for this assumption is implied from data such as that collected by Templin (1957), although her data were cross-sectional rather than longitudinal. Templin's data for all age groups combined showed that the most frequent errors were those of substitution (74 percent), followed by those of distortion (16 percent) and omission (10 percent). As the total number of errors decreased with age, substitutions maintained a relatively constant proportion over the three-to-eight-year age groups, but the proportion of distorted sounds fluctuated with no clear trend from the youngest to the oldest age. The proportion of errors of omission declined with increasing age. In other words, the number of articulation errors of all types was reduced with age, with the most dramatic reduction in errors of omission.

The review of data related to the type and number of articulation errors suggests that both these factors may be related to the judged severity of the disorder. This relationship was explored by Jordan (1960). He found that the variable that most highly correlated with a judgment of defectiveness was the number of single phoneme errors. Second in order of importance to a judgment of defectiveness was the proportion of misarticulations that were omissions, and the variable third in magnitude was the consistency of the misarticulated sounds. As separately contributing variables, errors of distortion and of substitution were of relatively little importance.

Listeners will consistently agree on the correct or incorrect judgments of phoneme productions but will not as consistently agree on the identification of error type (Norris, Harden, and Bell 1980). The function of the consonant in a syllable, if it performs a releasing (beginning position) or an arresting (final position) function, will have an effect on production accuracy (Kenney and Prather 1986). Sound context and syllable stress may also facilitate correct production (Kent 1982).

In summary, both the number and the type of errors are important considerations in judging adequacy of articulation skills. The consonant function in a syllable, the consonant context, and syllable stress all affect the number of correct productions. The variables most indicative of defective articulation appear to be the number of omission errors, the total number of single consonants misarticulated, and the consistency of misarticulations. Some inconsistency of articulation is to be expected, however, in the child's development of speech-production skills, and to some degree the inconsistency is predictable, for example, by syllable function and context.

AGE OF ACQUISITION

Another important consideration in the measurement of articulation skills is the type of test items used to measure these skills. There are approximately 43 phonemes in English; 25 are classified as consonants, and 18 are vowels or diphthongs. Some tests, which we have designated as single-phoneme tests, are constructed on the premise that a representative sample of speech must include all of the consonants and vowels and must usually test the consonants in initial, medial, and final word positions. The assumption implicit in a single-phoneme test is that the articulation of the test sound will be consistent and not significantly affected by context. Since context does make a difference, these tests cannot be construed as diagnostic as we have defined that term. Since most single-phoneme tests are interpreted according to age of acquisition, this information must be discussed before we review individual articulatory measures.

There are at least five sets of data reported on age of acquisition with a general agreement as to the order of sounds but with discrepancies as to the age at which children have acquired the production of the phonemes of English. The idea of "produced" compared to "acquired" may need some explanation. Several investigators (e.g., Irwin 1947; Miller 1951) suggest that by the time the child has reached approximately 18 months of age, he has produced all the sounds his oral mechanism is capable of making. This includes a variety of non-English sounds, but it does not suggest that the sounds have been used meaningfully or correctly in intended words. Consequently, "produced" as defined here means that the sounds have been used but not necessarily for intended expressions while "acquired" suggests that they are customarily and purposefully utilized a large percentage of the time.

Phonemes are minimal and nonmeaningful elements in all languages. They are defined by contrast and substitution and are concomitant bundles of features. Features, in the simplest definition, are partial acoustic, perceptual, and articulatory descriptions. For example, we have already divided the phonemes of English into vowels or consonants. By definition vowels have no obstruction of the airstream anterior to the vocal folds and have no narrowing of the vocal tract higher than the tongue position for the high front vowel /i/ or the high back vowel /u/. All vowels are voiced and continuant. Consonants are voiced or voiceless and have a secondary obstruction anterior to the vocal folds that obstructs or constricts the outgoing airstream through the oral cavity or diverts the airstream through the nasal cavity. Oral versus nasal, stop versus continuant, and similar descriptions are defined as "manner" of articulation, and the point of major obstruction in the vocal tract is defined as "place" of articulation. These descriptions are covered in more detail in the chapter on speech-sound discrimination, but the concept was introduced here to give credence or logic to the idea of an order of difficulty of speech-sound production. In an order of acquisition, the sounds with the least number of difficult features are expected to be mastered early while those sounds most complicated in their production will be the last to be mastered. It is not surprising then that Locke (1972) reported a positive correlation between adults' estimates of muscular ease of articulation and children's order of acquisition of speech sounds.

Some other data relative to both ease of articulation and type of error productions were reported by Singh and Frank (1972). Their data are in terms of sound features correctly maintained in children's articulation. The relative stability of each feature is given in the following listing as a percentage of correct production:

FEATURE	PERCENTAGE CORRECT
stop	99.69
nasal	98.75
voiceless	98.04
labial	97.26
voiced	96.92
alveolar	92.42
back	81.82
interdental	78.26

One generalization that Singh and Frank made from these data is that the earlier a feature is acquired the more stable it is and that the more stable features are likely to replace less stable features in articulation. In other words, we may assume that the speech sounds most frequently produced correctly are those phonemes that embody features at the top of this list and that production errors would most often occur on more difficult, less stable features.

As usually defined, acquisition or mastery is the age when a proportion of children correctly produce a given sound in all appropriate positions in a word. Usually the percentage is 75 to 100 percent at a given age level. All the children in the studies to be reviewed had normal hearing and at least normal intelligence.

The first of the five sets of data we wish to compare is by Wellman and others (1931), who tested 204 children ranging in age from two through six years. Test stimuli were pictured on 16 cards plus questions to which the children were asked to respond. The articulation test measured 133 sound units: 66 consonant elements (initial, medial, and final positions, where applicable), 48 consonant blends, 15 vowels, and 4 diphthongs. A sound was considered mastered when 75 percent of the children correctly produced the sound in applicable word positions.

Poole (1934) reported longitudinal data on 140 children over a period of three years with regard to their ability to articulate 23 consonant sounds in initial, medial, and final positions. Each child was tested at four-month intervals with single-word responses elicited by objects, pictures, and questions. Word-position data were pooled, and mastery was defined as approximately 100 percent correct production. That is, "sounds were considered established in the articulation habits of children at the age when the mean frequency of errors approached zero." One other difference in the data reporting of these first two studies is pertinent to mention: Wellman and others designated children under 2–6 as two years of age, children from 2–6 to 3–6 as three years of age, and so forth. Poole classified her 3–0 to 4–0 children as 3–6, the children from 4–0 to 5–0 years of age as 4–6, and so forth.

Templin (1957) administered a 176-item articulation test that included vowels, diphthongs, and single-phoneme consonants in initial, medial, and final word position to 480 children ranging in age from three to eight years. The sample included 30 boys and 30 girls at each half-year level from three through five years and each year level from five through eight years (3, 3½, 4, 4½, 5, 6, 7, 8). Mastery was defined as the age at which 75 percent of the subjects correctly produced the specific consonant elements in all applicable positions in a word.

Sander (1972) criticized the definition of "mastery" as it had been utilized because he thought it was overly stringent. He argued instead for what he termed "customary production" because of varying difficulty of production of a sound according to word position. For example, /t/ in the initial position of a word is produced correctly at a much earlier age than the medial /t/ in words such as "biting" or "city." He suggested that a more logical age placement for the consonant sounds would be the age at which 51 percent of the children tested correctly articulated the sound in at least two of three word positions. Not all sounds occur in all three word positions, however, so his first suggestion would provide for unequal treatment among the consonants. In order to standardize the treatment of consonants, he placed each sound at an age level where more than 50 percent correct production was achieved at an average of the combined word positions. Templin (1957) placed the sound of /dʒ / (the initial sound in "judge") at the seven-year level. The percentages of correct responses for the three positions for 3½-year-old children are 58 percent, 43 percent, and 22 percent for the initial, medial, and final positions respectively. The average of these three is 41 percent. Four-year-old children produced an average correct percentage of 69 percent for the three positions tested, and Sander would therefore place the /dʒ/ sound at the four-year-old level since it exceeds the 51 percent criterion. Sander did not collect new data from children; he resummarized the Wellman and others (1931) and Templin (1957) data with the 51 percent criterion as described.

Prather and others (1975) used a 75 percent correct criterion in testing the articulation skills of 147 children aged 24 to 48 months. The sample included groups of 21 children each at four-month separations: 24, 28, 32 months and so on. In this study, as in the Wellman and Templin studies, children were selected to represent different social classes. Test stimuli were 44 pictures selected from the *Photo Articulation Test* (Pendergast and others 1969) to represent only initial and final position single-phoneme consonants.

Table 3–1 summarizes the data from the five studies discussed. Note that the Sander data derived from the Wellman and Templin studies are quite similar to those collected by Prather and show earlier mastery ages than Poole's data. It should be remembered that Sander utilized a less stringent criterion judgment than Poole, and Prather tested only initial and final word positions.

We indicated earlier that single-phoneme tests may be called inventories since they sample speech sounds in a limited number of contexts. There are probably significant effects from even these limited contexts, however, and the data displayed in Table 3–1 can only be used to determine the general level of speech-sound development from the age-of-acquisition data.

The clinician may expect reasonably large variations in the speech-sound mastery of even a limited sample. In general, most children master speech sounds at a relatively early age. For example, Templin (1957) found that approximately 92 percent of the five-year-old children produced more than 75 percent of the tested sounds correctly in the initial position of words, and 85 percent produced these sounds correctly in the final position. Only the final position voiced /ð/ and /ʒ/, and unvoiced /hw/ in initial and medial positions were correct less than 50 percent of the time. In a later report on a five-year longitudinal study, Templin (in Smith and Miller 1966) commented:

Probably the most important observation that I have made up to this time is that the children with many misarticulations in kindergarten continue to have a considerable number of them when they are in the second grade. Because of the consistent findings from the cross sectional studies that mature articulation was achieved by seven- to eight-year-old children, it was originally planned to terminate the identification and longitudinal studies when the children at grade for their age had finished the second grade. This was not possible, however, because a larger number of children than anticipated had not yet achieved adequate production of the phonemes of English. The children who had poor articulation in kindergarten, while they improved considerably as a group, still had far from adequate articulation scores in second grade. (pp. 176–177)

TABLE 3–1   Comparison of the ages at which subjects produced specific consonant sounds

Sound	Prather	Sander	Templin	Wellman	Poole
m	2	–2	3	3	3–6
n	2	–2	3	3	4–6
h	2	–2	3	3	3–6
p	2	–2	3	4	3–6
ng	2	2	3	*	4–6
f	2–4	2–6	3	3	5–6
j	2–4	2–6	3–6	4	4–6
k	2–4	2	4	4	4–6
d	2–4	2	4	5	4–6
w	2–8	–2	3	3	3–6
b	2–8	–2	4	3	3–6
t	2–8	2	6	5	4–6
g	3	2	4	4	4–6
s	3	3	4–6	5	7–6
r	3–4	3	4	5	7–6
l	3–4	3	6	4	6–6
sh	3–8	3–6	4–6	[b]	6–6
ch	3–8	3–6	4–6	5	[b]
th	4	5	7	[b]	6–6
zh	4	6	7	6	6–6
dzh	4+[a]	4	7	6	[b]
th	4+[a]	4–6	6	[a]	7–6
v	4+[a]	4	6	5	6–6
z	4+[a]	3–6	7	5	7–6
hw	4+[a]	[a]	[a]	[a]	7–6

[a]Sound tested but not produced correctly by 75 percent of subjects at the oldest age level.
[b]Sound not tested or not reported.

Data are from Wellman and others (1931), Poole (1934), Templin (1957), Sander (1972), and Prather and others (1975). Poole used a 100 percent criterion level, Wellman and others and Templin used 75 percent. Poole, Wellman and others, and Templin used initial, medial, and final word positions in their tabulations. Sanders used Wellman and others and Templin data, averaged the percent correct, and used a 51 percent criterion. Prather used the average of only initial and final word positions and a 75 percent criterion. Ages expressed are in years and months; –2 indicates less than two years. Table adapted from Prather and others (1975).

If a single-phoneme articulation test is used, relative mastery of the speech-sound inventory should be expected at least by the age of five years in children of normal intelligence, normal hearing, and normal exposure to a linguistic environment. A child of four years should be readily intelligible, and by three years of age, all of the sound features of the adult language (including stridency, sound clusters or blends, liquids, etc.) should be observed. The blend or fricative may be wrong (e.g., /bw/ for /br/, /s/, for /sh/, or /f/ for /th/), but all of the features are represented in the child's productions.

ARTICULATION TEST RESULTS
AND INTELLIGIBILITY

The reliability of articulation testing and of specific articulation tests is more difficult to discuss than test responses, which require a relatively more gross judgment of yes or no, right or wrong. Assessing articulation and intelligibility is basically a perceptual judgment on the part of a listener (Moll 1968). The potential sources of variability that may affect the reliability (repeatability) of articulation tests results, according to Winitz (1969), can be attributed to the subjects, to the examiner, and to the test instrument, as well as to the interaction of the subject with the examiner.

Articulation testing usually includes the implicit assumption that the test result will somehow reflect the intelligibility and communicative ability of the one being tested. To a degree this assumption has validity, but it must be viewed cautiously. The ability of a speaker to communicate her intentions to a listener is obviously variable and less related to the listener's processing of the acoustic elements of speech than it is to the listener's understanding of the total context. Noll (1970) expressed the proposition this way:

> Since the concept of good speech really can be defined or determined only by the biases and standards of a human listener, articulation testing by the perceptual process of listening is the primary and basic means of assessment. (p. 284)

and further

> To communicate with a listener, a speaker must be able to use intelligible speech. If he has defective articulation, his intelligibility may well be reduced. One way, therefore, to measure articulatory skill is to assess how well the listener understands the message: the degree to which the speaker is intelligible. (p. 291)

A judgment of articulation skill would not be complete with only a reporting of test results; it must also include a statement of judged intelligibility. Probably the most frequently used definitions of intelligibility are from a choice of (1) easily intelligible, (2) understandable if the topic is known, (3) word intelligible now and then, and (4) unintelligible.

"Articulation" and "intelligibility" are related, but they are not identical. If a speaker distorts the sound elements but does so consistently, her speech may be easily intelligible because of the predictability of the errors. The consistency of the sound errors thus has an effect on intelligibility. As mentioned earlier, the number and type of errors will also influence a judgment of intelligibility, but there is at least one more factor in our judgment. According to Faircloth and Faircloth (1973), syllabic integrity is more critical to intelligibility than is phonetic integrity. They reported that speakers who closely approximate the appropriate number of syllables in a polysyllabic utterance and maintain the correct stress patterns, rhythm, and intonation are more intelligible than those who disrupt syllable integrity, regardless of whether the individual phonemes are correctly articulated.

The point to be made is that articulation testing is really done in the examiner's ear, and the specific test formats or test stimuli are only the vehicles for the examiner's judgment. Regardless of the test instrument or the means for making the evaluation, the examiner must bear in mind that intelligibility and articulation integrity are not necessarily the same thing and must decide whether he wishes to judge functional communication ability or phonetic accuracy or both.

The articulation tests to be discussed in the rest of this chapter are therefore assumed to be examples from which—according to his biases and purposes—an examiner may choose the phonetic or phonemic stimuli. The important judgments of functional adequacy and/or accuracy must still be made in the ear (and mind) of the beholder.

SINGLE-PHONEME ARTICULATION TESTS

The classification of tests as "single phoneme" is an approximation. It is perhaps more accurate to call them *primarily* single-phoneme tests because they include a few /s/, /l/, and /r/ blends. They appear to have been built on the rationale of gathering a phonetic inventory and generally have not been validated on other than the construct of age-of-acquisition norms. Examples include the *Bryngelson and Glaspey Articulation Test* (1951), the *Developmental Articulation Test* (Hejna 1955), and the *Photo Articulation Test* (Pendergast and others 1969, 1984).

The Bryngelson-Glaspey is important only as a historical base for the others. It includes 17 consonants (plus some examples of /s/, /l/, and /r/ blends) described as "most commonly misarticulated" and tested in initial, medial, and final word positions.

The *Developmental Articulation Test* provides picture stimuli for single consonants in all word positions and some two-consonant blends in the initial position of words. An adaptation of this test by Sanders (1970) utilized format designs from the *Developmental Articulation Test* and the *Photo Articulation Test* with each phoneme identified by the age at which 90 percent of Templin's (1957) test subjects had correctly produced the phoneme in the word positions tested.

We previously discussed the problems inherent in interpreting an age-of-acquisition test result, specifically, what age norms should be used and how a decision regarding the range of normal is to be made.

The primary difference between the *Photo Articulation Test* (PAT) and the Bryngelson-Glaspey and the *Developmental Articulation Test* is the use of photographs rather than line drawings. On the score sheet for the PAT, the stimuli are divided into "lip sounds," "tongue sounds," and vowels to aid in the determination of place of articulation as a variable. Test stimuli include 24 consonant singles in initial, medial, and final positions where they occur in words, a few /s/, /l/, and /r/

blends, plus 18 vowels and diphthongs. Sixty-nine of the test responses are elicited by use of the pictures. The remaining seven are obtained in response to questions.

The 1984 printing of the *Photo Articulation Test* includes error mean and standard deviation norms for children from 3–0 to 11–11 instead of the more usual eight-year-old upper limit found for other tests. The normative group included 684 white, middle-class children from the Seattle, Washington, area with 25 boys and 25 girls in each half-year separation from 3–0 to 5–11 and each year division from 6–0 to 11–11.

The mean error score for children in the mid age range of the PAT (5–6 to 5–11) is 6.5 with a standard deviation of 7.3. A one standard deviation range from this mean overlaps the mean of the 11–11 and the 4–4 to 4–11 age groups. In other words, although the age norms go up to age 12, there is very little difference between a 6-year-old and a 12-year-old in expected numbers of errors.

Validation reported in the 1984 printing was a comparison of responses to PAT items and *comparable* items from the Bryngelson-Glaspey and the *Templin-Darley Tests of Articulation*. That is, the issue addressed was whether the PAT photos generated the same responses as line drawings from the other two tests. No comparative information was furnished relative to the ability of the PAT to distinguish adequate and inadequate articulation skill. In a similar study, Madison, Kolbeck, and Walker (1982) compared the PAT with the *Goldman-Fristoe Test of Articulation* and the Templin-Darley. The essence of their findings was that children spontaneously identified the PAT photos more often than the Goldman-Fristoe or the Templin-Darley drawings. But again, this report did not address the issue of correct productions of sounds or the validity of the results. The "validation" did not investigate whether the test instrument was effective in differentiating between children with adequate or inadequate articulation skills. Instead, it was undertaken to determine if the photos were as efficient as line-drawings in eliciting the sounds in question.

Sampling techniques as well as stimuli may have an effect on test findings. Kenny and others (1984) compared three sampling methods for eliciting articulation responses from preschool children. The comparison was for imitation of real multisyllabic words, multisyllabic nonsense words (vowels in real multisyllabic words were changed to a schwa), and storytelling (spontaneous response condition). Slightly better articulation was observed in the word version, which is expected, since more articulation errors are found in syntactically more complex, more meaningful utterances, but the difference was not significant. The number and type of errors were consistent among the three types of testing.

The *Denver Articulation Screening Exam* (DASE) (Drumwright 1971) does not differ significantly in design or content from the other tests we have reviewed but has been included because of a difference in purpose. It was constructed as a screening examination for preschool economically disadvantaged children. The purpose was to set different adequacy criteria for these "culturally different" children in order to reduce the number of referrals of children for therapy whose speech-sound productions reflected dialectal differences, regional pronunciations, and foreign dialect. The standardization sample was 1,455 white, black, and Mexican-American preschoolers in the Denver, Colorado, area. All of the children were described as in the lower socioeconomic class. The 30 sound productions included on the test (primarily single phonemes in initial and final word positions and some two-element blends) were productions listed as correct by 85 percent of the six-year-old children studied by Templin. They were included in the DASE if 70 percent of the Denver inner-city six-year-olds were correct in these productions.

Raw scores for two-and-one-half to six-year-old children by half-year age groups were converted to percentile ranks, and the 15th percentile was selected as the adequacy criterion. It was suggested that referral should be based on this normal versus abnormal score plus a judgment of intelligibility. A child of three years or older was to be referred if he scored at less than the 15th percentile and was judged to be other than easily intelligible.

It must be remembered that the standardization population was limited to children from a lower socioeconomic level localized to the Denver inner-city area. The 15th percentile criterion, therefore, may not be appropriate to other regional, ethnic, or socioeconomic groups. If, however, you accept the argument of a lower standard of performance expected from the "disadvantaged" child, the test may be a useful tool for making decisions regarding "culturally different" versus "disordered" judgments expressed in the section in Chapter 1 on testing nonstandard populations. The unfortunate part of the validation procedure for the test was that the *Developmental Articulation Test* was used as the criterion measure for comparison to the DASE scores. The two tests are similar in content so scores might be expected to agree. However, we are unaware of any validation data for the *Developmental Articulation Test* so that questions regarding the validity of the DASE have not been addressed.

The *Arizona Articulation Proficiency Scale* (AAPS) differs in function and interpretation from other single-phoneme tests. It was published in 1960 (Barker), slightly modified in 1962 (Barker and England), and revised in 1970 (Fudala) and in 1986 (Fudala and Reynolds).

The purpose of the test is to provide a severity or intelligibility calibration of articulation skills. The distinctive characteristic of the test is the use of weighted values for phonemes based on their frequency of occurrence. Frequency-of-occurrence data were taken from a Bell Laboratory study (French, Carter, and Koenig 1930) that determined the frequency of occurrence of sounds from a corpus of the most commonly heard nouns, verbs, adverbs, and adjectives in 500 telephone conversations. These values were slightly modified by Denes (1963). The idea was to place a greater value on error productions of sounds that occurred more frequently and less value for less frequently occurring sounds.

The original version of the AAPS sampled 24 consonants in initial, medial, and final positions; several /s/, /l/, and /r/ blends; and 20 vowels, diphthongs, and vowel /r/ blends with the values for the consonants prorated across the three word positions. That is, each position was assigned the same value although different frequencies of occurrence for initial and final word positions would have made the assignment of different values appropriate. For example, the initial word position /t/ value was listed as 2.52, and final word position /t/ was 6.49. However, the value assigned to /t/ in all three positions was two points. Total value for all consonant productions on the test was approximately 55 points; total vowel value was 45 points.

The validation study reported with the 1960 publication included 45 children aged 6 to 12 years. Nine of the 45 were reported to be receiving therapy; two had no errors in production; and no description was provided for the other 34 children.

One-minute conversational samples were tape-recorded for each of the children, and two 10-second samples were taken from these tapes. One of the two samples was used for training judges, the second for testing. The judges were trained to assign one-to-nine–point values on an equal appearing interval scale from least to most defective on the basis of the first sample. That is, the judges were not taught what numbers to assign; they were only familiarized with the range of deficiency to be rated.

As part of the validation study, Barker computed the correlations between AAPS scores for the three-position, equal-valued phonemes and for initial and final positions (eliminating medial) according to their frequency of occurrence with the one-to-nine–point ratings of deficiency. Total values for the consonants were adjusted so that they would be identical (54.5 points) for each selected grouping of test items. Barker reported a very high ($r = 0.94$) correlation for each set of data and concluded that the test instrument was valid and that medial word position did not need to be tested.

From a procedural standpoint, the validation study must be interpreted cautiously because of the limited sample size and lack of consideration of age as a variable. With data of this type, it would be expected that a 12-year-old would perform better than a 6-year-old and that a 6-year-old would more likely be in therapy. The potent age effect and its interaction with articulation ability would need to be explored in order to assess the value of correlation between AAPS scores and ratings of defectiveness in establishing the validity of the test instrument.

The 1970 revision of the AAPS included a sentence version in addition to the original picture stimuli and initial and final *syllable* positions are identified (e.g., /v/ in *television* is identified as an initial syllable position rather than as a medial word position as in the previous version). Two other important revisions have been included. First, the 23 consonants plus /s/, /l/, and /r/ blends have been reduced from 65 to 48 items while retaining the total consonant value of 54.5. This was accomplished by eliminating the medial word position and establishing values for each item based on its frequency of occurrence rather than by a proration across the three word positions.

The second change is in the age-of-acquisition designations for the phonemes. In the 1960 version of the test, vowels and consonants were listed according to age-of-acquisition data from Templin (1957). For the 1970 edition of the test, the phonemes were listed according to the ages at which 90 percent of a group of 702 children in the Seattle, Washington, area produced the sounds. The age scores are not "averages" but rather points at which the 90 percent criterion are met. The sample included 25 boys and 25 girls at each half-year level from 3 to 5½ years and at one-year intervals from 6 to 12 years (11–11).

The AAPS Second Edition (Fudala and Reynolds 1986) expanded the age range (18 months to 13–11 years) and was standardized on 5,122 children, and it provides normalized T-scores. As in the earlier versions, the weighted value derived from the number of speech sounds produced correctly is meant to be interpreted as an intelligibility score. For example, a score of 75 indicates that the child is credited with a weighted value score of 75 points for 75 percent intelligibility on the phonemes tested (not 75 percent of the sounds tested). Fudala reported earlier that the average score for 3-year-old children was 84 points, and the average score for 3½-year-old children was 89 points. Both scores should indicate readily intelligible speech. She also reported (1970, p. 5) that "fifty percent of the children tested had AAPS scores of 100 by age five," which is in keeping with our earlier comments on intelligibility and general early mastery of the phoneme inventory. These kinds of numbers, however, do not speak to the validity of the concept of weighted values of phonemes on the basis of frequency of occurrence. Put another way, if the error sounds were less frequently occurring, the number of erred sounds could be the same but would result in a higher level of "intelligibility." The manual for the second edition reports that validity is best for children seven years and under, but Fudala and Reynolds do not clarify how that validity was established.

We have gone into considerable detail in the description of the AAPS because a mathematically derived score to represent a level of articulation proficiency and intelligibility would seem to be a worthwhile endeavor. Unfortunately, the validity of the derived scores on the AAPS is questionable. Haller (1978), in a review of the test, pointed out that an important shortcoming is that omission, substitution, and distortion errors are treated in the same manner. Jordan (1960), in a validation study of the *Templin-Darley Tests of Articulation*, demonstrated that these types of errors were not judged equally. His data suggested that although the number of single phonemes in error was the highest rated factor in a judgment of intelligibility, errors of omission were considerably more important than errors of substitution or distortion.

Shriberg and Kwiatkowski (1982b) have also developed a procedure for determining the severity of articulation deficits that is based on the percentage of consonants produced correctly in a five-minute sample of continuous speech. However, they too fail to offer compelling data to validate this procedure for developing a numerical index of articulatory proficiency.

In an unpublished study, Peterson (1968) found that AAPS results did not reflect differences in articulation skill, and articulation scores were not in judged agreement with severity. In that study the test sample consisted of 241 children 6, 7, and 8 years of age. The 6-year-old group included 76 children between 5–7 and 6–6; the 7-year-old group included 92 children from 6–7 to 7–6; and the 73 children in the 8-year-old group ranged in age from 7–7 to 8–6. The children were from 9 schools in the northern and central part of Illinois and lived in communities that represented a range of socioeconomic strata. All the children were receiving speech therapy and were judged as having mild, moderate, or severe articulation disorders. Judgments of severity were made by experienced speech pathologists employed in those schools. The severity judgment was on an 8-point scale with 7 as very severe, 1 as very mild, and zero as no problem. The articulation testing was done by experienced graduate and undergraduate students who also rated intelligibility according to ease of understanding of the subject's speech.

Without going into the rest of the details, data shown in Table 3–2 illustrate the correlations between the test measures listed and judged severity of the articulation problem. Since we would expect a change in proficiency with age (improved skill and reduced variability), it is also pertinent to note the performance of the three age groups in Table 3–3, which lists the means and standard deviations for the *Templin-Darley Screening Test*, the AAPS, the number of distortions, substitutions, and omissions on the 43 single-phoneme items of the Templin-Darley test, and the number of single-phoneme errors that were corrected following stimulation for the error items.

TABLE 3–2   **Correlations of articulation test measures with judged severity of speech deficiency for six- to eight-year-old children**

Measure	Six Years (*N* = 76)	Seven Years (*N* = 92)	Eight Years (*N* = 73)
Templin-Darley Screening Test	.770[a]	.595[a]	.611[a]
Arizona Articulation Proficiency Scale	.468[a]	.171	.207
Number of distortions (single phonemes)	.165	.201	.334[a]
Number of substitutions (single phonemes)	.681[a]	.598[a]	.669[a]
Number of omissions (single phonemes)	.587[a]	.330[a]	.429[a]
Intelligibility (0–3)[b]	.670[a]	.607[a]	.539[a]
Number of stimulable sounds (single-phoneme errors)	.421[a]	.427[a]	.623[a]

[a]Significant beyond the 0.01 level of confidence; df = 72; r = 0.23 < 0.01.

[b]Intelligibility judged by the test administrator: 0 = easily intelligible, 1= understood if topic known, 2 = word understood now and then, 3 = unintelligible.

Severity judgments were made by speech pathologists who were familiar with the children. Testing and intelligibility judgments were done by student clinicians familiar with the tests but not with the children.

From Peterson (1968).

In reference to the mean numbers shown in Table 3–3, the most appropriate comparisons would be between Templin-Darley and AAPS numbers. In terms of the other data shown in Table 3–3, the number of omissions, substitutions, and distortions are obviously proportionate numbers, and the accumulation of the three would be related to total number of errors. The meaningfulness of those numbers would be their relative proportions across the three age groups (and their relative agreement with severity judgments as shown in Table 3–2). The most stable of the three type-of-error means in Table 3–3 is the number of distortions. It is also obvious that the number of stimulable sounds would be related to the number of error sounds—that is, as more errors are made in the production of the single phonemes, more items would be tested for stimulability. Because of the reciprocal nature of these numbers, mean stimulability for groups of children would not be as meaningful as a description of the stimulability change for an individual child.

While the data in Table 3–2 and 3–3 are not comprehensive in that all the varieties of articulation tests are not compared, they do at least indicate that the AAPS was not related to the severity judgments of experienced clinicians as closely as types of errors (omissions and substitutions), and the AAPS score did not reflect an improvement in articulation skill with age as did the Templin-Darley. Numbers can validly represent severity of articulation disorders but apparently weighted values derived from frequency of occurrence of speech sounds cannot.

The *Weiss Comprehensive Articulation Test* (WCAT; Weiss 1978, 1980) is a relative hybrid of articulation test styles incorporating both age-of-acquisition and intelligibility based on frequency of occurrence. It has a picture identification format (for nonreaders) and a sentence format (for those who can read). It was designed to be used for children from age 30 months and has no specified upper age limit, although it is assumed that children of seven years will make no errors on the test.

The 1980 version derives a Weiss Articulation Score (WAS) based on fre-

TABLE 3–3   Means and standard deviations for articulation measures listed (ages are shown separately)

Measure	SIX YEARS		SEVEN YEARS		EIGHT YEARS	
	$\bar{x}$	SD	$\bar{x}$	SD	$\bar{x}$	SD
Templin-Darley Screening Test (number correct of 50)	27.46	13.33	32.97	12.88	37.10	9.76
Arizona Articulation Proficiency Scale	85.27	12.97	83.87	22.62	83.70	25.03
Number of distortions (on single phonemes)	2.92	3.32	2.20	2.10	2.21	2.29
Number of substitutions (on single phonemes)	9.25	6.31	6.78	5.60	4.46	3.99
Number of omissions (on single phonemes)	3.23	6.47	1.79	4.44	1.23	3.50
Intelligibility (0–3)	.53	.72	.43	.71	.31	.68
Number of stimulable sounds (from single-phoneme errors)	6.44	5.52	4.03	4.13	3.93	5.39

Intelligibility judged by the test administrator: 0 = easily intelligible, 1 = understood if topic known, 2 = word understood now and then, 3 = unintelligible.

From Peterson (1968).

quence of occurrence of English phonemes (similar to the *Arizona Articulation Proficiency Scale* but with different values for phonemes), and a Weiss Articulation Age (WAA) based on age-of-acquisition. For the WAS the value of the misarticulated items is subtracted from 100. In this interpretation, a seven-year-old child is expected to score 100.[1] The WAA credits correct productions based on age-of-acquisition with a 90 percent criterion level. Age-of-acquisition norms were reportedly from data collected by Weiss (but not separately identified) and by Prather et al. (1975), Templin (1957), and others. All consonants and centering diphthongs are expected to be mastered by 78 months, all consonant blends by 84 months. The "articulation age" was derived by beginning with the base age of 36 months and adding one month for each phoneme correctly produced in one of the tested (initial-medial-final) positions, and two months for correct production in two or more positions.

Weiss reports good reliability (repeatability of test item responses) for the test but begs the issue of validity. Rather than a report of how well the WCAT scores agree with some other measure—for example, a judgment of intelligibility—he reports (1978, p. 5) that he considers *content* validity to be satisfied since the test includes a representative sample of the phonemes of the language, but he does not address such issues as criterion-related validity or construct validity.

The *Goldman-Fristoe Test of Articulation* (1969, 1986) was designed to include three levels of complexity. Twenty-three single phonemes and blends for /s/, /l/, and /r/ combinations (73 items) are tested in words in response to picture

---

[1]The 1978 version used a different format for intelligibility. That version suggested taking a continuous sample of the child's speech, selecting 100 consecutive words from the sample and counting the number of *words* that were unintelligible. Subtracting that number from 100 supposedly yielded an intelligibility index. A four-year-old child was expected to be 100 percent intelligible.

stimuli. Nine pictures and two stories are used to test the same phonemes in what is identified as a "sentence" test (simulating conversational speech) for the second level, and sounds produced in error are tested for stimulability in the third level.

With the addition of data gathered for the *Khan-Lewis Phonological Analysis* (1986), error score percentile ranks are available for boys and girls separately from age 2 to 16 years. Although there are no specific validation studies, the normative data from the earlier version would appear to be representative since they were gathered from the 38,884 children who comprised the National Speech and Hearing Survey (Hull et al., 1971). No recommendations are provided by the authors, so the cutoff for the judgment of articulatory adequacy is probably the 15th percentile.

The *Fisher-Logemann Test of Articulation Competence* (1971) differs from other single-phoneme tests in the way that the error sounds are analyzed. The response sheet for the 25 single-phoneme consonants tested is separated according to voicing, manner, and place of articulation of the error sound. The test, therefore, is designed to record the feature classification of error sounds, rather than just the occurrence of an error. For example, if a /t/ sound were substituted for an /f/, the response sheet matrix would indicate the difference in features of the two sounds as an intruded stop for the intended fricative and tongue-tip alveolar position intruded for the intended labiodental position. The sounds are alike in voicing. The error productions would thus be described in terms of the features in error.

Instead of the usual initial, medial, and final word-position description, the three positions are described as prevocalic, intervocalic, and postvocalic. The stimulus words are also chosen to represent standard dialects. For example, the final (postvocalic) sound in the word "garage" is counted correct with either /dʒ/, or /ʒ/ and the voiced /w/ would be accepted as a correct alternative for voiceless /hw/ in a word such as "whistle." The test includes single phonemes, /s/, /l/, and /r/ blends, and vowels and diphthongs. Sentences that sample "all the consonants and vowels of English" are included with the *Fisher-Logemann Test of Articulation*.

There are no separate norms for interpretation of this test. The developmental ages of the single-phoneme consonants according to Templin (1957) are listed as information for the examiner, but as stated earlier, the primary intent of the Fisher-Logemann test is to describe the feature differences in the error sounds.

DIAGNOSTIC ARTICULATION TESTS

We began this chapter with a division of articulation tests into single-phoneme (inventory) and phonetically detailed (diagnostic) tests. It should be borne in mind, however, that the best representation of the tests as a whole would be on a continuum from inventories to phonetically detailed. We have described several single-phoneme tests and have considered their rationales and interpretations. Now we turn our attention to phonetically detailed, or diagnostic, tests. Two representative diagnostic tests are the *Templin-Darley Tests of Articulation* (1969) and the *Edinburgh Articulation Test* (Anthony and others 1971).

An earlier version of the *Templin-Darley Tests of Articulation* (1960) included a 176-item diagnostic test that contained 50 items identified as a screening test. The second edition (1969) has been shortened to a 141-item test while maintaining the 50 screening items. The reduction was accomplished primarily by eliminating the testing of many single-phoneme consonants in the medial position of words and by removing some infrequently occurring consonant clusters. The manual provides means and standard deviations for the 141-item diagnostic test for boys and girls separately, for both sexes combined, and for upper and lower socioeconomic separations for ages three to eight. The age means are separated by half-year levels from three to five years (3, 3½, 4, 4½, 5) and by one-year levels from five to eight (5, 6, 7, 8). Eight years is considered adult performance, so an older child's or adult's performance would be compared with the means for eight-year-old children.

To facilitate description of the articulation of the subject, overlays are provided to assist with the analysis of special groups of sounds. For example, overlays are provided to view the 50 screening items separately, 42 consonant singles, 22 initial-position consonant singles, 43 *Iowa Pressure Test* items, 31 /r/ and /ɚ/ clusters, 18 consonant and syllabic /l/ clusters, 17 /s/ clusters, 9 miscellaneous sound clusters, 11 vowel groups, and 6 diphthongs. The manual has means and standard deviations by age groups tabled for each of these clusters.

The 50 screening test items consist of 1 vowel (/ɝ/), 1 consonant glide plus vowel (/ju/), 22 single consonants (10 in the initial, 8 in the medial, and 4 in the final position), 22 two-consonant clusters, and 4 three-consonant clusters. The 50 items are those that have been identified as best discriminating between good and poor articulation in preschool and kindergarten children. Templin (1947b) studied the production of 113 speech-sound elements contained in the 176-item diagnostic test by 100 preschool and kindergarten children. From the total test results, the 27 percent of the children with the highest number of correct responses were classified as the "good articulation group," and the 27 percent with the fewest number of correct productions were classified as "poor articulators." Through the use of the Lawshe Nomograph technique of item analysis (Lawshe 1942), a discrimination value (D-value) was determined to identify those sounds that best distinguished the two groups of children. The D-value indicates the separation between mean percentages of correct production by the good and the poor articulating groups. None of the 50 sounds had a D-value of less than two. In other words, the sample averages were separated by at least two standard deviations on each of the 50 items constituting the screening test.

In addition to means and standard deviations that are available with the screening test, a cutoff score is included. The cutoff score can be used to separate adequate from inadequate articulation skill by age. These cutoff scores happen to be approximately one standard deviation below the mean for boys and girls combined at each of the age levels. Remember that the adequate-inadequate cutoff score and the mean score for the 50 items were determined by two different statistical treatments, so an exact correspondence is not expected. Recall from the discussion in Chapter 1 that one standard deviation on either side of the mean usually defines the limits of "normalcy." Insofar as the normal curve model is appropriate, the cutoff score on the test and the minus one standard deviation point should be expected to approximate.

A response form to illustrate a young client's performance on the Templin-Darley articulation screening and consonant-singles subtest items is shown as Figure 3–1. She was identified as T. G. and was 4–2 years of age when tested. She was referred because of a concern about articulation skill. T. G.'s mother could understand her, but she was unintelligible to other listeners if the topic was not known. Her mother's description of the problem was that T. G. omitted medial- and final-position consonant sounds from her speech. As is shown in Figure 3–1, T. G. correctly produced 3 of the 50 screening items. Mean performance for a girl of this age is 34.2 with a standard deviation of 10.6. The cutoff separating adequate from inadequate performance for this age is 23 correct productions. She correctly produced 16 of the 42 initial- and final-position single-phoneme consonants included in this test, as compared to an expected 31.7 correct of 42. T. G. was also given the *McDonald Screening Deep Test,* and the result will be shown later in this chapter.

The *Edinburgh Articulation Test* is similar to the Templin-Darley test and consists primarily of two- and three-element blends. The rationale for the selection of test stimuli was to represent a "balanced and comprehensive picture of the consonants and consonantal clusters occurring in English at various positions in the word structure in monosyllabic, disyllabic, and a few polysyllabic words." Picture stimuli are utilized to elicit 41 words containing 30 blends and 38 single-phoneme consonants. The test utilized item analyses from 371 normal and 153 speech-retarded children ranging in age from 2.5 to 6.0 years of age to establish norms. A conversion table is used for interpretation of test results interpolated with three-month divisions; that is, age groups of 3.75 years but less than 4.0, 4.0 but less than 4.25, and so on. Analysis of the data indicated that 5.5 to 6.0 years of age was the terminal level of the test, or approximately adult level. The standardization sample was reported to be proportionately representative of the boys and girls, social class, and familial status of the population of the Edinburgh, Scotland, area. Tabled values from the standardization of the test indicate slight differences for sex, social class, and family standing, but the differences were not statistically significant, and the norms do not distinguish among these variables.

The child's responses are scored correct or incorrect for the quantitative portion of the test. The number of correct productions is then converted to a standard score according to age quartile. The standard score is set at 100 with a standard deviation of 15. Fifteen points of this standard scale represent approximately one year, and a standard score of 85 or less at any age is considered the "danger level." The examiner is encouraged to look at the error responses in phonetic detail to determine if the child shows speech retardation that calls for therapy.

The reason for the inclusion here of an articulation test standardized on a group of children who speak a Scottish dialect of English is not the probability of your encountering many such children in your local clinic or school populations but the uniqueness of the Edinburgh test interpretation. The test manual includes a qualitative as well as the more usual quantitative scoring. Examples are listed of children's responses to the target phonemes as a degree of closeness to the correct production. The qualitative scale ranges from productions that are "locally acceptable" and "close to intended" to "highly unusual" as qualitative variations. No specific values are derived from the qualitative range, but an overall judgment of how close or how far from customary the intruded sounds are.

The test protocol is included here as a possible model for construction of "local norms" for interpretation of dialectical variations in speech production. This system has the advantage of a quantitative score (for comparison with "standard" English) and a qualitative yardstick for potential calibration ranging from "differ-

	Screening Test			Consonant Singles		

1. ɝ	3	26. br-	bw	Initial			Final	
2. ju	✓	27. tr-	stw	51. m	✓	52. m	✓
3. r(i)	w	28. dr-	g	53. n	✓	54. n	✓
4. r(m)	w	29. kr-	kw			55. ŋ	✓
5. l(i)	j	30. gr-	gw	56. p	✓	57. p	−
6. v(i)	b	31. fr-	f	58. b	✓	59. b	−
7. θ(i)	f	32. θr-	fr	60. t	✓	61. t	−
8. θ(m)	−	33. ʃr-	sw	62. d	✓	63. d	−
9. θ(f)	−	34. pl-	p˗	64. k	✓	65. k	−
10. ð(i)	✓	35. kl-	k˗	66. g	✓	67. g	−
11. ð(m)	✓	36. gl-	gw			68. l	w
12. ð(f)	−	37. fl-	f	69. f	✓	70. f	−
13. z(i)	−	38. sm-	m			71. v	−
14. ʃ(i)	5	39. sn-	n	72. s	✓	73. s	−
15. ʃ(m)	−	40. sp-	p			74. z	−
16. ʃ(f)	−	41. st-	f			75. ʒ	−
17. ʒ(m)	−	42. sk-	k	76. h	✓		
18. j(i)	−	43. sl-	sw	77. w	✓		
19. j(m)	−	44. sw-	fw			78. dʒ	−
20. tʃ(i)	ts	45. tw-	sw				
21. tʃ(m)	−	46. kw-	xw				
22. tʃ(f)	x	47. spl-	pw				
23. dʒ(i)	−	48. spr-	pw				
24. dʒ(m)	s	49. str-	zw				
25. pr-	p˗	50. skr-	kw				

Screening test no.correct __3__   Consonant singles __16__
                                     no. correct

Expected for age: Mean __34.2__   Expected for age: Mean __31.7__

Standard deviation __10.6__   Standard deviation __5.5__

Cutoff score (adequate) __23__

FIGURE 3–1 **Templin-Darley articulation screening and consonant singles subtest scores for T. G. (C.A. 4–2). (3 = correct production, X = distortion, the phonetic symbol is inserted for substitutions, – = omission)**
(Adapted from Templin-Darley Tests of Articulation, Articulation Test Form. Copyright 1968 by The University of Iowa. Used by permission.)

ent" to "disordered." For example, the child may produce a glottal stop where an alveolar or palatal stop was intended. If the Scots dialect were spoken in the child's home, your interpretation may well be different than if standard English were the language of his home and his peers. Or, your interpretation of the child's production of /f/ for an intended voiceless /th/ in a word-final position may depend on your knowledge of whether this was an acceptable local variation.

SPECIAL PURPOSE TESTS

The three tests reviewed in this section are set apart because of the different purposes for which they were designed. The *Iowa Pressure Test* consists of 43 items from the 176-item *Templin-Darley Tests of Articulation* that were determined (Morris, Spriestersbach, and Darley 1961) to best separate between adequate and inadequate velopharyngeal closure for cleft-palate speakers. The test items include eight single-phoneme consonants and two- and three-element blends consisting primarily of fricative and plosive consonants. There are means and standard deviations for ages three to eight published with the Templin-Darley (1969) test manual, but these "norms" in and of themselves do not indicate adequacy or inadequacy of the velopharyngeal mechanism. That judgment can only be made in terms of the nasality *perceived* with the error production of the intended consonant.

The *Predictive Screening Test of Articulation* (PSTA) (Van Riper and Erickson 1968) was constructed, as the name implies, as a predictor of future performance. The authors indicate that the basic purpose is to

> . . . differentiate children who will master their misarticulations without speech therapy from those who, without therapy, may persist in their errors. More specifically, the PSTA may be used to identify, among primary school aged children who have functional misarticulations at the first grade level, those children who will—and those who will not—have acquired normal mature articulation by the time they reach the third grade level. (p. 1)

The test was designed for school clinicians who have a large percentage of their caseload in the primary grades. The contention of the authors of the test was that a great number of children are scheduled for articulation therapy when maturation would solve their articulation problem. Consequently, it would be inefficient use of therapy time to work with children who would outgrow their errors; and it would also be inefficient not to schedule for therapy those children who would still have clinically significant misarticulations by the time they entered third grade.

A total of 111 experimental items were selected from a larger pool of suggested items assembled from the literature and from practicing clinicians. The 111 experimental items were administered to 167 beginning first-grade children in southwestern Michigan. Each of the children had been judged to have clinically significant misarticulations. At the end of a two-year period when the children were entering third grade, the 134 still available children were retested. Van Riper and Erickson (1968, p. 2) reported that 47 percent of the identified children no longer demonstrated misarticulations, and 53 percent continued to exhibit articulation errors. Item analysis reduced the 111 items to the current 47-item test. This smaller test was administered to a similar-sized sample of first-grade children, and again the approximate 50–50 division of children occurred. Forty-nine percent were free of misarticulations, and 51 percent continued to demonstrate some misarticulations at the third-grade level.

The first 17 items of the 47-item test sample the child's production of 10 single-phoneme consonants; the next 19 items are two-element /r/, /s/, and /l/ blends followed by one /spl/ and one /str/ blend. The remaining 9 items are not usually found in an articulation test. They consist of a sentence to be repeated; the continuation of an /s/ and a voiceless /θ/ consonant in isolation; the production of the syllables /seeseesee/, /zoozoozoo/, and /puhtuhkuh/; the production of the syllables /lalala/ while the child has the tip of her thumb between her teeth to test the child's ability to raise and lower the tongue tip independently of jaw movement; the discrimination of an /ɚ/ vowel from a schwa on the end of a word ("finger" vs. "finguh"); and the child's repetition of a clapping rhythm. Specific instructions are given for each portion of the test. All stimuli are elicited by imitation.

There are no norms as such included with the test. Rather, the manual includes tabled data to indicate the predicted adequacy—inadequacy of the child's articulation when she reaches the third grade. The selection of a high cutoff score by the clinician would predict that relatively few children who needed therapy would be falsely identified as adequate but that a relatively large number of children would be identified as inadequate for whom maturation would solve the problem. That would be termed a "false positive error." If, on the other hand, the cutoff were set low, the proportion misclassified as not needing therapy would be high ("false negative error"), but relatively few children scheduled for therapy would have self-corrected through maturation. Van Riper and Erickson (1968) suggest that school clinicians may wish to select their own cutoff score according to their particular circumstances. If there is more room in their clinic load, they could set the cutoff high and risk working with some children whose misarticulations would be corrected by maturation but better ensure working with all the children who would need their professional help. If they have a full clinic schedule, they may set the cutoff low to reduce the false positive error and risk not identifying some children who would need therapy at the third grade. The authors of the *Predictive Screening* Test of Articulation recommend a cutoff of 34, which would balance the false positive and false negative errors at about 30 percent of each population.

Table 3–4 illustrates some midrange cutoff scores with the proportion of children identified at each of the scores. It is important to remember that the scores generated are for beginning first-grade children as predictions of their success at the beginning of the third grade. At the time of this writing, there are no predictions available for first to second grade, or second to third grade, or any other age–grade circumstance. It should also be remembered that the predictions do not necessarily apply to children with hearing loss or other organic deficits and may not apply beyond the population sample on which they were gathered.

The *McDonald Deep Tests of Articulation* include both a "Deep Test" (1965b) and a "Screening Deep Test" (1968), which will be discussed separately because they are slightly different in format and design. Since the tests are based on a theoretical explanation of articulation, it is first necessary to discuss some of the basic concepts.

TABLE 3–4 **Among first graders with functional misarticulations, total proportion classified as requiring speech therapy; proportion misclassified as requiring speech therapy (false positive errors); and proportion misclassified as requiring no speech therapy (false negative errors)— when classifications are based on PSTA scores**

Cutoff Score	Proportion Classified as Requiring Therapy	False Positive Errors	False Negative Errors
39	.72	.59	.15
38	.67	.51	.19
37	.64	.49	.22
36	.61	.44	.23
35	.57	.40	.27
34	.54	.37	.30
33	.48	.34	.39
32	.44	.33	.46
31	.37	.26	.51
30	.31	.21	.61

From Van Riper and Erickson (1968).

McDonald (1965a) based his articulation testing on four concepts:

1. *Articulation is a process consisting of overlapping ballistic movements.*[2] The overlapping ballistic nature of the articulatory movements places varying degrees of obstruction on the outgoing airstream and also modifies the size, shape, coupling, and resonance of the articulatory cavities.

This means that the production of a phoneme will be influenced by the articulatory positions of the abutting phonemes. Said another way, the sound produced is influenced by the context in which it occurs. The amount and the distance of influence has been called coarticulation. Daniloff and Moll (1968), for example, stated that left to right or retentive coarticulation (the articulatory characteristics of a phone observed in later phones in the string) may extend to as many as four consonants, and right to left or anticipatory coarticulation (an articulatory characteristic of a phone observed during production of preceding phones) may extend to as many as three consonants. An example may help here—consider the word "construe." The only lip-rounded phoneme is the high back vowel /u/, but lip rounding has been observed before or during the production of /n/. A discussion of coarticulation is not appropriate for our purposes here, and the comment was made only to lend support to the premise of overlapping movements. A more extensive consideration of this topic is provided by Kent and Minifie (1977).

---

[2]You remember from basic physiology that there are three types of movements: (a) fixed—the opposed muscles are in balance; (b) controlled—a slightly more powerful contraction of one set compared to the other results in a relatively slow, purposeful movement; (c) ballistic—characteristic of all skilled movements and consisting of three stages: a deep stroke to begin the movement, a momentum stage, and an arresting motion to stop the movement.

2. *Audible phenomena produced by a series of ballistic movements are highly variable and influenced by the sequences in which they occur.* This concept is a more concise restatement of the comments concerning coarticulation.

3. *Movements that produce these auditory phenomena (the sounds) develop specificity as a result of the interaction of sensory motor activities in time.* Figure 3–2 illustrates what this statement implies. As the child matures, both sensory and motor skills improve from gross to fine abilities. With maturation, he is progressively more capable in terms of both motor and sensory skills to produce more complex sound combinations.

4. *More gross movements must be developed before the fine movements can be produced.* This is self-explanatory and logical. McDonald uses it to account for the child's expected articulatory progression from omissions, to substitutions, to distortions, to correct production. The data on mastery of speech sounds (e.g., Templin 1957) does indicate that young children make more errors of omission than older children. We also noted earlier that an error of omission was judged as more important than an error of substitution or distortion in terms of the severity of the judged defectiveness. Although it may be empirically logical, there is no longitudinal data, as such, to suggest that a child would routinely go through this progression.

Two main points in the development or variability of specificity of function may be summarized as the basis for the McDonald test:

1. Articulation is a developmental behavior. There is variability in children, and with maturation the behavior becomes more specific. In practical terms, this means that the mean number of correctly articulated sounds should increase with age, and the variability around the mean should decrease.

2. Some movement sequences are more conducive to correct production of specific sounds. Two implications are contained in this statement. One is that if the articulatory positions for two abutting sounds are close together and do not interfere, those two

FIGURE 3–2   Gross to fine development of sensory and motor skills with resultant sound productions

(Adapted from E. McDonald, *Articulation Testing and Treatment—A Sensory-Motor Approach.* Pittsburgh: Stanwix House, 1965, p. 94.)

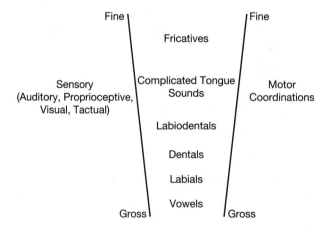

sounds may be more accurately produced than if the sequential positions are far apart. The other implication is that if we draw a continuum from sound productions being never or randomly correct to always correct, we would expect that the speaker would range on this continuum according to the complexity of the abutting sounds, and probably neither extreme of the continuum is valid.

Percent of correct productions

0%	50%	100%
(never)		(always)

To the degree that the above reasoning is valid, *McDonald Deep Test* results should provide a prediction of spontaneous improvement on the part of the child. For example, if a five-year-old child correctly produced 50 percent (maybe 30 percent or even less) of the /s/ contexts tested on the *Deep Test of Articulation*, it may be logical to expect her to correct misarticulations as well *without* therapy as with therapy. For a child placed in therapy, the implication would be to practice the child in the production of the sound combinations she already makes correctly. McDonald assumes that her production practice will make her more aware of how the sound is produced, and this knowledge will spread to other combinations and result in an easier carryover to correct productions.

It is obvious by now that the *Deep Test of Articulation* is designed differently from the other articulation tests we have been discussing. According to McDonald, the usual articulation test, with the initial, medial, and final word-position placement of the phoneme in a single-word stimulus, is not indicative of the typical speaking situation. The initial, medial, or final description would frequently imply an intrasyllabic test. If we assume that a conversational production of a statement such as "This is the house that Jack built" contains only one initial sound (the beginning /ð/ sound in "this") and the only final sound is the /t/ in "built," all other sounds in the sentence are medial and primarily intersyllabic (between syllables rather than within syllables). The *Deep Test of Articulation* does not purport to test every phoneme in every and all possible combinations, but it does place the sound tested in up to 30 intersyllabic positions with both an arresting function (final sound on the first of two syllables) and a releasing function (beginning sound on the second of two syllables). The sounds to be "deep tested" are determined by the examiner from conversation with the child or from another articulation test or any other means the examiner chooses. Both a picture test and a sentence test are available. The abutting consonants tested are keyed to the same response sheet in each version. The mechanics of test administration can be illustrated by the examiner's instructions to the child to name the pair of pictures presented to him—to make "one funny big word" out of the names of the two pictures presented rather than naming them separately. As mentioned before, this is an intersyllabic test. In English, for example, we have within-syllable combinations of /p/ plus /t/, as in the pronunciation of "capped" or "kept," but not /t/ plus /p/. In a between-syllable arrangement, as in conversational speech, the /t/ plus /p/ abutting would occur in a phrase such as "that point."

There are no norms for the Deep Test. The number of combinations produced correctly is converted to a percentage correct for each phoneme. The primary premise, as stated earlier, is that the sound productions are a function of the phoneme context, and some phoneme combinations will be more conducive to correct productions than other combinations. It should further be expected that there will be a common set of correct combinations, for example, among a five-year-old population. A six-year-old population of children should have that group of sounds plus others in correct combinations; the seven-year-old children should add still further to the common core of correct productions, and so on. Appleton (1969) has shown this to be true. Figure 3–3 shows a graph of the progression of percentage of correct responses for five-, six-, and seven-year-old children for the /r/ and /s/ phonemes in the various combinations. The children in Appleton's study were selected as having articulation skills at or above age level according to the *Templin-Darley Screening Test of Articulation* (1969).

The *Screening Deep Test of Articulation* restricts the testing to 9 phonemes that McDonald described as frequently in error, in each of 10 contexts. In other words, 9 consonants are tested in each of 10 contexts. While in the Deep Test all of the test sounds were placed in a medial (intersyllabic) position in the stimulus syllables, in the Screening Deep Test 30 of the 90 test phonemes are in initial or final (therefore, intrasyllabic) location. The picture stimuli are paired on a single card, and the instructions to the child are the same: "Make a funny big word" of the two pictures. Originally, there were no detailed norms published with the Screening Deep Test, so interpretation of the results was unclear. However, a later report (McDonald and McDonald 1974) provided longitudinal data on repeated testing of 521 children from beginning kindergarten to beginning third grade. The data reported are in terms of proportion of the children who correctly articulated the 9 consonants of each of the six test times (beginning and ending kindergarten and first grade; beginning second and third grade). McDonald and McDonald (1976a,b) reported cross-sectional data on children from prekindergarten to beginning first

FIGURE 3–3   Mean percentage articulation scores for five-, six-, and seven-year-old males in the production of the /r/ and /s/ phonemes in 46 phonetic contexts
(From Appleton [1969].)

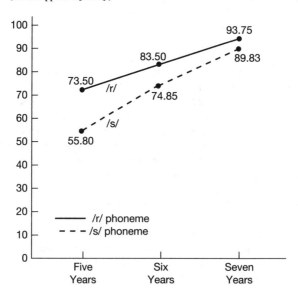

grade and a comparison of longitudinal and cross-sectional data on the Screening Deep Test. The cross-sectional report separates the data for boys and girls and shows a slight advantage for girls over boys in the earliest ages but a similar performance for boys and girls at the beginning of first grade. Table 3–5 shows an example of the type of data reported. Guidelines for interpretation are contained in the reports (1974, 1976a,b), but a general statement such as the following seems reasonable:

> ... any child who continues to produce fewer than 3 correct productions of any of these sounds from beginning kindergarten to the beginning of first grade should be considered a candidate for therapy at that time. (1974, p. 21)

When discussing the *Templin-Darley Tests of Articulation*, we included (as Figure 3–1) an example of a test result for T. G. and noted that she had been given the *McDonald Screening Deep Test* as well. That result is shown as Figure 3–4. Most of T. G.'s errors would be described as omissions of medial and final position sounds. Substitution errors were primarily simplification; for example, reducing two-element combinations to a single phoneme and replacing both /tʃ/ and /ʃ/ with the less marked fricative /s/. The only single phonemes not made correctly in any of the tested combinations or word positions (see Figure 3–4) were /tʃ/, /θ/, and /ʃ/.

The data from the Templin-Darley test and the McDonald screening test agree that T. G. is significantly below expected performance for a child of her age. Additionally, from both test protocols, she is consistent in her omission of consonants that serve an arresting function (final position) in most stimulus syllables tested. In other words, in planning therapy for T. G., it would be important to note that with few exceptions, the phonemes of English are, at least sometimes, correctly produced. In her case, the position (or function) of the phoneme would appear to be relatively more important than context per se.

TABLE 3–5   **Proportion of 2,125 beginning first-grade children correctly articulating each of the SDTA tested consonants in the indicated numbers of contexts**

	CONSONANTS TESTED ON THE SDTA								
	s	l	r	tʃ	θ	ʃ	k	f	t
10	.66	.75	.76	.88	.65	.81	.98	.83	.97
9	.13	.14	.09	.06	.10	.08	.01	.11	.02
8	.07	.07	.04	.02	.05	.03	.001	.05	.004
7	.04	.01	.02	.01	.03	.02	.001	.01	.001
6	.02	.01	.02	.01	.03	.01	.001	.001	.001
5	.01	.004	.01	.002	.02	.01	.002	.00	.00
4	.01	.003	.01	.01	.02	.01	.001	.001	.00
3	.01	.003	.01	.002	.01	.01	.001	.001	.00
2	.01	.01	.01	.001	.01	.003	.00	.001	.00
1	.01	.001	.01	.01	.01	.01	.00	.001	.00
0	.04	.001	.02	.01	.06	.01	.001	.001	.00

From McDonald and McDonald (1976a).

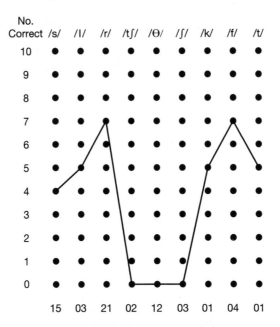

FIGURE 3–4   T. G.'s phonetic profile on the *McDonald Screening Deep Test of Articulation*. The graph line represents the number of correct productions of each of the 9 phonemes listed. The number at the bottom of each column is the approximate percentile rank that number of correct responses represents as compared to beginning-kindergarten-aged girls according to McDonald and McDonald (1976a).
(Adapted from E. McDonald, *Teacher's Record Sheet for a Screening Deep Test of Articulation*, Pittsburgh: Stanwix House, 1976. Used by permission.)

SUMMARY OF ARTICULATION TESTS

The articulation tests we have reviewed[3] to this point have varied in terms of the sounds tested and the value assigned to correct or incorrect productions. They cannot clearly be separated into categories, but in general, we described them as either phonemic inventories or phonetically detailed. Additionally, some were categorized as screening tests, some as diagnostic, and some as "special purpose." Results of testing were expressed as age-referenced scores, as standard scores, or as predictions of future performance. What they had in common was an implicit recognition of the phoneme as the minimal testable entity. Your choice of which test to use would be based on your purposes in testing and your construct of what an articulation test is supposed to do (bias).

The assessment procedures presented allow you to determine the number of correct (or incorrect) responses, which can then be compared to a choice of yardsticks. With the possible exception of the Fisher-Logemann test, these articulation

---

[3]A listing of the tests reviewed is included in Table 3–6 with age ranges and interpretation comments and norms.

tests do not define the error response. Rather, they identify a class of problems described as articulation disorders and perhaps do a better job of identifying children whose articulation is normal than they do of providing information about why the child's speech is abnormal. These tests are inadequate for determining *why* a child is unintelligible. Especially for children with extreme intelligibility problems, a second group of assessment procedures is necessary to describe what are termed phonological disorders.

ARTICULATION DISORDERS VERSUS PHONOLOGICAL DISORDERS

The distinction between an articulation disorder and a phonological disorder is at least partly theoretical. The term "articulation disorder" has historically implied that the child learned an inappropriate motor response. The term belonged to a sur-

TABLE 3–6   Summary of articulation tests

Test	Age range	Comment
Developmental Articulation	3–8 yrs	Age of acquisition–age range dependent on whose data you accept.
Photo Articulation Test	3–12 yrs	Expressed as errors for tongue, lip, and vowel sounds plus total; boys and girls separately.
Denver Articulation Screening	2½–6 yrs	Percentile rankings—for "culturally disadvantaged" children
Arizona Articulation Proficiency Scale	18 mos— 13–11 yrs	Percentage score to give intelligibility—based on frequency of occurrence of single phonemes
Weiss Comprehensive Articulation Test	30 mos–adult	"Intelligibility" Articulation Score (WAS) and Articulation Age (WAA)
Goldman-Fristoe	2–16 yrs	Percentile scores: boys, girls; words, sentences, stimulability
Fisher-Logemann	—	Features of sounds in error— interpreted also in age of acquisition
Templin-Darley Screening and Diagnostic Tests	3–8 yrs	Means and standard deviations, screening test has cutoff for "adequate"
Edinburgh Articulation Test	2½–6 yrs	Raw score converted to standard scale score; quantitative and qualitative
Iowa Pressure Test	3–8 yrs	Means and standard deviations ("pressure sounds" from Templin-Darley Test)
Predictive Screening Test	first grade	Probabilities of normal or defective by third grade; no other norms
McDonald Deep Test of Articulation	—	No norms—percentage of correct production for sounds tested
McDonald Screening Deep Test	K–3rd grade	Number of correct response for 9 sounds in 10 contexts with normative sample comparisons

face-level theory. Phonological disorder implies that the child has learned an inappropriate phonological rule. Language is a generative system—a rule-governed system, and the definition of "language" includes phonology, morphology, syntax, semantics, and pragmatics. A "phonological disorder" suggests that the child's heuristic rules of phonology are at variance with the rules of the adult community around him. Schwartz et al. (1980) stated that although there is not an isomorphic relationship between phonology and other aspects of language, a close relationship is expected.

The term "phonological disorder" does not have a consensus definition. Shriberg and Kwiatkowski (1982a), for example, use the term as a replacement for the historical category of "functional articulation disorder." Many authors appear to have replaced the generic term "articulation" with "phonological" when discussing disordered speech production. Some (e.g., Shelton and McReynolds 1979) reserve the term "phonological" for the underlying rules of behavior, while still others appear to ignore the issue of definition and simply discuss phonological processes.

McReynolds and Elbert (1981) have proposed qualitative and quantitative criteria to differentiate between what they term "surface" error patterns (articulation errors) and "underlying" patterns (phonological errors). Qualitatively, the sound affected by a phonological disorder must be found to be produced correctly and contrastively in at least some conditions. Quantitatively, a large enough sample must be taken to ensure the process is stable for a number of error sounds and occurs with a frequency that allows the examiner to feel confident that a process (that is, disordered rule) is present. A short example may help here. A child's final omission of /s/ in "bus" may be a function of a rule that calls for final consonant deletion in that context. Omission of the /s/ in the word "stick" would be termed a cluster reduction and would be a function of a different rule. Obviously, these rules are more specific and functional than a description of the errors as "omission of /s/."

In descriptions of rule-based phonological patterns, there appear to be differences in the functional definition of what constitutes a process. To some, the term is used to indicate all rule-governed articulation behavior. Others appear to reserve the term for those sound productions that are in error and at variance with the adult language system.

The Random House dictionary defines process as "a systematic series of actions directed toward some end, . . . a series of changes taking place in a definite manner," or, from a biological and anatomical standpoint, "a natural outgrowth." According to these definitions, both correct and incorrect speech-sound productions would be considered processes because they are the result of heuristic phonological rules. A rule is a formal device, and rule ordering sets up or encodes patterns.

Phonological process analysis then is a more comprehensive description of the child's articulation patterns than would result from an articulation test that lists correct and incorrect phonemes. This type of analysis is particularly useful when multiple speech-sound production errors are observed.

Although the terms in use are different, process analysis is generically similar to the distinctive feature descriptions of Chomsky and Halle (1968) and others that serve as part of a theory of generative phonology. The distinctive feature systems proposed by Jakobson (1962) and detailed by Chomsky, Halle, and others were a set of productions generated by deep structure rules and expressed through a series of rewrite rules. (For examples of application, see Compton 1970 or McReynolds and Huston 1971.) The important distinction for our present purpose is that distinctive feature descriptions (terms such as consonantal, vocalic, anterior, coronal, strident, etc.) are part articulatory (productive) and part perceptual. However, phonological process descriptions are all production descriptions. Therefore, they have more to do with articulatory productions of the child that are assumed to be an outgrowth of heuristically learned phonological rules than with the adult rules of phonology.

Process analysis describes what the child does that makes her productions of speech sounds importantly different from adult (normal) productions. As such, they describe the *raison d'être* for the omissions, distortions, or substitutions observed. Phonological process analysis provides a categorical description of what is to be suppressed or eliminated in order to make the child's productions more closely match the adult's.

PHONOLOGICAL ANALYSIS
WITH YOUNG CHILDREN

Several studies have investigated phonological development in children through the use of process analysis. Hodson and Paden (1981) described the phonological processes that separate unintelligible from intelligible speech in young children. Haelsig and Madison (1986) reported on the developmental progression of phonological processes. Khan and Lewis (1986) described a phonological system with 12 processes assumed to be normal in the developmental progression and 3 that are nondevelopmental, or not usual in children's mastery of the adult system. Shriberg and others (1986) have attempted to categorize phonological profiles as the basis for diagnostic subtypes.

Phonological process analysis procedures differ slightly in descriptive terms, the number of descriptions included, and the method of eliciting responses (imitation, spontaneous responses from the use of pictures or objects, culling words from spontaneous conversational samples). We include only a few examples of these analyses because they have evolved from a common theoretical base.

One of the first phonological process descriptions was developed by Ingram (1976). He included 18 processes that are listed and illustrated here.

deletion of final consonant	dog = dɔ
weak (unstressed) syllable deletion	candy = kæn
cluster reductions	stick = tɪk
stopping	see = ti
fronting	shoe = su
gliding (of liquids)	rabbit = wæbɪt
voicing processes (nonassimilatory)	bit = bɪd
initial consonant deletion	cat = æt
deaspiration	take = t°eɪk
reduplication	ball = bʌbʌ
glottal replacement	pig = pɪʔ

denasalization	nice = dæɪs
progressive assimilation	duck = dʌt
regressive assimilation	dog = gɔg
vocalization	bottle = batu
frication	yellow = zɛlo
nasal preference	bite = maɪt
backing	tap = kæp

Schwartz et al. (1980) included in their listings such descriptions as final consonant devoicing, labial assimilation, alveolar assimilation, velar assimilation, prevocalic voicing, and gliding of fricatives as well as many of the terms used by Ingram. They also charted the variability of these processes and included a category of consistent replacement (for the same words), which they termed nonoptional and inconsistent replacements, which were termed optional behaviors.

The *Khan-Lewis Phonological Analysis* (KLPA) was mentioned earlier in the discussion of the *Goldman-Fristoe Articulation Test*. They utilized the picture stimuli from the sounds-in-words subtest of the Goldman-Fristoe and administered the test to 907 children, approximately 200 at each full-year interval from ages 2–0 to 5–11. Children were stratified according to sex, race or ethnic group, and geographical location.

They defined 15 phonological processes, 12 of which were characteristic of normal speech development and 3 that were nondevelopmental—that is, infrequently or rarely occurring in normal-speaking children of these ages. The 12 normal developmental processes were deletion of final consonants, initial voicing, syllable reduction, palatal fronting, deaffrication, velar fronting, consonant harmony, stridency deletion, stopping of fricatives and affricates, cluster simplification, final devoicing, and liquid simplification. The 3 nondevelopmental processes were deletion of initial consonants, glottal replacement, and backing to velars.

The responses to the 44 stimuli were scored as correct or as reflecting one or more of the processes. The results could be interpreted as a normative score—percentile ranking by age as a function of the number of correct responses, as a speech simplification rating, and as an age equivalent. The simplification score is apparently treated as if it were akin to an intelligibility index. For the simplification rating, the number of instances of occurrence for each of the 12 phonological processes is tallied, and these numbers are converted to a zero-to-four rating, interpreted as insignificant to excessive. The sum of these ratings is a composite score that can be converted to a percentile rank and an age-score equivalent for each three-month age group from 2–0 to 5–11. The arrangement of phonological process descriptions on the response sheet is a listing of approximate rank order of suppression. In appendices to the Khan-Lewis test manual, the authors give examples of sound substitutions and process designations.

From the number of processes listed to this point from only three assessment descriptions, it is obvious that the examiner has some degree of choice in how best to describe a sound substitution. For example, if a child intruded a /t/ sound for /ch/, in process terms this substitution could be described as fronting, depalatization, deaffrication, or stopping. Is one more appropriate than the others? Is it all of these? It is probably best described as examples of all of these if our purpose is to describe what the child does. The number of phoneme errors per se is not the important datum. The usual procedure is to determine the percentage of times that a process occurs in relation to the number of times it is possible for it to have occurred.

Since the process designations and the eliciting procedures are arbitrarily, or at least empirically, determined, rather than review several slightly dissimilar procedures, let us report instead on two comparative studies. The determination we are looking for is the legitimacy of the variety of ways of collecting the child's responses and some judgment on which of the processes are the most useful descriptions of unintelligible speech.

Bankson and Bernthal (1982) compared the phonological processes identified through word and sentence imitation tasks. The test they used was Weiner's (1979) *Phonological Processes Analysis* (PPA). The PPA has 16 phonological process descriptions. Four of these are syllable structure processes (deletion of final consonants, cluster reduction, weak syllable deletion, and glottal replacement), 5 are harmony processes (labial assimilation, alveolar assimilation, velar assimilation, prevocalic voicing, and final consonant devoicing), and the other 7 are just called processes (stopping, gliding of fricatives, affrication, fronting, denasalization, gliding of liquids, and vocalizations). The PPA elicits 142 responses in imitation of words and 142 more with the key words included in imitation of sentences. The PPA protocol of testing is to intermix the two.

Bankson and Bernthal modified the procedure in testing 18 preschool children with the words and sentences separately to determine if both were necessary. Their data demonstrated no significant differences in the processes identified by either method and, in effect, suggested the examiner could save time by doing either the word or the sentence imitation.

A study by Paden and Moss (1985) compared the efficiency of 3 phonological analysis procedures. Their study included Shriberg and Kwiatkowski's (1980) *Natural Process Analysis* (NPA), Hodson's (1980) *Assessment of Phonological Processes* (APP), and the *Procedures for Phonological Analysis of Children's Language* (PPACL) by Ingram (1981). The NPA has 8 processes to be determined from a minimum of 5 minutes of conversational speech that are then transcribed and scored. The APP utilizes 42 responses to three-dimensional objects or pictures to determine 6 categories of processes (plus an "other patterns" category), and the PPACL has 27 process descriptions to be determined from a spontaneous sample— preferably from continuous speech.

Paden and Moss found that the processes identified were identical for the three procedures whether from one-word responses, elicited sentences, or a continuous conversational sample. The difference in the three procedures was then in the difference in time it took to test, transcribe responses, and interpret the results. The APP took approximately one hour, the PPACL about two hours, and the NPA nearly four hours.

What these comparisons suggest is that the imitation or spontaneous productions of words or sentences, as isolated instances or as culled from a conversational speech sample, apparently result in equivalent data. Obviously, the classes of consonant sounds (stops, fricatives, liquids, etc.), locations (pre- and post-vocalic, initial and final syllable position), and clusters of sounds must be present in sufficient redundancy to determine the range of processes employed and the consistency of the productions. Although not universally stated, the minimum number of possible occurrences appears to be 8 to 10.

Garn-Nunn (1986) and Garber (1986) report on the use of process analysis descriptions with "standard" articulation tests such as the Goldman-Fristoe or the *Photo Articulation Test.* The restriction in use of these procedures is that the stimuli from the tests must provide "enough" occasions for the processes to be reliably defined. That is, different articulation test stimuli may yield somewhat different results based on the number of possible occurrences available. The basic difference is that rather than looking only at the target phonemes specified for that test, the data for analysis would be the entire phonetically transcribed word.

Hodson and Paden (1983) defined 10 basic deficiencies and a set of percentage-of-occurrence criteria, as well as an added value for age of the child, on which to base a judgment of severity of the problem. If you use stimuli other than Hodson's APP, the percentage of occurrence may well differ, but the interpretive result may well be similar (at least according to the Garn-Nunn data).

The 1986 revision of the Hodson test (*Assessment of Phonological Processes–Revised*) eliminated or changed a few of the stimulus words and made some simplifying modifications in the analysis form, but the primary change we are interested in is the new formula for calculating severity ratings. A "phonological deviancy" score is derived from percentage-of-occurrence scores for the 10 basic omission and class deficiency processes. These 10 percentages are added together and divided by 10 to derive a phonological process average. If the child's average score is less than 15, no additional points are added for age, and it is assumed this child "would not be a candidate for a comprehensive phonological approach" (APP–R Manual, p. 15).

The 10 APP–R processes on which to base a severity judgment are shown here with data from a 3–1 child to provide an example.

PROCESSES	PERCENTAGE OF OCCURRENCE
Four segment omissions	
syllable reduction	10%
consonant sequence reduction	50
(formerly called cluster reduction)	
prevocalic singleton consonant omission	28
postvocalic singleton consonant omission	47
Six class deficiencies:	
stridency deletion	41
lack of velar stops	50
omission of liquid /l/	90
omission of liquid /r/	100
omission of nasals or substitution of	
nonnasals for nasal sounds	0
omission or substitutions	
for the glides /w/ or /j/	67
mean	47%

The child in this example was three years old. If she were older, you would naturally assume that these numbers represented a greater deviation from normal.

Hodson's (1986) deficiency score adds 5 points for a 4-year-old, 10 points for a 5-year-old, 15 points for a 6-year-old, and 20 points for a 7-year-old. In other words, if these date were gathered from a 7-year-old child, the child's score would become 67 rather than 47. Hodson also suggests that mental age may be a more appropriate base than chronological age for determining severity in mentally retarded children (p. 36).

The 1983 edition of the APP supplied four categories of severity (mild, moderate, severe, and profound) at apparently arbitrary 25 percent equally spaced increments. The APP–R *phonological deviancy* score was revised downward:

1–19 points	mild
20–39	moderate
40–59	severe
60 and above	profound

Hodson also suggested that the intervals can be further subdivided by designating the bottom five points as "low" and the top five points in each division as "high." That makes intuitive sense, although it is obviously still arbitrary. A child with an average deviation score of 35 is in the same (moderate) category as a child with a deviation score of 25 but probably has a greater problem and should have higher priority for scheduling therapy.

Garrett and Moran (1992) compared phonological deviancy scores (PDS), percent consonant correct scores (PCC) based on connected speech and on a list of single words, and perceptual judgments made by panels of graduate students in speech-language pathology and education. The high degree of intercorrelations (high 80s to low 90s) lends an assumption of validity to the results of phonological process testing.

In summary, the phonological process analyses described have a common theoretical base—that the productions are rule governed. Unlike distinctive feature analyses, all of the process descriptions are of production (articulatory gestures) rather than a combination of production and perceptual descriptions. The process analyses differ in detail but all have the same intent—to describe why the child is unintelligible. To that end, the recommended method of eliciting responses may differ—picture stimuli versus objects, imitative or spontaneous naming versus language sample—but the methods and the specific stimuli appear to be less important than the method used to provide a sufficient number of examples or opportunities for the processes to occur.

With the increasingly younger and greater number of pre–school-aged children being referred to clinics, schools, and so on, a phonological-process evaluation can be a very helpful addition to the clinician's armamentaria. Tests designed to demonstrate correct or incorrect productions of the phonemes of the language, as described earlier in this chapter, may well provide categorization of "adequate" or "inadequate" in the sense of age expectations, but they do not provide as detailed a base for therapy intervention. Phonological process analyses are intended to yield more than the number of correct and incorrect productions. They are intended to provide a description of why the child is unintelligible and also a calibration for measuring change. They are a description of the productive gestures the child displays that are different from the adult model. In other words, these are productive "processes" to be eliminated.

The descriptive purposes of articulation tests and tests of phonological processes are different. Garn-Nunn and Martin (1992) compared test outcomes for conventional articulation tests (the Goldman-Fristoe, the *Photo Articulation Test*, and the *Weiss Comprehensive Articulation Test*) with the *Assessment of Phonological Processes–Revised*, on a population of 20 children ranging in age from just over three years to nine years. All the children were considered to be phonologically impaired, but otherwise normal (normal classroom placement, normal hearing, and no structural or functional oral mechanism deviations). The researchers' concern was to determine whether or not there were differences in identification and therapy programming outcomes.

Basically, the results of the study were predictable. Standard scoring of the conventional articulation tests identified the children as having a problem—none scored within normal ranges (i.e., no score higher than the 4th percentile). The subjects in this study were primarily in the severe to profound range, and possibly different results may obtain with children in a more moderate range. The programming information, however, was much less clear. The phonological process format is designed to provide information on severity and nature of errors—quite logically these types of tests yield more information as to why the child is difficult to understand, and therefore do give greater programming direction.

Once again, note that previously stated caveat—your purpose in testing will be a large part of the decision as to what test procedure to use.

SPEECH SAMPLING

In the chapter on language assessment, we present material on gathering a speech sample and the various types of analyses of expressive language ability available from the sample. A speech sample provides important information as well about the relative articulatory facility of the child that supplements results from articulation tests.

Naturalistic sampling allows use of materials and topics that can be tuned to the child's level and interest and the sample can be obtained either within or outside the diagnostic setting. The child therefore demonstrates his speech perception and production capabilities as they naturally occur. It allows a more careful look at the syllables and word shapes used, stress at the word and syllable level, and intonation in utterances. Finally, the interaction of articulation with others parts of language and communication including pragmatics, syntax, semantics, and discourse strategies (new topics, on-topic responding, etc.) can be investigated.

The typical procedure is to gather approximately 50 utterances from the child. An audio recording usually is sufficient, but audio-video recording allows a view of the child's speech production system embedded in a context where other means of communication may be used (gesture, facial postures, etc.) and is preferred. Broad phonetic transcriptions of the sample are completed utterance by utterance. If, however, idiosyncratic patterns emerge (e.g., final vowel lengthening as a strategy for producing final consonants) or if the child has a disorder related to structure/function problems (nasal emission of fricatives, lateralization of /s/, dentalized /d/), narrow transcription may be required.

Differential diagnosis of articulation disorders differs between structured and more spontaneous speech sampling. They are similar in that articulatory information is gathered, organized, and analyzed for differential diagnosis. They differ in that structured tests require the permission of the child to collect the data and the level of cooperation may vary based on the child's motivation and age. Structured tests or follow-up controlled sampling are carried out to create opportunities to observe critical behaviors. Problems with these procedures are that the sounds may not be used within the productive lexicon of the child and may not elicit articulatory variability that may be a key feature of the disorder.

Typically data from the two types of data sampling procedures are analyzed separately. Each has advantages and disadvantages. Single-word and diagnostic tests typically are fast, have consistent use of sounds in positions, allow readministration, and guide identification of the target in unintelligible productions. However, they do not permit careful examination of variability, contextual complexity, vowel and consonant vowel productions, and intelligibility in connected speech and prosody, and most of the words are content words rather than functors. Spontaneous speech sampling allows the examiner to observe patterns of error, the interactions of segmental and suprasegmental features, and the effects of length of utterance and word complexity on segmental (speech-sound) production. Disadvantages of this type of sampling are that it is time consuming. Even when a relatively large sample (50 utterances) is obtained, the vocabulary items may be quite restricted. Finally, for the child who is moderately to severely unintelligible, transcription accuracy may be problematic.

A complete corpus of data for differential diagnosis of articulation disorders should include several kinds of sampling. Diagnostic articulation test data supplemented by controlled sampling (stimulability testing, repetition of words and short utterances containing target sounds) and naturalistic observation and analysis of connected speech will allow a more complete picture of the child's articulatory capability.

REFERENCES

ANTHONY, A., AND OTHERS, *The Edinburgh Articulation Test.* Edinburgh and London: E & S Livingstone (1971).

APPLETON, P., A study of the production of the /r/ and /s/ phonemes in forty-six phonetic contexts by five-, six-, and seven-year-old males. Unpublished master's thesis, University of Tennessee, Knoxville (1969).

BANKSON, N. W., AND J. E. BERNTHAL, A comparison of phonological processes identified through word and sentence imitation tasks of the PPA. *Lang. Speech Hearing Serv. Schools,* 13, 96–99 (1982).

BARKER, J. O., A numerical measure of articulation. *J. Speech Hearing Dis.,* 25, 79–88 (1960).

BARKER, J. O., AND G. ENGLAND, A numerical measure of articulation: Further developments. *J. Speech Hearing Dis.,* 27, 23–27 (1962).

BRYNGELSON, B., AND E. GLASPEY, *Speech Improvement Cards.* Glenview, Ill.: Scott, Foresman (1951).

CHOMSKY, N., AND M. HALLE, *The Sound Pattern of English.* New York: Harper & Row (1968).

COMPTON, A. J., Generative studies of children's phonological disorders. *J. Speech Hearing Dis.,* 35, 315–339 (1970).

DANILOFF, R., AND K. MOLL, Coarticulation of lip rounding. *J. Speech Hearing Res.,* 11, 707–721 (1968).

DENES, P. B., On the statistics of spoken English. *J. Acous. Soc. Amer.*, 35, 892–904 (1963).

DRUMWRIGHT, A., *Denver Articulation Screening Exam*. Denver: University of Colorado Medical Center (1971).

FAIRCLOTH, S. R., AND M. A. FAIRCLOTH, *Phonetic Science*. Englewood Cliffs, N.J.: Prentice Hall, Inc. (1973).

FARQUHAR, M. S., Prognostic value of imitative and auditory discrimination tests. *J. Speech Hearing Dis.*, 26, 342–347 (1961).

FISHER, H. B., AND J. A. LOGEMANN, *Fisher-Logemann Test of Articulation Competence*. Boston: Houghton Mifflin (1971).

FRENCH, N. R., C. W. CARTER, AND W. KOENIG, JR., The words and sounds of telephone conversations, *Bell Syst. Tech. J.*, 9, 290–324 (1930).

FUDALA, J. B., *The Arizona Articulation Proficiency Scale: Revised*. Los Angeles: Western Psychological Services (1970).

FUDALA, J. B., AND W. M. REYNOLDS, *Arizona Articulation Proficiency Scale, Second Edition*, Los Angeles: Western Psychological Services (1986).

GARBER, N., A phonological analysis classification for use with traditional articulation tests. *Lang. Speech Hearing Serv. Schools*, 17, 253–261 (1986).

GARN-NUNN, P. G., Phonological processes and conventional articulation tests: Considerations for analysis. *Lang. Speech Hearing Serv. Schools*, 17, 244–252 (1986).

GARN-NUNN, P. G., AND V. MARTIN, Using conventional articulation tests with highly unintelligible children: Identification and programming concerns. *Lang. Speech Hearing Serv. Schools*, 3, 52–60 (1992).

GARRETT, K. K., AND M. J. MORAN, A comparison of phonological severity measures. *Lang. Speech Hearing Serv. Schools*, 23, 48–51 (1992).

GOLDMAN, R., AND M. FRISTOE, *Goldman-Fristoe Test of Articulation*. Circle Pines, Minn.: American Guidance Service (1969, 1986).

HAELSIG, P. C., AND C. L. MADISON, A study of phonological processes exhibited by three-, four-, and five-year-old-children. *Lang. Speech Hearing Serv. Schools*, 17, 107–114 (1986).

HALLER, R. M., Review of *The Arizona Articulation Proficiency Scale: Revised*. In *The Eighth Mental Measurements Yearbook*, ed. O. K. Buros. Highland Park, N.J.: Gryphon Press (1978).

HEJNA, R., *Developmental Articulation Test*. Madison, Wis.: College Print and Typing Co. (1955).

HODSON, B. W., *Assessment of Phonological Processes*. Danville, Ill.: Interstate, Printers & Publishers (1980).

HODSON, B. W. *Assessment of Phonological Processes–Revised* Austin, Tex.: Pro-Ed (1986).

HODSON, B. W., AND E. PADEN, Phonological processes which characterize unintelligible and intelligible speech in early childhood. *J. Speech Hearing Dis.*, 46, 369–373 (1981).

HODSON, B. W., AND E. P. PADEN, *Targeting Intelligible Speech*. San Diego: College-Hill Press (1983).

HULL, F. M., AND OTHERS, The national speech and hearing survey: Preliminary results. *Asha*, 13, 501–509 (1971).

INGRAM, D., *Phonological Disability in Children*. New York: Elsevier (1976).

INGRAM, D., *Procedures for Phonological Analysis of Children's Language*. Baltimore: University Park Press (1981).

IRWIN, O. C., Infant speech: Consonantal sounds according to place of articulation. *J. Speech Dis.*, 12, 397–401 (1947).

JAKOBSON, R. *Selected Writings I*. The Hague: Mouton (1962).

JORDAN, E. P., Articulation test measures and listener ratings of articulation defectiveness. *J. Speech Hearing Res.*, 3, 303–319 (1960).

KENT, R., AND F. MINIFIE, Coarticulation in recent speech production models. *J. Phon.*, 5, 115–133 (1977).

KENNY, K. W., E. M. PRATHER, M. A. MOONEY, AND N. C. JERUZAL, Comparisons among three articulation sampling procedures with preschool children. *J. Speech Hearing Res.*, 27, 226–231 (1984).

KENNEY, K. W., AND E. M. PRATHER, Articulation development in preschool children: Consistency of productions. *J. Speech Hearing Res.*, 29, 29–36 (1986).

KENT, R. D., Contextual facilitation of correct sound production. *Lang. Speech Hearing Serv. Schools*, 13, 66–76 (1982).

KHAN, L., AND N. LEWIS, *Khan-Lewis Phonological Analysis*. Circle Pines, Minn.: American Guidance Service (1986).

LAWSHE, C. H., A monograph for estimating the validity of test items. *J. Appl. Psych.*, 26, 846–849 (1942).

LOCKE, J. L., Ease of articulation. *J. Speech Hearing Res.*, 15, 194–200 (1972).

MADISON, C. L., C. P. KOLBECK, AND J. L. WALKER, An evaluation of three articulation tests. *Lang. Speech Hearing Serv. Schools*, 13, 110–115 (1982).

MCDONALD, E., *Articulation Testing and Treatment—A Sensory-Motor Approach*, Pittsburgh: Stanwix House (1965a).

MCDONALD, E., *Deep Test of Articulation*. Pittsburgh: Stanwix House (1965b).

MCDONALD, E., *Screening Deep Test of Articulation*. Pittsburgh: Stanwix House (1968).

MCDONALD, E. T., AND J. M. MCDONALD, *Norms for the Screening Deep Test of Articulation*. ESEA Title III grant—Project number 73024 (1974).

MCDONALD, E. T., AND J. M. MCDONALD, *Articulation at Pre-Kindergarten, Beginning Kindergarten, End of Kindergarten, and Beginning First Grade on the Screening Deep Test of Articulation*. ESEA Title III grant—Project number 73024H, Report No. 2 (1976a).

MCDONALD, E. T., AND J. M. MCDONALD, *Comparisons of the Longitudinal and Cross-sectional Norms on the Screening Deep Test of Articulation*. ESEA Title III grant—Project number 73924H, Report No. 3 (1976b).

MCREYNOLDS, L. V., AND K. HUSTON, A distinctive feature analysis of children's misarticulations. *J. Speech Hearing Dis.*, 36, 155–166 (1971).

MCREYNOLDS, L. V., AND M. ELBERT, Criteria for phonological process analysis. *J. Speech Hearing Dis.*, 46, 197–204 (1981).

MILISEN, R., Method of evaluation and diagnosis of speech disorders, In *Handbook of Speech Pathology*, ed. L. E. Travis. Englewood Cliffs, N.J.: Prentice Hall (1957).

MILLER, G. A., *Language and Communication*. New York: McGraw-Hill (1951).

MOLL, K. L., Speech characteristics of individuals with cleft lip and palate. In *Cleft Palate and Communications*, eds. D. C. Spriestersbach and D. Sherman. New York: Academic Press (1968).

MORRIS, H. L., D. C. SPRIESTERSBACH, AND F. L. DARLEY, An articulation test for assessing competency of velopharyngeal closure. *J. Speech Hearing Res.*, 4, 48–55 (1961).

MORRISON, C. E., Speech defects in young children. *Psych. Clinic*, 8, 138–142 (1941).

NOLL, J. D., Articulation assessment. In "Speech and the Dentofacial Complex: The State of the Art," ed. R. T. Wertz. *ASHA Reports #5* (1970).

NORRIS, M., J. R. HARDEN, AND D. M. BELL, Listener agreement on articulation errors of four- and five-year-old children. *J. Speech Hearing Dis.*, 45, 378–389 (1980).

PADEN, E. P., AND S. A. MOSS, Comparison of three phonological analysis procedures. *Lang. Speech Hearing Serv. Schools*, 16, 103–109 (1985).

PAYNTER, E. T., AND T. C. BUMPAS, Imitative and spontaneous articulatory assessment of three-year-old children. *J. Speech Hearing Dis.*, 42, 119–125 (1977).

PENDERGAST, K., AND OTHERS, *Photo Articulation Test*. Danville, Ill.: Interstate Printers & Publishers (1969, 1984).

PERRIN, E. H., The rating of defective speech by trained and untrained observers. *J. Speech Hearing Dis.*, 19, 48–51 (1954).

PETERSON, H. A., SALI: Speech and Language Index. Paper presented to the American Speech and Hearing Association, Denver, Colorado (1968).

POOLE, I., Genetic development of articulation of consonant sounds in speech. *Elem. English Rev.*, 11, 159–161 (1934).

PRATHER, E. M., E. L. HENDRICK, AND C. A. KERIN, Articulation development in children aged two to four years. *J. Speech Hearing Dis.*, 40, 179–191 (1975).

SANDER, E. K., When are speech sounds learned? *J. Speech Hearing Dis.*, 37, 55–63 (1972).

SANDERS, L. J., (modification of Hejna's) *Developmental Articulation Test: D.A.T. in Procedure Guides for Evaluation of Speech and Language Disorders in Children*. Urbana, Ill.: Stenographic Bureau (1970).

SCHWARTZ, R. G., L B. LEONARD, M. K. FOLGER, AND M. J. WILCOX, Early phonological behavior in normal-speaking and language-disordered children: Evidence for a synergistic view of linguistic disorders. *J. Speech Hearing Dis.*, 45, 357–377 (1980).

SHELTON, R., AND L. MCREYNOLDS, Functional articulation disorders: Preliminaries to treatment. In *Speech and Language: Advances in Basic Research and Practice, Vol. 2*, ed. N. Lass. New York: Academic Press (1979).

SHRIBERG, L. D., AND J. KWIATKOWSKI, *Natural Process Analysis*. New York: John Wiley (1980).

SHRIBERG, L. D., AND J. KWIATKOWSKI, Phonological disorders I: A diagnostic classification system. *J. Speech Hearing Dis.*, 47, 226–241 (1982a).

SHRIBERG, L. D., AND J. KWIATKOWSKI, Phonological disorders III: A procedure for assessing severity of involvement. *J. Speech Hearing Dis.*, 47, 256–270 (1982b).

SHRIBERG, L. D., J. KWIATKOWSKI, S. BEST, J. HENGST, AND B. TERSELIC-WEBER. Characteristics of children with phonological disorders of unknown origin. *J. Speech Hearing Dis.*, 51, 140–161 (1986).

SIEGEL, G. M., H. WINITZ, AND H. CONKEY, The influence of testing instruments on articulatory responses of children. *J. Speech Hearing Dis.*, 28, 67–76 (1963).

SINGH, S., AND D. C. FRANK, A distinctive feature analysis of the consonantal substitution pattern. *Lang. Speech*, 15, 209–218 (1972).

SMITH, F., AND G. A. MILLER, eds., *The Genesis of Language, A Psycholinguistic Approach.* Cambridge, Mass.: MIT Press (1966).

SNOW, K., AND R. MILISEN, The influence of oral vs. pictorial presentation upon articulation testing results. *J. Speech Hearing Dis.*, Monograph Supplement, 4, 30–36 (1954).

TEMPLIN, M. C., Spontaneous vs. imitated verbalization in testing articulation in preschool children. *J. Speech Dis.*, 12, 293–300 (1947a).

TEMPLIN, M. C., A nondiagnostic articulation test. *J. Speech Dis.*, 12, 392–396 (1947b).

TEMPLIN, M. C., *Certain Language Skills in Children*, Institute of Child Welfare Monograph Series, No. 26. Minneapolis: University of Minnesota Press (1957).

TEMPLIN, M. C., The study of articulation and language development during the early school years. In *The Genesis of Language*, eds. F. Smith and G. A. Miller. Cambridge, Mass.: M.I.T. Press (1966).

TEMPLIN, M. C., AND F. L. DARLEY, *The Templin-Darley Tests of Articulation.* Iowa City: University of Iowa (1960, 2nd ed. 1969).

VAN RIPER, C., AND J. IRWIN, *Voice and Articulation.* Englewood Cliffs, N.J.: Prentice Hall (1958).

VAN RIPER, C., AND R. ERICKSON, *Predictive Screening Test of Articulation.* Kalamazoo: Western Michigan University (1968).

WEINER, F. F., *Phonological Process Analysis.* Baltimore: University Park Press (1979).

WEISS, C. E. *Weiss Comprehensive Articulation Test.* Boston: Teaching Resources Company (1978).

WEISS, C. E. *Weiss Comprehensive Articulation Test.* Allen, Tex.: DLM Teaching Resources (1980).

WELLMAN, B. I., AND OTHERS, Speech sounds of young children. *University of Iowa Studies in Child Welfare*, 5, No. 2 (1931).

WINITZ, H., *Articulatory Acquisition and Behavior.* Englewood Cliffs, N.J.: Prentice Hall (1969).

4

From Speech-Sound Discrimination and Perception to Central Auditory Processing

The problem to be overcome for theories of perception is the variable acoustic signal and an invariant identification.

H. S. Straight

INTRODUCTION

The testing of speech-sound discrimination has a historical base in speech-language pathology, but it is less often used in current practice. We briefly review what was being tested, and why, in order to put the demise of this testing procedure in perspective.

Tests for speech-sound discrimination were constructed on the assumption that speech-sound production confusions reflected confusions in speech-sound perception. The problem with the *tests* was that the discrimination contrasts tested did not often coincide with confusions in production. The problem with the *theory* (or the assumption) was that production confusions did not often predict perceptual (discrimination) confusions, and discrimination confusions did not often predict production confusions. So either the theory or the testing of the theory appears to be flawed.

Theories of speech perception in more encompassing terms have relied on phoneme (speech-sound) identification (data-driven or "bottom-up" theory) versus a higher order language-processing or "top-down" theory. The data-driven theory is basically one of discrimination and the top-down is an identification problem, not one of discrimination. Duchan and Katz (1983) interpret the available data to suggest that some of each is required in the processing of language. Our discussion ignores the details of those theories as outside the realm of this text. Instead, we discuss perception of speech and language from a more generic basis.

Just as an aside, theories of speech perception generally assume a single mechanism (of varying characteristics) for both the production and perception of speech. Straight (1980) suggested that instead of a single processor, there may be two information-processing mechanisms, one for the perception of auditorially presented stimuli and the other for the production of articularly realized responses. If this supposition were true, it would allow a more variable association between perception and production of speech elements.

As clinicians, we have a concern for theories not in and of themselves but primarily as a basis for our selection of tests and the interpretation of results. It is in that vein that this chapter is concerned with speech perception—phonemes or larger language units—and includes a discussion of the problem called "central auditory processing" and some tests used in its description and definition. Our discussion centers primarily on the types of tests and the types of information to be sought with less detail on specific test instruments.

THE HISTORY OF SPEECH-SOUND DISCRIMINATION TESTING

The basic assumption in the testing of speech-sound discrimination was that this skill tapped the base knowledge for speech-sound production. The primary problem for theoretical support was in how discrimination was tested and what forms were being tested. The different paradigms ranged from pairs of nonsense syllables (Travis and Rasmus 1931) and real words where the child's task was to judge "same" or "different" (Wepman 1958, 1973), to picture identification tasks (point to named picture) of two, three, or four choices (e.g., Goldman, Fristoe, and Woodcock 1970; Pronovost 1974; Templin 1957). Generally "live voice" presentations were used, but the *Goldman-Fristoe-Woodcock Tests of Auditory Discrimination* (1970) included tape-recorded signals to be presented under earphones so that a constant signal-to-noise ratio was maintained. This collection also included a test of selective attention that utilized tape-recorded signals with a background noise. That last mentioned paradigm (the inclusion of a signal-to-noise ratio) is frequently being used in testing for central auditory processing disorders (see later discussion).

Speech-sound discrimination scores generally increased with age, although rarely did these scores discriminate between ages. Data presented by Templin (1957) and Deutsch (1964) inferred that intelligence was also a factor in the agreement between speech-sound discrimination and speech production. Weiner (1967) cited age and intelligence as factors as well as a concern for the relative degree of articulation disorder or deficit. Performance scores infrequently discriminated between good and poor articulation groups who were matched on other important variables. In other words, even when the production and discrimination scores of groups of children did correlate, they probably reflected maturation more often than speech-production skill. You remember that correlation does not assign cause and effect, although the usual, implicit, interest in speech-sound discrimination testing was based on its being a basic skill on which speech-sound production was built.

The *Tree Bee Test of Discrimination* (Fudala 1978) is an example of a discrimination test that was apparently aimed more broadly, according to the test manual:

> Auditory discrimination as a pure function is fully developed in the average child by second or third grade. At that time auditory discrimination is no longer a basic function, but becomes a skill to be applied in learning phonics and in spelling. (p. 7)

There were no data given to support the validity of the Tree Bee test for identification of either discrimination/articulation disorders or discrimination/reading disorders. But then if we take the preceding quote as a rationale for the test, it would appear to have more concern for identification than for discrimination.

PHONEME FEATURES: ACQUISITION, DISCRIMINATION AND PRODUCTION

One other difficulty with the available test formats is that although the contrasts to be discriminated were routinely single phonemes, the phonemes sometimes differed by more than one feature. Phonemes are not minimal entities. Each phoneme is a concurrent bundle of acoustic and/or articulatory features. Pairs that differ by more than one feature should be more easily discriminated than single feature contrasts.

Crocker (1969) described an order of acquisition of speech sounds as a function of a hierarchy of acoustic features. The order of acquisition of distinctive features can be thought of as an order of articulatory and/or perceptual difficulty known as "markedness" theory (Chomsky and Halle 1968; Jacobson, Fant, and Halle 1955). For example, the phoneme /t/ should appear before /k/. The only feature different between the two is place of articulation—"front" for /t/ and "back" for /k/. The position "back" is considered to be "marked" or at a greater level of difficulty than "front." While /t/ and /k/ could be perceptually confused because of being only one feature apart, the /t/ for /k/ production substitution is logical (unmarked substituted for marked) but /k/ for /t/ is not logical (not developmental). Menyuk (1968, 1972), Singh and Black (1966), and others have suggested an order of acquisition of features that is similar across different language groups and could be predicted according to the relative "naturalness" (markedness) of the features.

Singh and Black (1966) studied the discrimination of consonant sounds by speakers of four language groups. Their results indicated that across groups the best discrimination scores were obtained by listeners for their own languages. In other words, listeners would best discriminate phonemes and sound features that are in their productive repertoires. Singh and Frank (1972) listed an order-of-feature acquisition and an order of probable errors in phoneme production based on the relative stability of the features involved. The more stable features (least likely erred) were those learned earlier. Koenigsknecht and Lee (1968) reported a similar order-of-acquisition difficulty for three-year-old children.

An additional variable to add then is the feature description and relative markedness of the phonemes to be discriminated. Some sound features are unmarked (easier to produce and/or perceive) in relation to other more marked sounds. For example, in the marking tradition, /s/ and /f/ are both fricative sounds but /s/ is longer in duration and louder than /f/, and the easiest way to produce a fricative is long and loud. Hence /s/ is unmarked for friction while /f/ is marked for friction. If /s/ and /f/ were confused, the /s/ for /f/ would be a believable though unlikely substitution, and /f/ for /s/ would be even more unlikely. A more likely example pair would be /f/ and /θ/. Both are marked for friction, but /θ/ is also marked for tongue position. A child may substitute the /f/ phoneme for an intended /θ/ because it is easier to produce. At the same time, in the postvocalic word position, /f/ may be produced where you expect /θ/ by an African-American speaker as a dialectical variation. That is, a speaker's sound productions may reflect language habits or motor movement habits rather than perceptual confusions.

The overriding problem with "standardized" speech-sound discrimination testing as it is usually accomplished was pointed out by Locke (1980a). His complaint was primarily that the confusions tested in the available discrimination tests included very few of the confusions made by children in their productions. He offered three alternative means of determining whether or not the child's productive confusion reflected a perceptual confusion (1980b). The first was a choice from the intended phoneme (identified as the stimulus), the child's production (response), and a nonconfused sound (the control). So if, for example, the child produced /f/ for /θ/ he would be asked to agree or disagree when asked: "Is this a [fʌm]?" (the response); "Is this a [θʌm]?" (the intended stimulus); and "Is this a [tʌm]?" (the control). According to Locke's report, all of his subjects accepted the stimulus, none accepted the control, and a small percentage accepted the response. In other words, most of the children tested by this means had no perceptual confusion to coincide with their production variation. For the children who did accept the response and the stimulus probes to be equivalent, you may conclude that their phoneme boundaries for /θ/ and /f/ overlapped—that the two sounds were allophonic variations of a single phoneme.

Locke's second alternative used an ABX paradigm where three sounds are presented. Take the example we used earlier with the /θ/ and /f/ contrasts. The triad could be /θ/-/f/-/θ/, /θ/-/f/-/f/, or /f/-/θ/-/f/, and the child's task is to indicate if the third sound is more like the first sound or more like the second sound. Again, by definition, a phonemic or categorical comparison is being requested.

The third alternative is an extension of the second. This one was borrowed from Pisoni (1971) and was termed 4IAX (four interval AX—same/different). Here the child is presented with two pairs (e.g., /f-f/, θ-f/) and his task is to decide if the first pair or the second pair is more alike. Where speech-sound discrimination testing is a matter of diagnostic interest, one of these three techniques would appear to have more validity than the published tests available.

RELATIONSHIP
OF DISCRIMINATION/PERCEPTION
TO SPEECH AND LANGUAGE PRODUCTION

It is a logical presumption that learning to use language requires perception of the units. It is not well agreed what the units of language perception are—whether the minimal units of perception are, for example, phonemes, syllables, or phrases—and/or the degree to which these "levels" of processing may interact. For explanations of that statement, Kuhl (1982) reviewed issues and theories of speech perception and concentrated primarily on the perception of phonemes; and Lemme and Daves (1982) reviewed theories of linguistic processing, with most of the discussion on larger units. Duchan and Katz (1983) also provide a review of "bottom-up" (phoneme-driven perception) and "top-down" (syllable- or phrase-driven perception) as well as a compromise resolution of the two apparently diverse theories. An interested reader may also wish to see, for example, Keith (1984), Lubert (1981), and Rees (1973, 1981) for discussions of auditory processing as a cognitive versus a linguistic disorder, how the reported "facts" fit the theories, and other such interesting topics.

That last heavily referenced paragraph is meant to suggest that auditory *discrimination*, *perception*, and *processing* are different concepts—and may well require different data or may acquire different interpretations with the same data. "Discrimination" means determining that an important (categorical) contrast exists; "perception" is often defined as mental awareness or as understanding; "processing" refers to the mechanics of understanding. "Cognition" should also be part of that collection of definitions as the assignment of value—or meaning—or knowing.

We should also remember that the acoustics of the sound productions (what someone once referred to as the "blooming, buzzing confusion" of the child's environment) will be stored only in short-term memory (a matter of a few seconds) and will very rapidly fade. What is maintained in long-term storage is not the sounds, words, or phrases but the meaning of the utterance. As diagnosticians our concern for testing *perceptions* of units or wholes (sounds, words, or meanings) would be related to our observations of a problem in production of language or a problem in language reasoning. Speech and language performance can be measured. Perception, when measured by the subject's performance, is only an inference.

Remember also that the units of a language (and their meaning) are arbitrary and assigned by users of that language. For example, Spanish has a prevoicing (voicing begins prior to the articulatory gesture), a simultaneous voicing, and a delayed voicing. English has only the last two distinctions—a simultaneous voicing and articulatory gesture—which we call a voiced sound, and a delayed voicing—which we identify as an unvoiced sound. An infant perceives (discriminates) among all three. A child of three years who does not hear the Spanish language in her environment, fails to distinguish between the prevoicing and the simultaneous voicing because the contrast (by then) is not deemed as linguistic (Oller and Eilers 1983). A child of four months of age distinguishes between a vowel of short duration from the same vowel with a long duration—a child of nine months does not (MacKain 1982). That distinction is important for a child learning Japanese where vowel duration is linguistic. When the child hears primarily English in her environment, vowel duration does not have linguistic significance, and she does not discriminate the two as being importantly different. The infant comes into this world with the capability to learn any language to which she is exposed communicatively. Those acoustic distinctions that are not part of the language in her environment are "lost" (Burnham 1986).

The point of this is a reminder that we are concerned with perception/discrimination of the sounds and elements of the language that carry meaning for the users of that language. The language the child hears at home, possibly with a different set of phonemes, may be an important variable to consider. And, again, our judgments of the child's *perception* when made from tests of speech and language *behavior* are based on inferences.

Perceptions of speech sounds (and meaning) can be directly measured as auditory evoked response potentials, although this methodology is not as routinely available as might be wished. Let us insert a short detour here for a brief explanation of evoked response potentials (ERP) as an explanation of directly measured perception, because we will include ERP measures later in our discussion of auditory processing.

THE MEASUREMENT OF CORTICAL RESPONSE

An electroencephalogram is a readout of the electrical activity of the brain using surface electrodes to record the activity at specific locations on the scalp. An "evoked" potential is a time-locked response of the brain's circuitry to an introduced event—such as a speech syllable, a word in a phrase, ongoing speech, a series of tones, or any similar event whose onset can be identified in time. Because it is difficult to separate the evoked response from the background (random) activity of the brain, evoked responses are averages of brain-wave activity to a number of like stimuli. Averaging of the time-locked evoked responses serves to "average out" the random background.

The overall time line of response for the ERP can be divided, for our purposes, into three divisions—early, middle, and late. Let's use a series of tones for this explanation and assume that 80 percent of the time these tones are high frequency (e.g., 1000 Hz) and randomly inserted into this series of tones is a 20 percent occurrence of low tones (e.g., 500 Hz). The early time line of neural response is from zero to approximately 10 milliseconds (msec) from the onset of the acoustic event and is localized in the brain stem (brain stem auditory evoked response). The information to be derived is a series of five waves (peaks of electrical activity that represent an accumulation of synaptic firings at junctures of structures within the brain stem) to measure auditory acuity—or "audition" at the level of the brain stem. The middle latencies (from 10 to approximately 100 msec) reflect passage of the electrically coded information through the midbrain and are not of primary concern in the current discussion.

The "late" responses begin at approximately 100 msec after onset of the signal and also have three general divisions in time. The expected neural result is a negative-going wave circa 100 msec (therefore N100), interpreted as "attention" and indicating that the "information" has reached the level of the cortex. To this point in time, the patterns of neural firing are a function of the internal machinery—unrelated to the acoustics or to the "value" of the signal.

The next point of interest is a positive-going wave in the neighborhood of 200 msec (P200) and generally represents the acoustics of the signal. In this region (from approximately 150 msec after onset of the signal) Molfese and Molfese (1985) report neural wave patterns of response that differ according to syllables (e.g., /ba/, /pa/, /da/, /ga/). They also reported that the infants in that 1985 study (averaging *12 hours* in age) who most consistently separated between syllables—according to their brain wave responses—showed better language skill at three years of age than those infants whose brain wave patterns showed less differentiation. This time line then represents a decoding of the acoustics or "perception" but obviously not "understanding" or "meaning" if it occurs in very young infants.

The third of the "late" time lines important for this discussion is called "P3"—for third positive wave—and is considered a "cognitive" response (Donchin and McCarthy 1979). This positive-going wave (circa 300 msec in 16-to-40-year-olds, closer to 700 msec in 3-year-olds; Corchesne 1977) is also identified as being a function of the informational value of the signal—that is, recognition that it is the target you are looking for if you were asked to count the infrequently occurring low tones mentioned earlier or the "surprise" of hearing the infrequent low tone or of hearing an unexpected word in a sequence (e.g., "the flowers smell tall" versus "the flowers smell sweet"—as in Hume 1984). The latency of the unexpected (therefore informational) response is related to neurological integrity and intellectual maturity. The amplitude of the response is "value" and attentional. That is, the infrequent odd-tone in a 60–40 ratio will evoke less amplitude of response than that to the infrequent event in an 80–20 ratio. If you ask a subject to count the odd tones, or to push a button when something happens, the intent is to assure closer attention to the task.

DISCRIMINATION VERSUS PERCEPTION

The reason for that brief detour was a reminder that the way in which we ask (test) a question may well influence the answer we get. Are we testing discrimination when we want to know about the perception of speech? The discrimination between /p/ and /b/ is not meaningful—phonemes are nonmeaningful elements. The discrimination of "bee" and "pea" should be available in context—to be wary of being stung versus eating one's vegetables. Are we testing discrimination or perception when we are concerned about production of speech or the appropriate understanding of speech and language information? Are we interested in the processing of language forms or of language content?

AUDITORY PROCESSING VERSUS LINGUISTIC PROCESSING

Lubert (1981) reviewed the literature concerning auditory perceptual impairments in conjunction with specific language disorders. However, the data cited were primarily concerned with adult aphasia. The references to children were largely speculative and dealt, for the most part, with the detection of sound features because "studies examining the relation between perceptual impairment and the severity of language deficit in children are nonexistent" (p. 9). Even in the Molfese and Molfese article cited earlier, the children were identified as higher or lower scoring in the language test used but these scores were not identified as being normal or delayed/deviant.

Rees (1973), in a review of auditory processing factors in language disorders, suggested that researchers have been using the wrong procedures in their search. Keith (1984) reported that there was no universally accepted set of criteria for determining a central auditory processing disorder. Lubert (1981) suggested that rather than a cognitive or "linguistic" deficit, the deficit may be in the perceptual detection of acoustic features of sounds.

Horst and Thatcher (in Otto et al., 1984), in discussing a rationale for using ERPs in aberrant developmental disorders, suggested that

> Current diagnostic categories are imprecise and over-lapping. Existing diagnostic tools are inadequate. ERP indices may allow us to decide whether or not a child's behavioral disorder has an organic basis in the brain. In addition, ERP measures may provide a means of discriminating clinically relevant clusters in groups of children with the same behavioral symptoms. (p. 319)

The reason behind the referral of a client may have been presented as a language problem, a language-processing problem, or an auditory-processing problem. The fact is that the presenting problems of two children may be the same but the referring label may be different. The tests administered may also be the same. What may be different is the interpretation by the examiner. In the previous chapter, we discussed a variety of tests for the measurement of articulation skill. In the following chapter, we discuss tests of both the form and function of language. Generally speaking, we assume that the basic forms of language (discrimination/identification) are mastered relatively early. Later, in the early school years, our concern may be the use (function) of language in acquiring information and in reasoning. The auditory *processing* of language assumes both an identification of pieces and assignment of functional value to the whole.

CENTRAL AUDITORY PROCESSING (CAP)

Some of the testing paradigms utilized for auditory processing were originally constructed for other purposes. Some of the auditory-processing armamentaria are deliberately concerned with acoustic events without meaning; others are purposefully concerned with linguistic processing, that is, the understanding of meaningful signals. Some test packages are apparently unconcerned that language facility is a variable in language processing.

Willeford (1985) and others have reported that some children with central auditory processing problems have language/learning disorders and some do not. Some children with language/learning disorders have an auditory-processing problem and some do not. This distinction may be some function of the test batteries used, but it also may be a function of the theoretical preference of the examiner.

Test batteries for determination of a central auditory processing disorder may include general listening behaviors; identification of syllables, words, and phrases with or without a noise background; competing messages as in dichotic tasks; tone pattern identification; and occasionally evoked response potentials.

Willeford (1981, 1985) developed an *Auditory Behavior Rating Scale*, which was a series of observations to be completed by a classroom teacher. They were essentially a set of judgments made on a five-point scale (always to never) that deal with whether the child is a good listener, pays attention to instructions, is disturbed by background noise, and so on. There are 10 items in total on which to determine a child's "good" or "poor" auditory behavior. This procedure appears to have a face validity and to reflect a logical concern—whether or not the child attends and performs. At the same time, it is logically a conclusion the teacher would draw after she has decided that the child is not performing well and may or may not be the basis of that behavior.

Smoski, Brunt, and Tannahil (1992) constructed the *Children's Auditory Processing Performance Scale* (CHAPPS), which included listening behaviors in noise, in quiet, under ideal listening conditions, and with multiple inputs. Tasks included auditory memory and sequencing and auditory attention span, and performance on these tasks was rated on a six-point scale. The referring educators were asked to provide a case history and social/behavioral history.

Child subjects in the CHAPPS study had been referred for CAP testing because of perceived academic problems. This 1992 report was concerned with the results of children referred as having a CAP disorder. The performance of these children differed widely, depending on listening condition and/or function. Educational history varied widely—half of the subjects had some trouble reading at grade level, half functioned as expected. The social/behavioral performances of the referred children were similar to those of non-CAP children. The CAP testing included Katz's (1962) *Staggered Spondaic Word Test*, dichotic digits, competing sentences, and a three-tone pitch pattern identification (as in Pinheiro and Musiek 1985). Of the 20 control subjects, two failed this CAP testing.

Essentially, these results infer that "listening behaviors" as defined here do not differentiate—that is, a judgment of poor listening behaviors on the part of educator or parent need not mean a CAP disorder. Keep this in mind too: Half of the children were having a problem in reading (subjects were 7–1—11–8 with mean age 9–3) and half were not. Basically you may assume that reading is parasitic to oral language. The separation of a language or language-learning problem from an auditory-processing problem may be a very difficult call, especially in a child under second or third grade. Early primary-grade reading skill appears primarily to be an identification of symbols—letters and words. Later reading skill is more probably judged as identification and retention of ideas.

There are a group of tests to assess what is identified as binaural interaction. In these types of tests, part of the message, not sufficient for interpretation, is presented to each ear separately, and the listener is expected to be able to fuse the two inputs into a cohesive message. For example, the left ear may receive part of the acoustic spectrum through a low pass filter, and the right ear receives only a high passed signal. Neither is sufficient by itself, but the message—when fused—becomes intelligible. Or, in *rapidly alternating speech* (RAS), a connected sentence is played through earphones with parts of a word in the left ear and parts in the right ear. If one were to perceive only the odd numbered units or only the even numbered units, it would not be enough to reproduce the integration of the signal.

The formation of the perceptual event would require an integration of the parts. Those tests are commonly utilized by audiologists as part of the determination of integrity of the auditory system. They will not be discussed in more detail here because they require specialized equipment. For more detail on tests of this nature, the interested reader may see Tobin (1985). The purpose in those test formats, and the point for our discussion, is a concern for auditory processing—not language processing.

One of the tests that is frequently used, and that was originally designed as relating to the integrity of the auditory system or site of lesion, is Katz's (1962) *Staggered Spondaic Word Test* (SSW). Spondaic, or equally stressed two-syllable, words (such as baseball, railroad, uptown), are presented to the two ears with and without competition. That is, there is a lead syllable without competition presented to one ear (monotic); the second syllable of the first word is presented simultaneously with the first syllable of the second word (i.e., there are dichotic or competing signals to the two ears), and the second syllable of the second word is presented without competition. For example, the two spondaic words "uptown" and "downstairs" would be presented in the following format:

NONCOMPETING	COMPETING	NONCOMPETING
left ear	right ear	
	left ear	right ear
up	town	
	down	stairs

Results are interpreted as a function of a variety of scores such as percent correct responses for right and left ears; competing and noncompeting scores; omissions; distortions and reversals; and lead and trailing ear scores. Raw scores are adjusted, and the result is interpreted as auditory competence rather than linguistic facility.

Available norms and interpretations of patterns of responses (Arnst and Katz 1982) are for 11- to-80-year-old subjects in terms of the performance scores previously noted and are used primarily for the determination and location of central nervous system lesions. The SSW is frequently used as part of the testing for CAP or language/learning disorders, but there are no concise norms for comparison with children under 11 years of age. There are some tentative norms (e.g., White 1977), but the interpretation of results with a population not suspected of having a central nervous system lesion is tentative at best, and scores are likely to be influenced by language facility. This test, as well, is usually administered by an audiologist and requires special training and either a two-channel audiometer or a stereo tape player with good channel separation and earphones.

SPEECH SIGNALS WITH COMPETING NOISE

Other tests more frequently used by speech-language clinicians include the *Goldman-Fristoe-Woodcock Selective Attention Test* (GFW-SA) (1970) and the *Flowers Auditory Test of Selective Attention* (FATSA) (Flowers 1983). The GFW-SA is basically a four-choice picture-identification task with the stimulus words presented in a calibrated and increasing signal-to-noise ratio. The FATSA is also a picture-identification task—the child is asked to point to a selected picture only when a key word is paired with the name of the picture (sort of a "Simon says" routine) and has a variety of auditory distractions during the task. In that sense, both tests require auditory selective attention.

Glass, Franks, and Potter (1986) have reported a comparison of the GFW-SA and the FATSA on a sample of thirty 8- to 12-year-old children with poor reading skills but at least average intelligence, on the assumption that at least some of these children would have poor auditory-processing abilities as a basis for their poor reading skill. The criterion measure used to separate good and poor "auditory profiles" was a relatively high or low (good or poor) score on the Willeford scale mentioned earlier. The Glass et al. data showed a low but significant correlation between the GFW-SA and the FATSA ($r = 0.44$), indicating relatively little commonality between the two instruments. Neither of the two measures separated between the good and poor listeners, and neither showed a significant agreement with the Willeford. It would seem as if these three instruments (identified as selective attention and judgments of attention) have little in common—or possibly the experimental population was too heterogeneous to be combined in this way.

Condon (1984) compared the results of a small group of 7- to 10-year-old children on the SSW and on the Selective Attention and Memory for Sequences subtests of the GFW. The children were not described as having any auditory dysfunction and were "in normal classrooms and with normal hearing." There was no other description of language skill, reading or academic skills, or listening habits. Condon reported a low but significant correlation between the GFW-SA and the right competing raw score of the SSW and a moderate but significant correlation between the Memory for Sequences subtest and the left competing raw score of the SSW.

Baran and Gengel (1984), in another study with a small group of 5- to 11-year-old children, which bears on the interpretation of Condon's results, reported poor (nonsignificant) test-retest reliability of the GFW-SA subtest, and moderate but significant ($r = 0.56$) reliability for the Memory for Sequences subtest. Examination of individual scores revealed that 11 of the 20 subjects improved their performance on the Selective Attention retest, suggesting some practice effect. In other words, both the reliability and the validity of the instruments are questioned.

DICHOTIC TESTING

Dichotic testing with syllables, numbers, or sentences (the two ears receive two different, therefore competing signals) is also frequently used in auditory-processing testing. Speech-sound discrimination tasks are diotic, since both ears receive the same signal. Testing with a speech signal in one ear and noise in the other ear is also, to a degree, concerned with competing tasks but designed to test an attentional skill more than processing of linguistic material. The intent of a dichotic task is generally to show an ear preference and, with normal bilateral hearing function, also has a language facility variable.

There are two well-supported observations regarding results of dichotic listening tasks. First, it is generally agreed (Berlin, 1972; Kimura 1961; Shankweiler

1971; Studdert-Kennedy and Shankweiler 1970) that within the brain the contralateral (opposite side) pathway from ear to processing brain center is more efficient than the ipsilateral (same side) pathway. The right ear is a preferential pathway to the left hemisphere for processing of speech (linguistically relevant) information, and the left ear (right hemisphere) is apparently more efficient in processing such things as musical tones. The second assumption is that for most normal adults the auditory-processing areas most important for language are located in the left hemisphere of the brain (Penfield and Roberts 1959). The area on the right hemisphere of the brain analogous to the left hemisphere language area appears to be primarily concerned with making judgments about spatial relationships. The acoustic events most important for communication are consonant sounds, and consonants are handled most efficiently in the left hemisphere in most people. Most left-handed people are assumed to have a left-hemisphere dominance for speech but probably have less one-sided dominance of language processing than right-handed people.

That is not to say that language is processed only on one side of the brain— both sides are actively involved. The laterality effect is meant to say relatively more brain activity on one side—a dominance is assumed to be more efficient in terms of the processing requirement. As it happens, females are less lateralized in their language function (both the left and right sides of females' brains show more neural activity for cognitive tasks than do males' [Gur et al. 1982]) but that is another story, although it may be kept in mind when concerned with laterality of processing or ear preference.

It is also assumed that dichotic listening procedures indicate hemispheric dominance for speech and language functions (Berlin 1972; Berlin and Lowe 1972; Berlin and others 1972; Wada and Rasmussen 1960). In addition, laterality of brain function[1] as determined by ear preference scores may be considered to be established as early as four years of age (Kimura 1963).

McDuffie (1975) tested ear preference for dichotic speech signals with five- and six-year-old children with varying degrees of speech and language skill to determine what effect, if any, language skill had on dichotic listening performance. Speech signals consisted of the stop consonants /p, b, t, d, k, g/, each paired with the vowel /a/. For the dichotic listening tasks, each of the six consonant-vowel (CV) syllables was paired with each of the other syllables, resulting in a total of 15 stimulus pairs. Each of these 15 competing pairs was randomly presented six times, for a total of 90 dichotic items. McDuffie also included a dicotic listening task composed of 15 random-order presentations of each of the six CV stimulus syllables, for a total of 90 stimulus items. The children indicated their responses by pointing to one of six pictures that had been identified for them (and practiced to a criterion level) as representing the stimulus items. The data obtained from each of

---

[1]For clarification, "laterality of brain function" refers to the relative efficiency of linguistic processing. Shadden (1979a,b) and Shadden and Peterson (1981) demonstrated that a left-ear advantage may be expected for reaction time to a nonlinguistic task. Stimuli that require linguistic processing would generate a right-ear advantage in most linguistically facile subjects. For example, speech-sound stimuli such as "pah" or "bah" presented to subjects instructed to respond as quickly as possible after presentation of the stimulus would show a left-ear advantage probably because a linguistic judgment is not required. If the subjects were instructed to identify what they heard from options such as "pah," "bah," and so on, and if these syllables were identified as names of pictures, then a linguistic judgment is required, and a right-ear advantage would be expected. In other words, the task more than the stimuli is important to a laterality effect.

the 10 subjects consisted of a discrimination score for the dicotic listening task and a right-ear, left-ear, and error score for the dichotic listening task. The child's task was to point to the picture that he heard best.

The "good" and "poor" articulation group designations were based on the children's *Templin-Darley Screening Test of Articulation* scores. "Good" articulation children all scored at or above the expected mean for their age; the "poor" articulation children were all below the cutoff for adequacy at their age.

Analysis of the results indicated that there was no significant difference between the two groups on the dicotic test but that there was a significant difference (beyond 0.01 level) between the two groups in the dichotic discrimination task. Both the good- and poor-language group children showed a right-ear preference but the good-language group showed a greater right-ear preference than did the poor-language group children.

A number of the sources cited previously have noted an expected improvement in ear-preference scores with chronological maturity. What this study showed was an improvement with linguistic maturity.

An addendum to this discussion of ear preference is warranted in the use of dichotic testing as part of the central auditory battery. Minor (1977) utilized the same stimulus materials as McDuffie with two groups of children similarly defined. The focus of her study was to determine the trainability of the right-ear preferences. Following the procedure to determine baseline performance, the poor-articulation group children were trained to pay attention to the right-ear signals. With the dichotic tape, you will recall, there were six sets of 15 pairs of CV syllables comprising the 90 stimulus presentations. The first set of 15 was used for training in which the children (tested individually) were told which syllables would be presented to the right ear by the examiner pointing to the appropriate picture immediately before each of the dichotic presentations. The second randomized set of 15 was used as a test vehicle (responses recorded but no cues given), the third set for training, the fourth set for testing, and so on through the six sets on the 90-item tape. By the end of the second complete tape (180 items with six training and six test sections), the poor-articulation children, as a group, performed equally as well as the good-articulation children. As an ad hoc comparison, two of the original 12 poor-articulation children were retested one month later. Both children performed approximately at their pretraining level. In other words, it is relatively easy to train a right-ear response in children of this age, but what was apparently "trained" was attention to an immediate task. The ear preference as a correlate of articulation facility was not significantly altered. Hence, a reminder that the instructions to the child—what her task is—may be an important variable. Also, remember that if you are testing a child in this way, having her tell you (rather than point to) what she hears may be a test of your perception rather than the child's.

TONE PATTERN PERCEPTION

Musiek and Pinheiro (1985) reviewed the assessment of central auditory processing and reported two types of testing as most productive in their view. They were the dichotic speech testing and the use of a nonlanguage (tone) patterning task that separated between good and poor performers. The theoretical underpinning of the tone pattern (nonspeech) task is that both speech processing and patterning of nonspeech tasks are assumed to be left-hemisphere functions.

Musical tones are generally assumed to be processed in the right hemisphere. If, however, you are a musician it is probable that you process music in the left hemisphere—the assumption is that as a musician you analyze what you hear instead of just listening. Mazziotta and Phelps (1985) reported a positron emission tomography (PET) study in which subjects were asked to listen to pairs of sequences of two-to-five tones per pattern and identify which of the tones in the sequences were different. The subjects who reported having a strategy for solving the task showed more left hemisphere activity. Subjects who did not report having a strategy for the task showed more right hemisphere activity. In other words, the importance of that study for our processing curiosity is not the tones (the stimuli) but the task—*pattern* perception is the magic word.

The tone sequences used by Musiek and Pinheiro had three tones—two alike and one different. The subject's task was to reproduce and to identify the sequence (e.g., high, low, high). When the subjects were asked to reproduce (hum) the tones, the task performance did not differ between good and poor processing groups. The identification task did. That is, apparently the ability to identify which of the three were high, or which of the three were low was facilitated by the subjects' constructing a pattern for the tone sequences.

EVOKED RESPONSE POTENTIALS AND TESTING OF CENTRAL AUDITORY PROCESSING

There is a considerable literature on the P300 or cognitive response measurement related to age, stimulus materials, task, and such variables. A number of aberrant adult populations have been studied and reported, but relatively fewer studies have been done with clinical children. Jirsa and Clontz (1990) reported longer P300 latencies and lesser amplitude of cognitive response in children identified as having auditory processing problems, and Jirsa (1992) reported a significant decrease in P300 latency along with an increase in P300 amplitude in a CAP disorder group following a therapeutic intervention program.

Ludlow (1979) discussed the need for studies using ERPs with language-impaired groups:

> If ERP phenomena such as the P300 wave are studied in conjunction with subjects' responses, we can better interpret their responding difficulties. Without such phenomena, we have no way of knowing whether subjects are not responding correctly because they are not attending to the signals, cannot identify those attributes of signals which are being tested, or are having difficulties responding to the stimuli although they have identified the targets. (p. 189)

In other words, when we are concerned with auditory processing, and whether or not that concern is separable from language processing, we should probably utilize ERP testing to an odd-ball tone (e.g., 80 percent frequent and 20 percent infrequent—or "odd") because that paradigm has been sufficiently researched to at least have some reasonable expectations in terms of latency and relative amplitude for frequent and infrequent (target) stimuli. In addition, the ERP responses to language stimuli, for example, an anomalous word in a sentence (Hume 1984), categories of animals or of male and female names (Donchin and McCarthy 1979), known and unknown real and nonsense words (Molfese 1989, 1990), would yield direct (not inferred) data on language processing.

Of interest would be the laterality of response (it is expected that the left parietal region—approximately overlying the brain's auditory association area—should show greater amplitude of response), the latency of response and the difference in amplitude between target and nontarget stimuli, expected versus nonexpected word, or belonging to or not belonging to the primary category. These sorts of data may demonstrate a possible difference between auditory-processing capability (recognition of patterns) and language-processing facilities.

Let us introduce a young man of 9–6 who was referred because of a suspected central auditory processing disorder. We will call him T. R. This young man is not necessarily representative of the population, but his data are included here for illustration and discussion. His physician diagnosed him as having an attentional deficit disorder; his classroom teacher reported that he had trouble reading and that he was normal in intelligence. His speech was easily intelligible. His mother reported that he did not appear to understand speech when someone called him on the telephone. In our interview, he did not respond to talkers when he could not see their faces. Bilateral hearing was normal according to audiometric results. CAP testing results indicated the following:

> Monotic testing:
> > Low pass filtered speech—results were normal for his age.
> > Pitch pattern perception—inconclusive. Pretest training
> > > for pitch identification could not be achieved.
>
> Dichotic:
> > *Staggered Spondaic Word Test*—normal for age.
>
> Binaural:
> > *Rapid Alternating Speech Sentences* (Willeford 1977)—left
> > > ear first and right ear first—normal for age.
> > *Selective Auditory Attention Test* (Cherry 1980)—normal
> > > for age.

Figure 4–1 represents T. R.'s ERPs. The test stimulus was an odd-ball tone sequence. Testing was accomplished in a sound-isolated room. He was seated in a comfortable chair and asked to listen to the tones presented through an overhead speaker approximately one meter over his head. Stimulus intensity was approximately 70 dB at ear level. To help reduce head and eye movement artifacts, a series of slides approximating the movement of the minute hand on a clock was projected on the wall in front of him. Electrodes were placed on his scalp at left and right frontal, left and right temporal, and left and right parietal locations. He was asked to count the low tones (17 out of the 100 tones).

Figure 4–1 represents the left parietal electrode location (approximately auditory association area). Amplitudes (peak amplitude here is approximately 10 microvolts) were not importantly greater than the homologous right hemisphere location, which may suggest that T. R. was not perceiving the tones as patterns. A few other

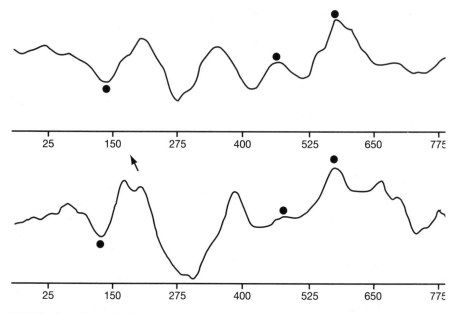

FIGURE 4–1   The top half of this graph is an average of T. R.'s responses to the high (frequent) tone, and the bottom half of the graph represents his averaged brain wave responses to the low (infrequent) tones. The first dot from the left margin represents N1 or the negative-going wave denoting attention. The second dot on the graph marks the third positive-going wave (P3) and the third dot is identified as the "cognitive" response—here as P4.

points in T. R.'s responses may be important. They include the negative-going wave at approximately 120 msec (N1) interpreted as attention—this is in an acceptable time line. The latency of the third positive wave (P3 at approximately 460 msec) is within normal limits for his age but is expected to be the point of greatest amplitude. Instead P4 (570 msec) appeared to be greatest in amplitude. Even more surprising, the frequent (high) tone generated about as much "surprise" as did the infrequent (low) tone. He had been asked to count the low tones. He reported that there were 83—he had apparently been counting highs rather than lows. Remember that on the pitch pattern perception test the results were inconclusive because he did not train to sufficient accuracy to be tested. From the looks of his response sheet, however, he did not routinely reverse high and low identifications. The ERP response is expected to be of greater amplitude to the infrequent tone whether or not he is attending to it. What is important is that he apparently was not attending to the stimuli as if it were patterned. Look back at the Ludlow comment earlier in this section.

Once again you are reminded that our task as diagnosticians is to describe behaviors and to interpret what we see and hear in order to plan an intervention strategy. Our suggested strategy for T. R. was for patterning or categorizing activities—"what happened?," "what do you expect to happen next?"

If you are concerned with auditory function, keep in mind the subject's language skill as measured in the preceding chapter (articulation) and the following chapter (language). Linguistic skill is a variable in the concern for language processing. Speech-sound discrimination testing except in the formats suggested by Locke (1980b) would be a waste of time. When you want to test auditory processing, it is helpful to know that you are not testing identification of form.

REFERENCES

ARNST, D., AND J. KATZ, eds., *Central Auditory Assessment: The SSW Test, Development and Clinical Use*. San Diego: College-Hill Press (1982).

BARAN, J. A., AND R. W. GENGEL, Test-retest reliability of three G-F-W subtests. *Lang. Speech Hearing Serv. Schools*, 15, 199–204 (1984).

BERLIN, C. L., Critical review of the literature on dichotic effects, 1970. In *1971 Review of Scientific Literature on Hearing*. American Academy of Ophthalmology and Otolaryngology, 80–90 (1972).

BERLIN, C. L., AND S. S. LOWE, Temporal and dichotic factors in central auditory testing. In *Handbook of Clinical Audiology*, ed. Jack Katz. Baltimore: Williams and Wilkins (1972).

BERLIN, C. L., AND OTHERS, Central auditory deficits after temporal lobectomy, *Arch. of Otolaryng.*, 96, 4–10 (1972).

BROWN, R., *A First Language, the Early Stages*. Cambridge, Mass.: Harvard University Press (1973).

BURNHAM, D. K., Developmental loss of speech perception: Exposure to and experience with a first language. *App. Psycholing.* 7, 207–240 (1986).

CHERRY, R. S., *Selective Auditory Attention Test*. St. Louis: Auditec of St. Louis (1980).

CHOMSKY, N., AND M. HALLE, *The Sound Pattern of English*. New York: Harper Row (1968).

CONDON, M., Performance of normal-hearing children on the SSW, GFW noise subtest, and the GFW memory for sequence subtest. *Lang. Speech Hearing Serv. Schools*, 15, 192–198 (1984).

COURCHESNE, E., Event-related brain potentials: Comparison between children and adults. *Science*, 197, 589–591 (1977).

CROCKER, J. R., A phonological model of children's articulation competence. *J. Speech Hearing Dis.*, 34, 203–213 (1969).

DEUTSCH, C. P., Auditory discrimination and learning: Social factors. *Merrill-Palmer Quarterly*, 10, 277–296 (1964).

DONCHIN, E., M. KUCOBY, M. KUTAS, R. JOHNSON, AND R. HERNING, Graded changes in evoked response P300—amplitude as a function of cognitive activity. *Percept. Psychophys.*, 14, 319–324 (1973).

DONCHIN, E., AND G. MCCARTHY, Event related brain potentials in the study of cognitive processes. In *The Neurological Bases of Language Disorders in Children: Methods and Directions for Research*, eds. C. L. Ludlow, and M. Doran-Quine. NINCDS Monog. No. 22. Washington, D.C.: U.S. Dept. of Health, Education and Welfare (1979).

DUCHAN, J. F. AND J. KATZ, Language and auditory processing: Top down plus bottom up. In *Central Auditory Processing Disorders*, eds. E. Z. Lasky and J. Katz. Baltimore: University Park Press (1983).

EILERS, E. R. AND D. K. OLLER, A comparative study of speech perception in young severely retarded children and normally developing infants. *J. Speech Hearing Res.*, 23, 419–428 (1980).

FLOWERS, A., *Flowers Auditory Test of Selective Attention*. Dearborn, Mich.: Perceptual Learning Systems (1975).

FUDALA, J. B., *Tree-Bee Test of Auditory Discrimination*. Novato, Calif.: Academic Therapy Publications (1978).

GLASS, M. R., J. R. FRANKS, AND R. E. POTTER, A comparison of two tests of auditory selective attention. *Lang. Speech Hearing Serv. Schools*, 17, 300–306 (1986).

GOLDMAN, R., M. FRISTOE, AND R. W. WOODCOCK, *Goldman-Fristoe-Woodcock Test of Auditory Discrimination*. Circle Pines, Minn.: American Guidance Service, Inc. (1970).

GUR, R. C., AND OTHERS, Sex and handedness differences in cerebral blood flow during rest and cognitive activity. *Science*, 217, 659–661 (1982).

HOLM, V. AND L. KUNZE, Effects of chronic otitus media on language and speech development. *Pediatrics*, 43, 833–839 (1969).

HORST, R. L. AND R. W. THATCHER, A rationale for using ERPs in aberrant development research. In

Developmental Aspects of Event-Related Potentials, eds. D. Otto and others. *Annals New York Academy of Science*, 425, 319–323 (1984).

HUME, C. B., Neurophysiological correlates of meaningful and non-meaningful sentence processing. Doctoral dissertation, University of Tennessee, Knoxville (1984).

JACOBSON, R., C. G. M. FANT, AND M. HALLE, *Preliminaries to Speech Analysis*. Cambridge Mass.: M.I.T. Press (1955).

JASPER, H. H., Report of the committee on methods of clinical examination in electroencephalography. The ten-twenty electrode system. *Electroenceph. Clin. Neurophysiol.*, 10, 371–375 (1958).

JIRSA, R. E., The clinical utility of the P3 AERP in children with auditory processing disorders. *J. Speech Hearing Res.*, 35, 903–912 (1992).

JIRSA, R. E., AND K. B. CLONTZ, Long latency auditory event-related potentials from children with auditory processing disorders. *Ear and Hearing*, 11, 222–232 (1990).

KATZ, J., The use of staggered spondaic words for assessing the integrity of the central auditory nervous system. *J. Auditory Res.*, 2, 327–337 (1962).

KATZ, J., The effects of conductive hearing loss on auditory function. *Asha*, 20, 879–886 (1978).

KEITH, R. W., Central auditory dysfunction: A language disorder? *Topics in Lang. Dis.*, 4, No. 3, 48–56 (1984).

KIMURA, D., Cerebral dominance and the perception of verbal stimuli, *Can. J. Psych.*, 15, 166–171 (1961).

KIMURA, D., Speech lateralization in young children as determined by an auditory test. *J. Comp. Physio. Psych.*, 56, 899–902 (1963).

KOENIGSKNECHT, R., AND L. LEE, Distinctive feature analysis of speech-sound discrimination in three-year-old children. Paper presented at American Speech and Hearing Association Convention, Denver, Colorado (1968).

KUHL, P. A., Speech perception: An overview of current issues. In *Speech, Language, and Hearing, Vol 1, Normal Processes*, eds. N. J. Lass, L. V. Reynolds, J. L. Northern, and D. E. Yoder. Philadelphia: W. B. Saunders Co. (1982).

LEMME, M. S., AND N. H. DAVES, Models of auditory linguistic processing. In *Speech, Language and Hearing, Vol. 1, Normal Processes*, eds. N. J. Lass, L. V. McReynolds, J. K. Northern, and D. E. Yoder. Philadelphia: W. B. Saunders (1982).

LOCKE, J. L., The inference of speech perception in the phonologically disordered child. Part I: A rationale, some criteria, the conventional tests. *J. Speech Hearing Dis.*, 45, 431–444 (1980a).

LOCKE, J. L., The inference of speech perception in the phonologically disordered child. Part II: Some clinically novel procedures, their use, some findings. *J. Speech Hearing Dis.*, 45, 445–468 (1980b).

LUBERT, N., Auditory perceptual impairments in children with specific language disorders: A review of the literature. *J. Speech Hearing Dis.*, 46, 3–9 (1981).

LUDLOW, C. L., Research directions and needs concerning the neurological bases of language disorders in children. In *The Neurological Bases of Language Disorders in Children: Methods and Directions for Research*, eds. C. L. Ludlow and M. Doran Quine. NINCDS Monog. No. 22. Washington, D.C.: U.S. Dept. of Health, Education and Welfare (1979).

MACKAIN, K. S., On explaining the role of experience on infants' speech discrimination. *J. Child Language*, 9, 527–542 (1982).

MAZZIOTTA, J., AND M. E. PHELPS, Human neurophysiological imaging studies of local brain metabolism: Strategies and results. In *Brain Imaging and Brain Function*. ed. L. Sokoloff. New York, Raven Press (1985).

MCDUFFIE, A., Dichotic listening task performance of five- and six-year-old males with different levels of language skill. Unpublished master's thesis, University of Tennessee, Knoxville. (1975).

MENYUK, P., The role of distinctive features in children's acquisition of phonology. *J. Speech Hearing Res.*, 11, 138–146 (1968).

MENYUK, P., *The Development of Speech*. Indianapolis: Bobbs-Merrill (1972).

MINOR, D., A study concerning the training of dichotic right-ear discrimination ability of five- and six-year-old males. Unpublished master's thesis, University of Tennessee, Knoxville (1977).

MOLFESE, D. L., Electrophysiological correlates of word meanings in 14-month-old human infants. *Develop. Neuropsych.*, 5, Nos. 2, 3, 79–103 (1989).

MOLFESE, D. L., Auditory evoked responses recorded from 16-month-old human infants to words they did and did not know. *Brain and Lang.*, 38, 345–363 (1990).

MOLFESE, D. L., AND V. J. MOLFESE, Development of symmetrical and asymmetrical hemispheric responses to speech sounds: Electrophysiological correlates. In *Central Auditory Processing Disorders*, eds. E. Z. Lasky and J. Katz. Baltimore: University Park Press (1983).

MOLFESE, D. L., AND V. J. MOLFESE, Electrophysiological indices of auditory discrimination in newborn infants: The bases for predicting later language development. *Infant Beh. and Devel.*, 8, 197–211 (1985).

MUSIEK, F. E., AND M. L. PINHEIRO, Dichotic speech tests in the detection of central-auditory dysfunction. In *Assessment of Central Auditory Dysfunction—Foundations and Clinical Correlates*, ed. M. L. Pinheiro and F. E. Musiek. Baltimore: Williams & Wilkins, (1985).

OLLER, D. K., AND R. E. EILERS, Speech identification in Spanish- and English-learning 2-year-olds. *J. Speech Hearing Res.*, 26, 50–53 (1983).

OTTO D., R. KARRER, R. HALLIDAY, R. L. HORST, R. KLORMAN, N. SQUIRES, R. W. THATCHER, B. FENELON, AND G. LELORD, Developmental aspects of event-related potentials. *New York Academy of Science*, 425, 319–337 (1984).

OWENS, R. E., Jr., *Language Development*, 2nd ed. Columbus, Ohio Charles E. Merrill (1990).

PENFIELD, W., AND L. ROBERTS, *Speech and Brain Mechanisms*. Princeton: Princeton University Press (1959).

PINHEIRO, M. L., AND F. E. MUSIEK, Sequencing and temporal ordering in the auditory system. In *Assessment of Central Auditory Dysfunction*, eds. M. L. Pinheiro and F. E. Musiek. Baltimore: Williams and Wilkins (1985).

PISONI, D. B., On the nature of categorical perception of speech sounds. *Status Report on Speech Research (SR-27)*. New Haven, Conn.: Haskins Laboratories, (1971).

PRONOVOST, W., *Boston University Speech-Sound Discrimination Test*. Cedar Falls, Iowa: Go-Mo Products (1974).

REES, N. S., Auditory processing factors in language disorders: The view from Procrustes' bed. *J. Speech Hearing Dis.*, 38, 304–315 (1973).

REES, N. S., Saying more than we know: Is auditory processing disorder a meaningful concept? In *Central Auditory and Language Disorders in Children*, ed. R. W. Keith. San Diego: College-Hill Press (1981).

SANDERS, E., When are speech sounds learned? *J. Speech Hearing Dis.*, 37, 55–63 (1972).

SHADDEN, B. B., Ear differences in reaction time as a function of processing task and mode of stimulation. Unpublished Ph.D. dissertation, University of Tennessee, Knoxville (1979a).

SHADDEN, B. B., Reaction time measures of laterality: Task, competition, and attentional variables. Paper presented at the convention of the American Speech-Language-Hearing Association, Atlanta, Georgia (1979b).

SHADDEN, B. B., AND H. A. PETERSON, Reaction time measures of laterality: Task, competition, and attentional variables. Paper presented at American Speech-Language-Hearing Association Convention, Atlanta (1979).

SHADDEN, B. B., AND H. A. PETERSON, Ear differences in simple reaction time: The influence of attentional factors. *Brain Lang.*, 14, 181–189 (1981).

SHANKWEILER, D., An analysis of laterality effects in speech perception. In *The Perception of Language*, eds. D. L. Morton and J. J. Jenkins. Columbus, Ohio: Chas. E. Merrill (1971).

SINGH, S., AND J. BLACK, Study of 26 intervocalic consonants as spoken by four language groups. *J. Acous. Soc. Amer.*, 39, 372–387 (1966).

SINGH, S., AND D. C. FRANK, A distinctive feature analysis of the consonantal substitution pattern. *Language and Speech*, 15, 209–218 (1972).

SMOSKI, W. J., M. A. BRUNT, AND J. C. TANNAHILL, Listening characteristics of children with central auditory processing disorders. *Lang. Speech Hearing Serv. Schools,* 23, 145–152 (1992).

STRAIGHT, H. J., Auditory vs. articulatory phonological processes and their development in children. In *Child Phonology, Vol. 1, Production*, eds. G. H. Yeni-Komshian, J. F. Kavanagh, and C. A. Ferguson. New York: Academic Press (1980).

STUDDERT-KENNEDY, M., AND D. SHANKWEILER, Hemispheric specialization for speech. *J. Acous. Soc. Amer.*, 48, 579–594 (1970).

TEMPLIN, M. C., *Certain Language Skills in Children*. Minneapolis: University of Minnesota Press (1957).

TOBIN, H., Binaural interaction tasks. In *Assessment of Central Auditory Dysfunction*, eds. M. L. Pinheiro and F. E. Musiek. Baltimore: Williams and Wilkins (1985).

TRAVIS, L. E., AND B. RASMUS, The speech-sound discrimination ability of cases with functional speech disorders. *Q. J. Speech*, 17, 217–226 (1931).

WADA, J., AND T. RASMUSSEN, Intracarotid injection of sodium amytol for the lateralization of cerebral speech dominance: Experiments and clinical observation. *J. Neurosurg.*, 17, 166–182 (1960).

WEINER, P. S., Auditory discrimination and articulation. *J. Speech Hearing Dis.*, 33, 19–29 (1967).

WEPMAN, J. M., *Auditory Discrimination Test*. Chicago: Copyright by J. M. Wepman (1958, 1973).

WHITE, E. J., Children's performance on the SSW test and Willeford battery. In *Central Auditory Dysfunction*, ed. R. Keith. New York: Grune & Stratton (1977).

WILLEFORD, J., Assessing central auditory behavior in children: A test battery approach. In *Central Auditory Dysfunction* ed. R. W. Keith. New York: Grune Stratton (1977).

WILLEFORD, J., An auditory behavior-rating scale. Unpublished (1981).

WILLEFORD, J., Assessment of central-auditory disorders in children. In *Assessment of Central Auditory Dysfunction*, eds. M. L. Pinheiro and F. E. Musiek. Baltimore: Williams & Wilkins (1985).

5

Language Testing

'Twas brillig, and the slithy toves
Did gyre and gimble in the wabe;
All mimsy were the borogroves,
And the mome raths outgrabe.

Lewis Carroll
Through the Looking Glass[1]

INTRODUCTION

As listeners, we make three assumptions when we hear a language. We assume that
the noises or sounds we hear make sense, that the sounds are nonrandom, and that
what we hear is truth. Taken together, these three assumptions suggest that language is a system—a system that we can use to learn about the world. It is the sys-

[1]Lewis Carroll, *Alice's Adventures in Wonderland and Through the Looking Glass*. Copyright ©
1962 by Macmillan Publishing Co., Inc. Used by permission.

tematic nature of language that allows us to recognize that the jabberwocky lines of Lewis Carroll are grammatical. A definition of "grammatical," in this sense, would include the fact that the lines can be translated. Translation does not only mean that the words can be replaced by more conventional words but that the syntactic structure, the relationship among the words, is evident. For example, the "slithy toves" is obviously the subject of the second half of the conjoined sentence in the first couplet, and "slithy" is a modifier or qualitative description of whatever a "tove" is; and the predicate ("did gyre and gimble") describes the action of these "toves" and the location.

The study of language or, for our purposes, the description of language abilities is divisible into three levels and more technically into five aspects. Table 5–1 illustrates these divisions, the relationships, and the definition of the elements.

Descriptions of the language at the *sound* level are concerned with the phonemes and permissible phoneme combinations. In Chapter 3, we discussed testing articulation skills in children. Speech-sound discrimination assessment, in theory, tests the child's perceptual identification of phonemes. Assessment of the understanding of the rules of phonology, the child's knowledge of what sounds are combinable in English, was suggested by Whorf (1956), who identified this knowledge as "implicit phonology." Phonological knowledge was assessed by Messer (1967) and Whitacre, Luper, and Pollio (1970). They demonstrated that children with good articulation and language-performance skills also have a better understanding of which sounds are combinable (permissible) as words in English than children with articulation skills delayed in development for their age.

"Grammar" is defined as the relationship of sound to meaning. Morphemes are the smallest meaningful units; a change in morphemes is a change in meaning. We will include one test of morphology by Jean Berko, but our tests of syntax also assess the child's use of morphological endings to indicate appropriate pluralization, possession, verb tenses, and so on. "Syntax" is the relationship among the words in a sentence. By analogy, sentences have a structure in the same way that a bridge has a structure. Elements of the sentence, like the bridge, must fit together properly to perform the desired function. In the mid-sixties, largely because of the work of Chomsky (e.g., *Aspects of the Theory of Syntax*, 1965), *syntax* was the focus of research. In the seventies, the emphasis moved to *semantics*, which was in turn replaced by *pragmatics* because theories with "meaning" as a base appeared more productive than theories of language with syntax as a base.

TABLE 5–1   The levels, aspects, and elements of language

Levels	Aspects	Elements
Sounds	Phonology	Phonemes
Grammar	Morphology	Morphemes
	Syntax	Words
Meaning	Semantics	Words in context
	Pragmatics	Sentences in context

FORM VERSUS FUNCTION

Tests of phonology, morphology, and syntax are generally tests of language form. Tests concerned with semantics and pragmatics are tests of language function. You must realize that these are operational terms and that "form" means "primarily concerned with form" and that "function" suggests "primarily function." Obviously, the language cannot accomplish the intended "function" unless the "forms" are interpretable for the function.

Procedures that test the child's use of morphological endings indicating the understanding of verb tenses, possession, agentive versus instrumentative case grammar functions, and so on are tests of language form. What is primarily necessary for the correct interpretation of the meaning of the utterance is an understanding of the value of the individual elements and/or the structure. Tests of language function are those procedures that require the child to understand the meaning of the utterance in context, for example, to decide the difference in meaning between "a man out standing in his field" versus "a man outstanding in his field."

The *meaning* level of our tripartite description is less well defined. We measure meaning to some degree in vocabulary but more so in the meaning of an utterance. The swing to semantics (e.g., Bloom 1974; Brown 1973; Fillmore 1968; Schlesinger 1971a,b; and others) was based on the assumption that the semantics held more answers to the question of language learning than did syntax. "Pragmatics," likewise, represents the "bigger picture." For additional information, see Bates (1976), Duchan (1984), or Schlesinger (1974).

The five aspects of language shown in Table 5–1 may be thought of as concentric circles. Pragmatics is the outside circle, and each smaller circle within is progressively more defined. At each of the several levels, the meaning of the elements or units is defined by contrast and substitution. That is, contrast and substitution determine whether a change in a sound, word, arrangement of words, and so on constitutes an important difference or whether one unit can be substituted for another and maintain the same meaning or intent. At one level, this may be whether the substitution of /t/ for /k/ is important; at another level, it is the difference between "outstanding" and "out standing."

"Pragmatics" refers to the meaning of words, phrases, and sentences in context. The metaphor that someone is "as big as a house" would not be interpreted literally because our knowledge of the world and the relative sizes of people and houses would force us to assume that the speaker had added emphasis, not that the speaker was untruthful. Similarly, if your friend told you that someone was "a real cool cat," your interpretation would not likely be a description of a frigid feline. Here the example is meant to include knowledge of the vernacular. This means that your grandmother, if restricted to the slang of her day, might not understand this phrase. Social contexts are necessary to understand the meaning of an utterance in terms of pragmatic considerations. The example also illustrates a maturational/ development level. A seven-year-old asked to explain what "being cool" means may well describe a child in the snow without her mittens. It requires a more abstract interpretation to arrive at a psychological rather than a physical meaning. A pragmatic understanding refers to an other-than-literal translation, which is why idioms are frequently used to test language understanding with older children and adults. "The spirit is willing but the flesh is weak" is not intended to translate as "the whiskey is good but the meat has gone bad."

One other example of what constitutes pragmatic understanding is what Bates (1976) termed "paralinguistics." It refers to the fact that the meaning of the message is carried not only in the words but also in the social context of the situation (facial features, intonational contours, etc.). If you refer to your friend with a term that translates as questioning the legitimacy of his ancestry but say it with a smile, you may get a chuckle in return rather than a punch in the nose.

The point to be made is that the child's understanding of the use of language, as well as the forms of language, is maturationally and experientially developed. Piaget based this understanding on cognitive levels. Children from 7- to 12-years-old, according to Piaget, operate at a concrete level, which implies literal translation of words. Children 12 years and older are supposed to operate at a level of formal operations, which includes figurative translation. That is why tests for older children frequently include interpretation of idioms (e.g., Nippold 1991). Nippold and Martin (1989) reported test results of 14- to 17-year-old subjects in their interpretation of idioms in isolation and in context and arrived at what they called a qualitative analysis.

Pragmatics, however, is not restricted to an age level. To Bates (1976), all of language is pragmatic to begin with, and the acquisition of pragmatics begins before speech development. The infants' attention to her mother's face, the turn taking in babbling, the looking away to break off a "conversation," and so forth are precursors to the linguistic means of communication. According to Bates, we choose our meanings to fit contexts and build our meanings onto those contexts. In her words, "the two are inseparable, in the same way that 'figure' is definable only in terms of 'ground.'" Semantics emerges developmentally and logically from pragmatics in much the same way that syntax emerges from semantic knowledge.

Bates's reasoning is not unrelated to *speech acts theory* (Searle 1969), which assumes that every utterance has both a propositional meaning and an intention that the speaker wishes to convey. Pragmatics relies on presuppositions between speaker and listener—the information that is shared, contexts of utterances, social mores, and so on.

PERSPECTIVE

Our descriptions of test protocols for determining the child's relative mastery of phonology, morphology, syntax, semantics, and pragmatics are separated in this chapter as an editorial convenience. They are developmental aspects or facets of language that are, as in our earlier example, embedded one within the other—concentric circles where each of the larger circles encompasses and utilizes the information or elements of the smaller circles. They may also be viewed as representing a hierarchy with "intent" as the basic proposition (Schlesinger 1971a) or deepest level and the production of phonemes as the most superficial (surface structure) level. The "deeper" the error, the greater the impedance to communication. When you look at the picture from this angle, you would not find it surprising if a tested child's errors in production or understanding overlapped adjoining circles.

Most children develop their language skills according to highly predictable developmental patterns (e.g., Brown 1973). Some 5 to 10 percent of normally intelligent children are delayed in their development of speech and language skills. A five-year-old child's grammar acquisition is 90 percent complete (Owens 1984), and virtually all the phonemes of the language are made correctly by at least 50 percent of five-year-old children (Sander 1972). Certainly some errors of syntax, morphology, and articulation may still occur into the early school years, but most "developmental delays" have been remedied by intervention of speech-language pathologists or have "spontaneously" been cleared by eight years of age.

Generally speaking, these developmental delays were assessed as errors in the *forms* of language (phonology, morphology, and syntax). Semantics and pragmatics require identification of the language forms; but more than that, they require the use of logic and reasoning with language. For example, "The chickens are ready to eat" is an ambiguous sentence that is resolved by context. "Chickens" is either the deep structure subject or the deep structure object of the verb "to eat." Likewise, the possible ambiguity of "She dropped the plate on the table and broke it" is resolved by the hearer's knowledge of tables and plates in general—or more particularly by knowledge of a specific plate and a specific table.

As we have said before, language is a patterned and rule-governed system. If this were not so, and the elements of the language were randomly and haphazardly sequenced, languages could not be learned. In order to learn a language, the hearer must have identified the meaningful elements, the important aspects of contexts that make a difference in meaning, and strategies for perceiving the speaker's intent.

The rules of the language are derived (learned but not generally taught) by children as listeners to the language patterns in their environment. "Culturally different" or "limited English proficiency" children (e.g., Adler 1991), that is, those whose exposure is primarily non-mainstream language patterns who may have learned a different set of form and patterns, are not different in their ability to reason with language—although their linguistic as well as their cultural habits may affect their language use. And idioms are culturally based. The caution to the clinician in this case is to evaluate the form and function regularities exhibited by the child and compare these to the child's language environment *as well as* to the mainstream environment in which we wish to educate the child. In terms of that last implied choice, the professional and cultural biases that you hold may influence your judgment as a diagnostician and as a planner of direction, goal, style, and choice of intervention.

Cognition—One More Detour

Coupled with the recent attention to pragmatics has been increased interest in the relationship between cognition and language. For example, Slobin (1973, 1979) posited cognition as the base for language. The child uses language to express what he knows about the world. Because of imperfect command of the forms in his early forays into the world of language, he uses old words to express new concepts and new words to express old concepts. Piaget (e.g., Piaget and Inhelder 1969) assumed a generalized development of cognitive abilities as the base for language development. Bates (1976) defined cognition as separable knowledges rather than the

Piaget-type general sensorimotor stages. Schlesinger (1974, 1977) assumed an interaction of cognition and language in children's development.

"Cognition," as defined by Snyder (1984), is native ability or capability, which approximates a definition of intelligence. If this limited definition is extended to mean understanding of the world in the sense of "how language works to allow communication and convey information," then we are not primarily concerned with determining a causal relationship between cognition and language but rather with the functional interrelationships between language and cognition in determining a child's skill in communicative function. That is, our purpose is to determine the need and the direction for intervention. Teaching language forms without an understanding of the concepts would be meaningless.

FORMAL VERSUS INFORMAL TESTING

A primary problem with structured formal testing is the restrictiveness of the test situation. We hope to observe what the child *can do* rather than what she *does do* in this conversational context. In contrast, the problem in informal testing of the "eavesdropping" type is that we may observe what the child *does* which is less than what she is *capable of doing*. The hazard is in interpreting what she does as if it were what she can do and making our judgments accordingly.

Both formal and informal testing can be appropriate and meaningful. Your choice of methods between these two polar alternatives may depend on what you are more interested in knowing for your description purposes.

TESTING PRAGMATICS IN "NATURAL" CONTEXTS

Those who argue most strongly for informal testing express an overriding concern with pragmatics. Duchan (1984), for example, argued for informal assessment in natural contexts since it was the only means of determining how well the language-disordered child made sense of what was going on around him and how well he managed conversational interactions in the real world. In Duchan's words, how your definition of pragmatics relates to the rest of language is a deciding factor in how testing of linguistic function is approached:

> Like Buffalo chicken wings, pragmatics can be bought in its mild, medium or hot versions. The mild version takes pragmatics as a new aspect of language which needs to be assessed along with our traditional assessment approaches. . . . Those with medium tastes see pragmatics as more pervasive, . . . which requires them to evaluate their children's language in natural contexts, even when the language problem is one of phonology or syntax, or has as its source a cognitive deficiency. . . . The hot version of the pragmatics movement is forwarded by the movement's revolutionaries, who opt for overthrowing our previous conceptions that language is what we are assessing, and propose that we move toward a new conceptualization which examines communication and context, and if called for, the language within it. (1984, pp. 177–178)

THE ASSESSMENT CONCEPT—AGAIN

The preceding discussion, heavily weighted on semantics, pragmatics, and cognition, aimed at providing a broad-based perspective on components of communication, since judgments on all three levels (sound system, grammar, meaning) are necessary to determine the pervasiveness or concentration of the problem. Before we place a child in therapy to remediate a problem, we need to define the parameters of the problem. A test score is at best only a comparative yardstick and not a description. The pattern of responses along with our recognition of the relative demands and restrictions of the test situation should be the interpretive basis of our assessment. As noted by Siegel and Broen (1976):

> Assessment is a broad concept that includes and goes beyond formal tests. Before an adequate assessment program can be devised, the clinician must have a general notion of what is to be subsumed by language. . . . [S]uccessful assessment always requires that the clinician go beyond the bounds of specific procedures to the basic language dimensions themselves . . . [and] . . . the most reliable and useful language assessment device is a clinician who has a good grasp of language in its various aspects and a willingness to probe and be inventive in creating new approaches to language assessment. (p. 118)

In 1986, *Asha* published an annotated bibliography of 133 books, articles, and presentations on language disorders. Even a brief review of the assessment procedures and tests of language function in children would be a monumental task. The language tests reviewed here are limited and have been included because they illustrate different purposes and styles of testing.

LANGUAGE TEST MEASURES

We begin our discussion with tests that serve as measures of verbal output. Following descriptions of procedures for determining length and complexity, we discuss vocabulary testing, tests specific to grammar (morphology and syntax), broad-based tests of language function, and finally tests designed to measure pragmatic function.

Mean Length of Response (MLR)

The idea of using length of response as a criterion for a child's progress in speech was suggested at least as early as 1925 by Margaret Morse Nice. She divided speech development into four stages:

a. single words
b. early sentences (an average of more than one but less than three words)
c. short sentences of three to four words
d. complete sentences of six to eight words

Nice assumed that 30 or more sentences would comprise an adequate sample. McCarthy (1930) elaborated on this general idea, collected 50 responses per child, and developed mean-length-of-response norms for children at six-month separations from 18 to 54 months. McCarthy (1954) and later Templin (1957) modified the critical descriptions of what would be considered a word and how responses were to be determined. Templin reported norms for children from three to eight years of age. Both McCarthy (1930, 1954) and Templin (1957) reported alternatives to the mean length of response, such as the mean of the five longest responses, the number of independent clauses, and so on, but these too were just quantitative counts of words. Minifie, Darley, and Sherman (1963) reported mean length of response to be the most reliable of the seven measures they compared.

Winitz (1959) suggested tape-recording the responses for greater accuracy and also recommended that at least 60 responses be recorded. The first 10 responses were to be discarded on the assumption that early in the interview the child might be reluctant to talk and you might not get as representative a sample as from the next 50.

A considerable amount of time is required to elicit 50 responses from most children, and for at least this reason, the clinical usefulness of such a measure is offset by its awkwardness. To determine if reliable information could be obtained from fewer than 50 responses, Darley and Moll (1960) collected 50 responses from 150 children and calculated the MLR from 5, 10, 15, 20, 25, 35, and 50 responses. They determined that 25 responses were adequate for most descriptive purposes, although the highest reliability was obtained from 50 responses.

Even with 50 responses, MLR is only an approximate measurement. The norms published with 50 responses do not discriminate between age levels nor, apparently, between good and poor language skill groups. Shriner (1969) concluded that:

> response length does not appear to be a significant indicator of expressive language for children who are approximately five years of age or older, because of increased response variability. . . . Whether or not one sampling of 50 responses is representative of a "true" MLR for children below the age of approximately five years has not been determined. (p. 66)

Mean length of response is no longer a frequently used measure, although some of the research done with a MLR format is pertinent. For example, 50 responses continue to be the usually suggested sample size for an evaluation of a child's conversational language skills. One of the peripherally reported findings of a study by Hahn (1948, p. 365) was that "the [length of the] child's response and completeness of his sentence structure depend more on the immediate situation and the topic. Skills, as we measure them here, are high when speaking is fun." In other words, it is important to remember that the child is likely to perform better on a speaking task if we appreciate her performance and show that we are interested in what she is saying. Under pleasant circumstances and before an appreciative audience, she is more likely to provide a good sample of what she can do.

The elicitor and the setting of the language sample may also be important variables for consideration. Olswang and Carpenter (1978) compared language samples collected by mother and by clinician for young language-impaired children. They reported that the children's samples generated similar lexical, grammatic, and semantic data for the two elicitors (mother versus unfamiliar female clinician) but that mother generated more utterances within the restricted time period in the clinical setting. Scott and Taylor (1978), on the other hand, reported that mother (at home) was likely to generate more complex language structures than was a clinician in the clinical setting. This difference in favor of the home and mother was primarily true of "good-language" children with utterance lengths that average three or four or more morphemes. They reported that:

> Clinical sampling underestimates the frequency of complex utterances, questions, modals, and volitional verb forms and predisposes the child to talk about ongoing or imminent activity and the location of things. (p. 494)

Mean Length of Utterance (MLU)

The distinction between response and utterance is not in the definition of the word meanings but in the way the terms have been used. A mean length of utterance (MLU) is counted in morphemes rather than in words and is probably a more valid index of linguistic maturity. There are no norms per se for MLU by age. Roger Brown (1973) described the stages of language development with MLU ranges to mark off five arbitrary stages. In the early stages, from one to four and five morphemes, he stresses that children differ in age of acquisition but show considerable consistency in the morphemic elements used with stages of progression. The numbers usually quoted then are not normative but suggestive. Although they are not normative, approximations to Brown's data are shown in Table 5–2.

As an example of the difference between a word count and a morpheme count, "The deer were running" has four words but seven morphemes. An MLU count would credit "deer" for plurality, "were" for past tense, and "running" as progressive and would give the child appropriate credit for more linguistic complexity than would a word count.

Structural Complexity Score (SCS)

McCarthy (1930) was probably one of the first to suggest an analysis of children's utterances in terms of linguistic complexity of the response. Williams (1937) used measures comparable but not identical to McCarthy's, and assigned weights of 0 to 4 according to response complexity. Templin (1957) modified the definitions slightly and also assigned weights of 0 to 4:

0. incomplete responses, including those that are functionally complete
1. a simple sentence with or without phrases
2. a simple sentence with two or more phrases or a compound subject or predicate with a phrase
3. a compound sentence
4. complex and elaborated sentences

Templin published norms for three- to eight-year-old children (age 3, 3.5, 4, 4.5, 5, 5.5, 6, 7, 8) and noted that while the performance increased from age three through age eight, the increments from age to age were not as stable as they were for most language tests. The norms are based on 50 responses, each of which is valued on the 0 to 4 scale, making a possible score of 200. Similar to the MLR exam-

TABLE 5–2   Approximate divisions for early language stages

Stage	Mean	MLU Range	Approximate Age
I	1.75	1.0–2.0	12–26 months
II	2.25	2.0–2.5	27–30 months
III	2.75	2.5–3.0	31–34 months
IV	3.25	3.0–3.75	35–40 months
V	4.0	3.75–4.5	41–46 months

Stage I: Single-word utterances and early two-word combinations.
Stage II: Early grammatical morphemes, semantic relations (e.g., modifier plus head).
Stage III: Simple sentences (subject + verb + object), yes/no and wh questions, negatives.
Stage IV: Early embedded sentences (e.g., *The boy who fell cried*).
Stage V: Compound sentences (e.g., *Jack fell down and Jill ran after*).

ple of an expected score for a five-year-old child, on the SCS score with Templin's (1957, p. 82) norms, the mean for a child of five years is 56.9 with a standard deviation of 21.5. The three-year-old mean is 34.3 (SD 18.3), and for an eight-year-old child the mean is 77.7 (SD 33.8). It can be seen that one standard deviation on each side of the mean SCS given for a five-year-old is clearly within the range of normal performance for both the three-year-old and the eight-year-old children on this measure.

Darley and Moll (1960) also investigated the reliability of the SCS. Their data showed that while 50 responses were a sufficient sample for the MLR in terms of reliability, 50 responses were not sufficient to give an equally reliable measure of structural complexity.

The advantage of the SCS, over what was then available, was the fact that it supplied a qualitative measure of language complexity—not just sentence length but the linguistic complexity of the utterance. In that sense, both the *Developmental Sentence Scoring* and the *Length Complexity Index* to be described next have some beginning in the SCS.

Developmental Sentence Scoring (DSS)

Developmental Sentence Scoring (Lee 1974; Lee and Canter 1971) was developed to analyze the syntactic growth of children who are at the stage where at least 50 percent of their utterances are complete. If less than 50 percent of the utterances are complete, the *Developmental Sentence Types* (Lee 1966, 1974) is a more appropriate instrument. In *Developmental Sentence Scoring*, 50 consecutive complete utterances are selected for analysis. "Complete" in this sense means a subject and predicate relationship is expressed and not necessarily that the sentence is grammatically complete by adult standards. That is, "Me go" or "Daddy broke car" are both considered complete. A modifier plus a noun, such as "red car," would not be complete, but an imperative such as "Go" or "Don't" would be complete because in the adult standard an imperative sentence can omit the implied subject.

As in the MLR procedure, the clinician is advised to discard the first few sentences as "warm-up" and then take 50 consecutive responses beyond that point, preferably selecting that portion of the total discourse that represents the child's highest level of language skill. Repeated utterances are scored only once, so if a child says "I know, I know, I know," the second two repetitions are discarded and not scored. Unintelligible responses are also usually omitted from scoring. An exception to this rule is if an unintelligible word occurs in a sentence but its function is obvious. For example, in "He chased the ____ and the lion," the unintelligible word might reasonably be interpreted as a noun, and the sentence could be included. Exact imitations of the clinician's sentences are also omitted from analysis. As utterances are omitted, further consecutive responses are added to obtain the suggested 50.

Segmenting utterances is logical but somewhat discretionary. As in the MLR, intonational and inflectional cues are useful in separating utterances, as are pauses in the child's ongoing commentary. Conjunctions, such as *and* occurring as the initial word in a sentence are usually excluded. Initial-position conjunctions that introduce dependent clauses are included: "When I grow up, I'll be a fireman" or "If I want to, I can have another cookie." The conjunction *and* may be included any number of times in a series listing: "Sam and Andy and Betty and Jack went to the store," but *and* between series of clauses may be omitted at the clinician's discretion. For example, "And I went to the store and I got some candy and then we went to the zoo and I saw a tiger and . . . ." The first *and* would be omitted, the first sentence would be presumed to have ended with ". . . some candy"; the next *and* would be omitted; and the second sentence for analysis would begin with "Then we went . . ." Conjunctions other than *and* are usually maintained, but other "run-on" sentences as the one illustrated may be separated at the clinician's discretion. Sentence tags are given sentence status: "It's a red car, I think."

Scoring for DSS. The 50 sentences selected for scoring are copied onto a record form. Scores are entered on the record form for each of eight grammatical categories: indefinite pronouns or noun modifiers, personal pronouns, main verbs, secondary verbs, negatives, conjunctions, interrogative reversals, and wh-questions. Words in each of these categories are valued from 1 to 8 points. For example, the conjunction *and* is given 3 points; *but, so, or,* and *if* are given 5 points credit; *because* is 6 points, and so forth. Structures are credited only if they meet the adult standard for correct usage. A sentence point is given if the sentence meets all semantic, syntactic, and morphologic requirements of the adult grammar. Total points for the 50 sentences are summed and divided by 50; the resultant mean score constitutes the DSS. The child's performance can be compared with norms provided for children from 2–0 to 6–11 at six-month levels. Norms are in terms of percentiles, with the 90th, 75th, 50th, 25th, and 10th percentiles charted.

The subjects for the normative data were 200 normally developing white children between 2–0 and 6–11 years, with 5 boys and 20 girls between 2–0 and 2–11, 3–0 and 3–11, and so on. All but 3 of the 200 children were from middle-income families, and all were from monolingual homes where standard English was spoken. The normative data indicate a progressive increase of DSS with increasing age and a statistically significant ($p = < 0.01$) separation between all five one-year age groups.

Developmental Sentence Types (DST)

The DST was proposed by Lee in 1966 and was then discussed in more detail in 1974 as the classification procedures were refined. When discussing the DSS, you will recall that it was suggested for use when at least 50 percent of the child's utterances contained a subject–predicate relationship. If fewer than 50 percent of the sentences were complete in that respect, the DST was suggested as an alternate tool. The DST was designed as a measure of the "presentence" stage in language development, those sentences which have only partial subject–predicate relationships expressed.

The DST chart for "clinical" children's utterances contains three horizontal levels: (1) single words, (2) two-word combinations, and (3) multiword constructions that are not complete sentences. The vertical dimension has five segments: (1) noun phrases, (2) designative phrases, (3) predicative sentences, (4) subject–verb sentences, and (5) fragments. The *fragment* designation includes all utterances that are mere appendages to the three main sentence types: the designative, the predicative, and the subject–verb sentences.

The DST classification is a linguistic description of the child's utterances but does not generate a score and as such is not a measurement device in the sense that we have been discussing them. The kinds of data that result from a DST analysis are the proportion of the utterances that were single words, the proportion that were two-word combinations, and the proportion that were elaborated as different sentence types. In other words, the chart is an informational source for tracking a child's progress in the acquisition of syntax but does not provide a calibration or a numerical value.

Length-Complexity Index (LCI)

The *Length-Complexity Index*, as the name implies, is based on both length and complexity. It was developed by Shriner and Sherman (1967) and was modified and elaborated by Miner (1969). Using language samples from 200 children ranging in age from 2–6 to 12–0 years, Shriner and Sherman obtained an equation for predicting language development as measured by psychological scale values. The initial battery used *Mean Length of Response* (MLR), *Mean of Five Longest Responses* (M5L), *Number of One-Word Responses* (N1W), *Standard Deviation of Response Length* (SD-RL), *Number of Different Words* (NDW), and *Structural Complexity Score* (SCS). The measures retained as the best predictors included M5L, N1W, NDW, and SCS. MLR was not maintained in the final equation although it correlated more highly with the dependent variable than did any other single predictor variable. According to Shriner and Sherman (1967, p. 46), its lack of significant prediction in the equation may be because it also correlated highly with each of the retained predictor variables.

From this base, Miner assigned score values to phrases or constructions in terms of their length and complexity. He assigned values of 1–7 and 1–6 respectively to noun phrases and verb phrases according to inclusion of modifiers, morphological endings, use of auxiliary words, and verb tenses. Additional points were scored for negatives, interrogatives, and conjunctions.

Segmenting of responses follows the same general rules as the MLR and

DSS. There are some arbitrary rules for counting words, such as hyphenated words, compound words, and proper nouns being counted as single words and not counting prepositions when they appear as the last word in a sentence ("I want to"), but generally these rules are similar to those followed in MLR, SCS, and DSS scoring procedures. From the typescript protocol of a child's responses, slash marks are inserted to mark off responses, and the sentence responses are numbered consecutively and transferred to a scoring sheet. Major sentence components (NP_1 and NP_2, VP_1, VP_2) plus the extra point categories (conjunctions, negatives, and additional points) are then considered for scoring. An example (Figure 5–1) may help to visualize these categories.

After the sentence has been transferred to the score sheet, the NP_1 (subject of the sentence) is underscored with a single line and the VP_2 (predicate) is underscored with a double line. The number designations illustrate that the marking is from left to right. VP_2 is the predicate that dominates VP_1 and NP_2. In the examples given, NP_1 (the black cat) is an article plus modifier plus noun and is credited with 3 points; NP_2 is an article plus noun and is given 2 points. VP_1 is a past tense verb and is given 2 points. The total credit for the sentence is then $NP = 3$ ($NP_1 = 3$) and $VP = 4$ ($VP_1 = 2$ and NP_2 dominated by $VP_2 = 2$) or 7 points.

Three measures can be computed from these analyses: a noun phrase index ($NPI = NP_1$ points divided by the total number of NP_1s); a verb phrase index ($VPI = VP_1$ points divided by the total number of VP_1s); and the length complexity index ($LCI = NP_1$ points plus VP_2 points plus additional points divided by number of sentences).

In terms of identification of children with delayed language development, the DSS norms provide a numerical comparison that the LCI does not. The LCI, on the other hand, like the DST or the DSS, can provide the clinician with a description of the child's language usage that would be essential to therapy planning.

As an example of the types of information generated by a child's language sample, the following examples are inserted from a boy we will identify as L. B., who was five years, six months old at the time of testing. A short sample of 35 utterances was elicited from L. B. in response to pictures and from conversation with the examiner. The mean length of response for the 35 responses was 3.87, and the mean length of utterances was computed as 4.84. Templin's 1957 norms for a child of 5–0 years show an MLR of 5.7 words with a standard deviation of 1.5. L. B.'s MLR is just outside the −1 SD point by that comparison. The MLU is not normed.

FIGURE 5–1

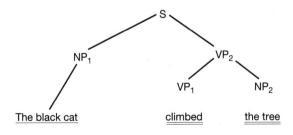

L. B.'s responses were also scored on the LCI and the DSS. For purposes of comparison on those two measures, the 35 responses were reduced to 18 that were grammatically complete. The remainder of L. B.'s responses were functionally complete as answers to questions but were grammatically incomplete and thus eliminated from the analysis. Figure 5–2 lists the 18 scored responses and their value on the LCI. Figure 5–3 identifies the same responses by number and how they were valued according to the DSS. The LCI, as you recall, is not normed so no comparisons can be made against a hypothetical normal group. The DSS computation gave a score of 8.50. Lee's DSS norms show a mean of 9.19 for children of chronological age 5–6. The 25th percentile is 7.89, and the 10th percentile point is 6.72. If we assume the −1 SD point to be approximately the 16th percentile, then the two normed measures of the four utilized are in relative agreement. By most standards of comparison, L. B. would not be considered to have a language problem—or no more than a mild delay in his expressive language or grammatical skills.

VOCABULARY

Earlier we defined "semantics" as including word meanings. Vocabulary testing usually includes primarily "referent" (lexical) words or words that create images and avoids "nonreferent" (nonlexical; function words) items. In practical terms, that means it is more likely to expect a child to recognize a picture of a dog or a horse or a chair or an action such as sitting or eating than a picture of *the* or a picture of *is*. Vocabulary recognition tests are not "semantic" tests as we have defined them here. That is as good a reason as any why we would not expect to find high correlations between picture vocabulary recognition tests and the other language tests to be discussed.

The Peabody Picture Vocabulary Test–Revised

The *Peabody Picture Vocabulary Test* (PPVT) was originally published in 1959, expanded in description in 1965, and revised in 1981. It has consistently been one of the most used tests of receptive vocabulary.

Earlier versions of the PPVT provided tables for converting the raw score to a "mental age" or "intelligence quotient." It is frequently true of intelligence tests that the vocabulary subtest score correlates highly with the total score, but intelligence is more than vocabulary, especially with children who have hearing impairments or who may not be in the mainstream of the culture. Most speech-language pathologists, recognizing that vocabulary is more a function of language (and cultural) exposure than it is of native ability, translated these terms of mental age and intelligence to the more functional "vocabulary age score" and reported the results as percentile ranks and standard scores. Now the test makers have done the same. The results are reported as age equivalent and standard score equivalent values.

In light of our earlier discussion, the PPVT–R is neither a cognitive (intelligence or ability) test nor a receptive language (semantic) measure. It is a test of vocabulary recognition that measures the child's ability to match words spoken by the examiner to a choice of four pictures. It is expected, however, that the test result

Sentence #	NP		VP		AP		
	NP$_1$	NP$_2$	VP$_1$	VP$_2$	Con.	Neg.	?
1. He used to be two,	1	1	3	4	1		
now he's one.	1	1	1	2			
2. I don't know.[a]	1	0	2	2		2	
3. Yeah, I got two brothers,	1	3	2	5			
one of them' s Eric	3	1	1	2	1		
and one of them's Bobby.	3	1	1	2			
4. Eric's this much	1	2	1	3			
(holding up three fingers).							
5. Yeah, I'm this many (five fingers).	1	2	1	3			
13. We got animals and tigers and raccoons and Idon't know and lions and all the animals.	2	10	1	11	5		
19. I seen this at the store.	1	4	2	6			
25. He's waving 'bye.	1	1	3	4			
26. There's a tweety-bird.	1	2	1	3			
27. Tweety-bird hit on the cat.	1	3	1	4			
28. They like this.[b]	2	1	1	2			
29. He's trying to catch that tweety-bird.	1	2	4	6			
30. It's snowing there.	1	1	3	4			
31. He's trying to catch that tweety-bird. again	1	3	4	7			
32. He's cooking a pie.	1	2	3	5			
33. He's snowing again.	1	1	3	4			
34. He's got his trunk caught and	1	3	4	7	1		
tweety-bird went with her.	1	3	2	5			
35. He's talking.	1	0	3	3			
[a]Do is a modal, part of VP	28	46	47	93	8	3	—

[b]For example: They like this
$\underbrace{\text{They}}_{\text{N+P1}}$ $\underbrace{\text{like this}}_{\text{V + N}}$

$$L.C.I. = \frac{NP_1 + VP_2 + AP}{\# \text{ Sentences}} = 7.33$$

FIGURE 5–2 **A short language sample from a 5–6-year-old boy scored according to the length complexity index (LCI).**

(We are indebted to Dr. Lynn E. Miner for checking the accuracy of the LCI values.)

	Indef Pro	Pers Pro	Main Verb	Secon Verb	Neg	Conj	Inter Rev.	Wh Ques.	Sent Pt.	Total
1	3,3	2,2	2,1	5					a	18
2		1	4		4				1	10
3	3,3,3	1,3,3	$-1,1^{b}$			3			–	21
4	1,7		1						–	9
5	1,7	1	2						–	11
13	3	3	$\_^{b}$		c	3,3^{c} 3,3			–	18
19	1	1	–						–	2
25		2	1						1	4
26		1							1	2
27			1^{d}						–	1
28	1	3	1						1	6
29	1	2	1	5					1	10
30	1		1						1	3
31	1	2	1	5					1	10
32		2	1						1	4
33		$\_^{e}$	1						–	1
34		2,2,2	$7^{f},2$			3			1	19
35		2	1						1	4
										153

[a] no sentence point because not semantically accurate
[b] got not acceptable for have   DSS = 8.50
[c] and I don't know excluded from scoring
[d] verb hit has no past tense marker
[e] he is wrong pronoun—not credited
[f] has got caught credited as passive

FIGURE 5–3   **The language sample displayed in Figure 5–1 is shown as scored by the developmental sentence scoring (DSS) procedures. Sentence numbers refer to the listing as on 5–1.**
(We are indebted to Professor Emeritus Laura Lee who graciously consented to score this sample for DSS values.)

will agree more closely with intelligence and academic performance than it will with articulation or language test results.

The PPVT–R utilizes two alternate forms (L and M), each containing 175 plates with four pictures per plate. The earlier version of the PPVT utilized 150 plates with the same set of pictures used for both A and B versions. The extension to 175 plates should provide more precision, especially at the extremes of the age range. The manual reported that two-thirds of the original pictures were redrawn or replaced to remove dated words ("weiner" a.k.a. "hot dog" was a casualty) and words with sex, geographic, ethnic, or racial bias.

Eight plates are included for each year of development. Plates are placed at age levels where 40 to 60 percent of the standardizing population correctly identified the intended picture. Pictures are grouped on a page with (obviously) one correct choice, one most common error foil that the child would be expected to respond to if he correctly identified part of the concept intended, and two less likely choices. With four choices available on each page, the child would logically respond correctly one time in four or two times in eight by chance alone. Plates are arranged in ascending order of difficulty. That is the rationale for the base level of eight consecutive correct responses and the ceiling of six errors in eight consecutive responses. The total raw score is the highest correct response minus the number of errors. All items below the base level are credited as correct.

The raw score is converted to a standard score, percentile rank, and stanine score. Mean performance is again set at a standard score of 100 with a standard deviation of 15. The normal range (approximately two standard deviations) is usually considered to be from 75 to 125 points. Comparison scores listed in the manual show the PPVT–R scores as slightly lower than for the PPVT (7 to 17 "I.Q." points for the 3-to-12 year age range and 3 to 22 points for the 13-to-18 year age range). This suggests that the older PPVT norms may have exaggerated the vocabulary abilities of today's children as compared to the 1950s standardizing population of children. Choong and McMahon (1983) compared the PPVT and the PPVT–R on a sample of 80 children 3–6 to 4–6 years old. Their data showed significantly higher scores (nine months) for the PPVT than for the PPVT–R, with the PPVT–R scores more closely approximating chronological age.

One other improvement in the revised PPVT is the restructuring of the conversion tables. Tables are now listed by three-month rather than by six-month separations, which increases the precision of score interpretation. In addition to the nine stanine (half-standard deviation) separation conversions for the standard score, a range of "true scores" is provided for each obtained score. For example, a standard score of 105 shows a confidence band of +/– seven points (the standard error of the mean); hence, the true score is assumed to be between 98 and 112—a "high average score."

The standardization sample for the PPVT–R included approximately 200 children at each six-month level from 2–6 years to 19 years and just over 200 adults at five-year separations from 20 to 40 years, geographically, racially, and socioeconomically representative of the U.S. population (1970 census).

Vocabulary Comprehension Scale (VCS)

The *Vocabulary Comprehension Scale* (Bangs 1975) is a restricted vocabulary test. It assesses the understanding of pronouns and words of position, size, quality, and quantity in children two to six years of age. Objects, rather than pictures, are utilized in the assessment; that is, the child is requested to "push the car around the tree" rather than to identify a picture of "around." Materials used include a tea set and two dolls (for pronouns); a "garage set," which includes toys such as ladder, fence, trees, and cars; a sponge; and wooden and metal cubes. The child is required to name or point to all the objects used before the scale is administered.

Normative data were collected from 60 children: 10 at each six-month age separation from two to six years of age (2–0 to 2–5, 2–6 to 2–11, etc.). The children for the standardization population were all from middle-income families of mixed ethnic backgrounds and were enrolled in preschool programs in Houston, Texas. Selection criteria included a judgment by the teacher that the children presented no obvious language deficits and that each child scored at or above her age level, or no more than six months below her age level, on the *Peabody Picture Vocabulary Test*.

The primary purpose of the VCS is not to determine a vocabulary age per se but to demonstrate to the examiner which specific pronouns and words of position, size, quantity, and quality are understood by the subject. The 61 words on the scale include 17 pronouns (I, my, mine, they, their), 6 quantity words (more, less), 6 words of quality (hard, soft), 6 of size (big, little), and 26 words of position (around, next to, beside). The manual lists each of the stimulus words with the percentage of the standardization sample at each age level that demonstrated understanding of that word. A criterion of 80 percent was selected as "mastery" level.

The test subject's performance is marked on a scoring form (+ for pass, – for fail, and blank for not administered). The scores on this form are then transferred to a summary section that has the stimulus words listed in developmental order. A summary of the results could yield a vocabulary index for classes of words, an overall vocabulary age, and information for planning instructional activities. The manual for the VCS does contain suggestions for classroom activities to be utilized in teaching pronouns, positional words, and so on, but it does not contain any statistical data for reliability or validity.

Test of Word Finding (TWF)

The *Test of Word Finding* (German 1986) is not a test of word knowledge or expressive vocabulary but a test of accuracy and speed of word retrieval. The words are assumed to be in the expressive vocabulary of the children tested, and it is, therefore, a test of word finding. The words to be retrieved, when prompted by visual and auditory stimuli, are common nouns and verbs found within the reading material of the first through sixth grades to be tested.

There are six sections to the test: Picture Naming Nouns, Sentence Completion Naming, Description Naming, Picture Naming Verbs, and Picture Naming categories; the sixth section is a Comprehension Assessment with two levels of difficulty. The same five areas are assessed within this section, but the child is requested to select a picture from a choice of eight ("The cloth flowing down Superman's back is a red ____"), or, if he fails to supply the word by pointing to the correct picture in this sentence-completion example, he is requested to point to something specific ("Point to the cape"). Items tested in the Comprehension Assessment are only those that the child failed to supply correctly in the first five sections. The Comprehension Assessment is administered only to be sure that the words are in the child's vocabulary.

The test is designed for children 6–6 to 12–11 in first through sixth grades. Eighty items are included on a primary form (first and second grades) and 90 items on an intermediate form (third through sixth grades). Most of the items are common to the two forms but with different beginning and ending plates.

The primary score obtained is the number of correct one-word responses. The raw score (accuracy) is converted to a percentile rank and standard-score derivative for comparison by age and by grade. Speed is of secondary importance and is determined by the examiner's recording of the total time required to complete each section. Total time for the five sections is then judged as "fast" or "slow" as compared with the standardization sample, so the child's responses are listed as being in one of four categories: (1) fast-accurate, (2) slow-accurate (which was most representative of the normal population), (3) fast-inaccurate, or (4) slow-inaccurate.

The TWF is one of the new breed of tests that publish statistics on the mechanics and the rationale of how and why the test was assembled. Reliability is adequate, and validity is demonstrated primarily by construct and content descriptions. Construct validity, measured as the ability to retrieve words expected in the vocabulary of children in these age groupings, was demonstrated by agreement with clinicians who made judgments of word-finding problems in the children. Scores for the standardizing sample appropriately separated between normal-language children and those with word-finding problems according to clinical judgments of experienced speech-language pathologists.

As an indication of content validity, words were included on the final version of the TWF that were successfully supplied by at least 95 percent of the normative sample (95 percent of the first and second graders and 99 percent of the third through sixth graders comprehended 95 percent of the TWF items). In terms of accuracy, scores lower than one standard deviation below the mean for the standardizing population were considered suspect, making the adequacy cutoff at approximately the 16th percentile.

The standardization sample consisted of 1,200 children from 18 states, including approximately 100 boys and 100 girls at each of the six age (grade) groups with regional and ethnic balance representative of the 1980 U.S. population. The children were judged to be normal in language functioning and school performance with the exception of 40 children included as "linguistically handicapped" and representative of the population to be identified.

The test is intended for children with reading, language, fluency, and language/learning disorders. Although it has not been demonstrated that the test identifies children from each of these groups equally well, the test does appear to be effective at measuring a child's semantic skill and in identifying children with word-finding difficulties.

Test of Adolescent/Adult Word Finding

The *Test of Adolescent/Adult Word Finding* (German 1990) is an expansion of the TWF and is designed for middle school and secondary school students and beyond. There are norms for ages 12–0 to 19–11—grades 7 through 12. There are also norms for the 20–40, 40–60, and 60–80 age groups. Categories include the same five sections as in the elementary version—Picture Naming Nouns, Sentence Completion Naming, Description Naming, Picture Naming Verbs, and Naming Picture—and, as before, section 6—Comprehension Assessment—ensures that the words are in the subject's receptive vocabulary. There is also a "brief test" of approximately one-third of the items in each section designed for those who are expected to tire easily. Once again the concern is not size of vocabulary but speed and accuracy of word retrieval.

Vocabulary words were selected from a variety of children's dictionaries and "core" vocabulary lists from first through sixth grades. Raw scores are converted to standard scores, percentile ranks, and standard score SEMs for ages and for grades separately.

TESTS OF GRAMMAR

In the tripartite description of language, which we defined earlier, "grammar" consisted of morphology and syntax. For the tests discussed in this section, we use a rather broad definition of syntax.

Morphology

"Morphemes" were earlier defined as the smallest units with meaning. "Morphology" is, therefore, a study of the rules by which morphological units are applied to indicate the intended meaning function of words. Berko (1958) reasoned that if a child were asked, for example, to give the plural of chair or glass or cat, her correct response of adding a /z/ to chair, /Iz/ to glass, and /s/ to cat could have been because she had been taught those specific responses and may not indicate knowledge of rules to apply in the three instances. These would be examples of known elements in known circumstances. One alternative to this paradigm would be to place unknown items in known circumstances, which is what Berko did. (If we were to place unknown elements in unknown circumstances, the subject would not know what rules to apply, so little knowledge of a rule system would be gained.)

Berko constructed 27 brightly colored picture cards described by elliptical sentences. The sentences contained both real words and nonsense words. For example, the child is shown a picture of a birdlike creature and below it on the same page a picture of two of the creatures. The examiner says: "This is a picture of a wug (/w ʌ g/). Here is another one. Now there are two ____." The child is expected to say "/w ʌ gz/." On another plate, a man is pictured balancing a plate on his nose, and the examiner says: "Here is a man who knows how to rick (/rIk/). He is ricking. He did the same thing yesterday. What did he do yesterday? Yesterday he ____." The child's response should be that the man "/rIkt/."

Sentence-completion tasks, such as these, were generated to test the child's knowledge of plurals, singular and plural possessives, past tense, present progressive, comparative and superlative forms of adjectives (quirky, quirkier, and quirkiest for a dog with spots, more spots, and even more spots), and derived compounds (a wug-house as the name of a house where a wug lives).

Berko administered this test to a control group of 12 college graduates who were native speakers of English. The answers given by 100 percent of the adults were assumed to be the correct responses. In practical terms, that also means that only regular endings would be included on the morphology test.

The *Berko Test of Morphology* was published as the *Berry-Talbot Exploratory Test of Grammar* (1966). For the Berry-Talbot version, the pictures were redrawn, but no norms were published. The Berko percentages of correct responses may be viewed as an approximate order of difficulty among the morphological elements tested, at least for preschool and first-grade children, but they are not normative.

Validity. Validity for the Berko test paradigm appears to be questionable (or at least equivocal). Templin (1966) followed 435 children from preschool age through the second grade and charted the changes in their morphology scores and related the scores to articulation skill. Sylvester (1969) found significant differences in morphology test scores between good and poor articulation first-grade–age children, but these and other studies using samples of children with normal intelligence cannot apparently be generalized to retarded populations. Newfield and Shlanger (1968) investigated the Berko morphology test responses and a group of meaningful words paralleling Berko's nonsense words with a group of 30 educable mentally retarded children and with a group of 30 normal children. The normal children performed better on both tests of morphology than did the retarded children, and although the retarded children paralleled the normal children's performance in many respects, the retarded children showed a greater inability than the normal children in generalizing rules from familiar to unfamiliar words. Dever (1972) made a stronger statement. He tested the ability of the Berko test paradigm to predict errors made by retarded children while speaking. He found that although many children who scored 100 percent correct on the test also showed 100 percent correct usage in their speech, many other children scored 0 percent correct on the test and 100 percent correct in their speech.

The interpretation of these last two studies would suggest that we may not be able to use the Berko test results as a basis for what is to be taught in a language-intervention program. On the other hand, Ramer and Rees (1973) used a modification of some of the Berko items with African-American children and reported that the responses were an adequate representation of forms used in their dialect.

Northwestern Syntax Screening Test (NSST)

The *Northwestern Syntax Screening Test* was developed by Lee (1969, 1971) and was intended as a screening instrument only. It should not be considered a general language measurement, or even an "in-depth" evaluation of syntax. Therefore, it should be accompanied by other measures of language development. It was patterned after the Imitation-Comprehension-Production (ICP) paradigm used by Fraser, Bellugi, and Brown (1963), who reported an increasing degree of difficulty, in terms of reduced percentage of correct response, when the children were asked to repeat the stimulus sentence (imitation), identify a picture associated with the stimulus sentence (comprehension), or, having been given a choice of descriptions, produce the sentence (production) that best described the indicated picture.

The NSST contains both receptive and expressive portions with identical syntactic forms on the two parts of the test. The receptive portion contains 20 plates with four pictures per plate, two of which are to be identified on each page. The vocabulary items on each plate are controlled, with minimal distinctions to be made between pictures. For example, plate number one has four pictures with a cat and a chair, and the critical distinction is the preposition denoting the relationship of the two elements. (The cat is in front of, on, under, or behind the chair.) With the plate of four pictures before the child, two of the four pictures are described, but the specific pictures are not identified. For example, the examiner may say: "On one of these pictures, the cat is behind the chair, on another, the cat is under the chair. Show me '*The cat is behind the chair.*'" (Wait for a pointing response.) "Now show me '*The cat is under the chair.*'"

The range of syntactic structures tested includes prepositions; personal pronouns; singular and plural noun–verb agreement; present versus past tense; singular and plural possessive; present progressive versus future tense; *who, what, where* contrasts; *this* and *that* designators; active versus passive constructions; and subject + verb + indirect object + direct object (The mother shows the baby the kitty) versus subject + verb + direct object + indirect object (The mother shows the kitty to the baby). The clinician is cautioned not to emphasize the critical distinctions between stimulus items or to give exaggerated intonational patterns for questions. There are demonstration items included to help illustrate what is expected. The NSST is not intended as a measure of speed of comprehension nor as a test of memory, so Lee allows the examiner to repeat the sentence more than once if necessary.

The syntactic structures illustrated on the 20 pages are in an increasing order of difficulty, which means that if the child were to fail on the first 10 items, it would be logical to terminate the test. With scattered errors, however, it is probably safest to continue testing. The entire test is not expected to take more than 10 to 15 minutes to administer.

The expressive portion of the test contains the identical structures but with different pictures. There are two pictures on each of the 20 plates for the expressive portion. The two pictures are described, and the child is asked to listen carefully and then to copy the exact words of the examiner. For example, the first plate contains a picture of a baby who is asleep and a picture of a baby who is awake. The clinician would say: "The baby is sleeping. The baby is not sleeping. Now, what's this picture?" (Examiner points to one of the two pictures.) "Now, what's this one?" If the child were to say: "The baby is awake," she would be grammatically and syntactically correct, but her response would not reflect use of the negative. If this type of response were to occur on the first few plates, it might be wise to assume that the child had forgotten the rules of the game. Remind her again that she is to say "exactly what you say," and try the plate a second time. Responses that are different from your stimulus, even though they are grammatically correct, are to be considered errors for the purpose of testing these syntactic constructions.

Scoring.   There are 2 correct identifications on each of the 20 receptive-portion plates and 2 correct responses on each of the 20 expressive-portion plates. Each response is credited as correct or incorrect, which yields 40 possible points on each half of the test.

Norms are provided for five age-year levels: 3–0 to 3–11, 4–0 to 4–11, 5–0 to 5–11, 6–0 to 6–11, and 7–0 to 7–11. Tabled norms are expressed in terms of percentile scores (90th, 75th, 50th, 25th, and 10th percentile) and are based on a total of 344 children. Norms are for receptive and expressive scores separately to allow for the expected higher numerical performance on the receptive portion compared to the expressive portion of the test. The means and percentile rankings are also shown on a graph provided in the manual, which allows the clinician to find an interpolated point on the graph for evaluation of a child who is at either extreme of the age categories given. For example, if a child were 4–11 or 5–0, it would be more appropriate to compare his score to a point midway between the vertical lines indicating the four-year-old and the five-year-old groups. An additional line on this chart indicates a point two standard deviations below the mean, which would be equivalent to the 2nd or 3rd percentile for the age groups.

Validity. Ratusnick and Koenigsknecht (1975, p. 59) reported that the NSST "assessed consistently the syntax and morphology used by children with atypical language development." They used tests of internal consistency in evaluating the responses of 20 preschoolers with normal language development, 20 with severe expressive language impairments but normal intelligence, and 20 mentally retarded children. The normal and the language-delayed children did not significantly differ on the receptive portion of the test but did differ on the expressive portion. The retarded children differed from the normal intelligence groups on both expressive and receptive portions. Prutting, Gallagher, and Mulac (1975), using a normal intelligence, language-delayed sample of approximately the same age, determined that the expressive portion of the NSST did not present an accurate representation of the children's language performance. They indicated that 30 percent of those syntactic structures incorrectly produced on the NSST were correctly produced spontaneously in the language sample gathered for comparison.

Arndt (1977) criticized the NSST on the basis of what he termed "serious inadequacies" in its meeting of psychometric standards. Specifically, the complaints dealt with the small and socially restricted normative population sample, the inability of some items to consistently separate between adequate and inadequate language skill in children, and the relatively small difference in scores expected between ages (especially at the high end of the age range).

Ratusnik, Klee, and Ratusnik (1980) published a short form of the NSST. They reduced the length of the original test from 20 expressive and 20 receptive items to 11 items on each with 95 percent of the test score variance captured. In other words, they reduced the test length by 45 percent, reduced the time of administration by approximately half, yet lost relatively little of the test capability. Included in their population sample were 900 children from 3–0 to 7–11 years from Chicago, northern Indiana, and the Madison, Wisconsin, area, with an SES balance; sex balance; and urban, suburban, and rural representation. Although this was a more representative sample than the original completed by Lee, it was still regionally restricted.

Burns (1982) objected to the explanation of improved efficiency proposed by Ratusnik et al. He repeated many of Arndt's objections and declared that reducing the number of items should have increased the variability of the test scores. Burns questioned the validity of the NSST design in its long or short form. Klee and Ratusnik (1982), in a rebuttal to Burns, reported that 99 percent of the children identified on the long form were identified by the short form.

The reports that have been critical of the NSST have cited the incidence of false negative findings. That is, children may perform better in their conversational samples than on the NSST, or they have been identified as language deficient according to performance on the NSST but not by some other measure. No studies have been reported (Lee 1977) in which language-delayed children were falsely identified as normal on the NSST. In light of these critiques, it is probably appropriate to caution the clinician to use the NSST as a screening device, as it was intended, and not to assume that it is a diagnostic instrument. The format of pictures demonstrating context for the descriptions to be identified or elicited at least has an advantage over the noncontext sentence repetition of some other test protocols. The test appears to be more discriminating below the age of seven, and it is probably safe to assume a greater likelihood of a false positive finding (identified as needing therapy when the child does not need therapy) than there is of a false negative finding (identified as normal when the child has a language problem). Either way, the test is a screening measure and is not an adequate description of syntactic skills.

Carrow Elicited Language Inventory (CELI)

The Carrow Elicited Language Inventory (1974) is a sentence-repetition task (one phrase plus 51 sentences) with the stimuli ranging in length from 2 to 10 words. Carrow described it as a diagnostic test. It was designed to assess linguistic structures through repetition of sentences rather than eliciting spontaneous language samples from the child for clinician analysis.

Linguistic theories frequently assume that children's imitation of sentence structures is a fair representation of their linguistic skill. Children as young as two years (Brown and Fraser 1963; Slobin and Welsh 1973) and three years (Fraser, Bellugi, and Brown 1963) will frequently imitate nonsense words in a sentence they do not understand (but the words have been assigned a grammatical function by location in the utterance), providing the sequence is short enough. Young children will spontaneously utter sentences they cannot imitate (Slobin 1968) and will generally repeat sentences from their own production cues rather than from the adult model. Smith (1973) has reported that in repetition tasks with ungrammatical utterances, children frequently err by making the sentences grammatical when the grammatical forms are part of their repertoire. Slobin and Welsh (1973, p. 487) reported that "number of words, or number of morphemes is clearly not a relevant measure of how much of a sentence a child can imitate."

From these and other data, there is general agreement in the psycholinguistic literature that children understand utterances they cannot accurately repeat and that if a child can repeat an utterance it is probably safe to assume she has the linguistic structures in her repertoire. It is also true, empirically, that some children will repeat (to the limits of their retention span) utterances they do not understand. Frequently, these repetitions will be monotonic or mechanical sounding. In that sense, sentence-repetition tasks, such as the CELI, will be assumed to have some descriptive value concerning syntactic skill for most children. McDade, Simpson, and Lamb (1982) have suggested requiring a three-second time lapse between your model and the child's repetitions in these imitative tasks. Their data were gathered with one-second, three-second, and five-second pauses prior to the child's production, and the three-second–delay productions were most likely to include the forms and constructions the children used in their conversational speech. In other words, to guard against spurious results tainted by memory skill versus language skill, you more probably may depend on the validity of the results if you delay the child's response by three seconds. That sort of instruction is not included in the CELI, the NSST, or other sentence-imitation tasks, but the imitative-sentence–test format is not intended to be a memory task. The CELI provides norms for children 3–0 to 7–11 years.

Administration and Scoring.   None of the 52 stimuli are embedded or coordinated sentences. Of the 51 sentences, 47 are in the active voice, 4 are passive; 37 are affirmative, 14 are negative; 37 are declarative, 12 are interrogative, and 2 are imperative. The grammatical categories and features included in the test are articles, adjectives, nouns, noun plurals, pronouns, verbs, negatives, contractions, adverbs, prepositions, demonstratives, and conjunctions. The test is administered by the clinician reading the sentence and asking the child to repeat. Carrow suggested that a high-quality tape-recording be made of the child's responses for more accurate scoring. The clinician's task is to mark any errors in production on the score sheet. The average time for administration, transcription, and scoring is approximately 45 minutes. In addition to the total error score, subscores are obtained for each grammatical category and error type (substitution, omission, addition, transposition, or reversal). With few exceptions, only one error per word would be tallied.

Normative comparisons can be made with total error scores, grammatical category scores, and error types on percentile rankings according to age. Carrow attempted to fit the error scores to a year–month score, and those data are reported in an appendix to the manual. It is interesting to note that in the comparison of age-by-month with error scores, errors decrease to about age 6–7 years and then *increase* steadily to the 7–11 limit of the test. According to those data (1974, p. 31), expected number of errors at the 7–11 age are approximately equal to the number expected at 5–3. A curvilinear relationship between age and language score is not to be expected. The percentile rankings do not show these curvilinear relationships, possibly because they are plotted by whole-year divisions rather than by one-month divisions. The clinician should probably pay more attention to the grammatical category descriptions of the child's errors and relatively less attention to the "normative" comparisons, especially for children above the 6–6 year level.

Other Reliability and Validity Data.   Carrow reported that the test-retest reliability or stability of the CELI was high. In terms of validity, she assumed that a progression of scores with increasing age demonstrated the validity of the CELI. She also reported a statistically significant agreement between CELI error scores and clinician judgment and a high correlation between CELI error scores and the *Developmental Sentence Scoring* procedure. The reports (1974, p. 9) did not indicate the age or the number of comparison subjects. In summary, the CELI would at least appear to have good construct validity and may be a more valid measure of grammatical skill with younger (children 6–6 and younger) than with older children.

Assessment of Children's Language Comprehension (ACLC)

The *Assessment of Children's Language Comprehension* (Foster, Giddan, and Stark 1973) is a four-part receptive language test. The four parts include a short vocabulary section and three sections in which the vocabulary pieces are combined into two, three, and four critical-element statements. The vocabulary items (section A) are presented first. There are 10 plates with five pictures per plate in this section, for a total of 50 words. Thirty of the pictures identify common nouns; 10 are action verbs; 5 are adjectives; and 5 are prepositions. Sections B, C, and D of the test require two, three, and four critical-element identifications respectively. In a linguistic description, these elements would serve *functions* as agents, actions, objects, relations, and attributes. For example: The boy (agent) is sitting (action) on (relation) the big (attribute) chair (object). The purpose of the ACLC is to assess the child's core vocabulary and his comprehension of the elements in increasing element contexts. The ACLC is described by its authors as "diagnostic" in the sense that it should indicate to the clinician the level of difficulty at which performance breaks down. The authors also state that one consistent problem they have found with language-impaired children is poor auditory memory span (Foster and others 1973, p. 14), and the ACLC is heavily weighted to assess auditory memory span. Specifically, it is "designed for the purpose of identifying individual children who have difficulty processing auditory information" (1973, p. 31).

Administration and Scoring.   The ACLC takes approximately 10 minutes to administer. The vocabulary portion (Part A) is administered first, and all 50 items are to be identified as the examiner names them. There is not a specific cutoff for the test, but it would obviously be a futile effort to continue if the child missed a large proportion of the vocabulary items. Part B, two critical elements, has two-word combinations such as agent + action (a horse standing, from a choice of a swan flying, a swan standing, a horse standing, and a horse running); attribute + noun (dirty box); or noun + noun (chair and horn). Part C has three elements, for example, attribute + agent + action (happy lady sleeping) or agent + action + object (boy riding the horse). Part D has four critical elements that allow more complex combinations such as attribute + attribute + agent + action (happy little girl jumping) or agent + action + relation + object (monkey sitting on the fence). In all the pictured stimuli, the vocabulary is balanced. Each of the incorrect choices has only one element in error. For example, with the stimulus *monkey sitting on the fence*, the choices in order on the page have a monkey sitting on a chair, a monkey sitting in front of the fence, a monkey sitting on the fence, a monkey standing on the fence, and a boy sitting on the fence. The score sheet allows the examiner to mark if the first, second, third, or fourth element was in error.

Part A has 50 points possible, one for each of the 50 words; Parts B, C, and D have 10 points each, one correct answer for each of the 10 plates per part. Four scores are determined, one for each of the four parts. Part A score is expressed as a number correct; Parts B, C, and D, as the percent correct for comparison with the norms.

The normative data published with the 1973 (experimental) edition are mean scores only for boys and girls separately at six-month separations from 3–0 to 6–5. There are no percentile rankings or standard deviations provided. A minor revision from the 1972 manual changed some of the pictures that were found to be ineffective, and this actuation would be likely to have an effect on the mean scores expected. There are no reliability or validity data published with the 1973 edition, so at least for now, the mean scores provided should be treated as suggestive rather than as normative.

Another comparative example may be helpful here. Remember T. G., the little girl (chronological age 4–2) whose articulation test data were used in chapter 3? As part of her diagnostic testing, she was also tested in language skills. As reported earlier, she was so difficult to understand that an expressive-language sample was not analyzed. Language comprehension was tested, however. On the *Peabody Picture Vocabulary Test*, she scored beyond her age-level expectations. On the receptive portion of the *Northwestern Syntax Screening Test*, her score was approximately at the 50th percentile for children her age with 22 correct picture identifications of the 40 chances. Errors were in identification of *in–on* prepositions, singular–plural designations, inflected endings, *who–what* and *this–that* designators, present–past tense, and passive constructions. There was also some question of her identification of the correct concept but the wrong picture. For example, for the plural designation "The deer are running," she correctly pointed to the picture of the two deer; for the singular designation "The deer is running," she pointed to one of the two deer on the same picture. The same type of error occurred in her choices for "The boy sees the cats/the cat." Her understanding of the concept appeared to be correct, but her choice of pictures was incorrect. As would be expected, more errors occurred on the more complex linguistic structures. As discussed earlier in the section on the NSST, T. G.'s score may be a minimal estimate of her language skill, but there does not appear to be a problem.

As a further example, T. G. was also given the ACLC test. In this receptive measure, she correctly identified 45 of the 50 vocabulary pictures (Part A), erring on three of the five prepositions tested and two present progressive verb forms. It is always at least possible in a picture-identification test that the child's errors may be a function of the pictures rather than the concept purportedly represented, but the *in–on* error was in agreement with her NSST responses. In the two-, three-, and four-critical element sections (B, C, D), she correctly identified all the items tested, including those that she missed on the vocabulary section.

For the record, her hearing was normal according to pure-tone screening responses; oral-peripheral structure and function, pitch, voice quality, and fluency were also judged to be normal.

GENERAL TESTS OF LANGUAGE

Under the rubric of "general" tests are included a diverse selection of measures. They range from the *Test for Auditory Comprehension of Language*, which appears to define language primarily in terms of morphology and syntax, to tests such as the *Clinical Evaluation of Language Fundamentals*, which are still "language form" but are more concerned with the use or function of language. In other words, the test formats vary partly by their underlying theory—in some cases the underlying theory may be less well defined. The *Illinois Test of Psycholinguistic Abilities* is included because it is unique in the linguistic model after which it was patterned—and there is some concern about whether or not the model is appropriate. Also included are some examples that are more generally developmental rather than specific to language. To add further to the diversity, the *Basic Concept Inventory* is included as an example of a criterion-referenced test.

Test for Auditory Comprehension of Language—
Revised (TACL-R)

The *Test for Auditory Comprehension of Language–Revised* (Carrow-Woolfolk 1985) has gone through a number of printings and at least two major revisions since its first publication (1968). The 1985 edition is similar to the earlier (1973) version but has more balanced internal coverage, an ordered level of difficulty of items, and an expanded age range. The intent of the test is to assess auditory comprehension (interpreted as language performance) and to provide differential determination of problem areas.

Auditory comprehension is measured as a three-choice picture identification task for common nouns, verbs, adjectives, and adverbs (section 1), grammatical morphemes (section 2), and elaborated sentence structure (section 3). In the revised version, items are arranged by age groups as suggested starting points. The first four items correctly identified in an age group comprise the basal level; the ceiling is three errors in a row. The raw score is the number of correct responses, including those below the established basal.

Raw scores (numbers of correct picture identifications) for the three sections separately and for the summed total are converted to percentile ranks, age equivalent scores, and standard scores for ages 3–0 to 9–11 and grades from kindergarten to sixth. The normative population of 1,003 children included approximately 100 boys and 100 girls at each of the half-year age levels from three to six years and one-year levels from seven to ten years. The normative group was reported to be representative of the U.S. population in terms of parental occupation, geographic location, and ethnic background. Reliability and validity data were gathered from normal children and adults as well as from speech-language disordered children, hearing-impaired children, mentally retarded children, and seven adult asphasics. Results appear to be consistent with other tests representing similar constructs.

The validity judgment of the earlier version was reported on the basis of the test score separating normal from language-deficient children (Carrow 1973; Carrow and Lynch 1973; Weiner 1972) and normal from articulation-deficient children (Marquardt and Saxman 1972). A comparison of test items on the two versions of the test appears to show not only better balance between the areas tested but more items in face-validity agreement with the construct being tested.

Bankson Language Screening Test (BLST)

Another test with relatively broad coverage is the *Bankson Language Screening Test* (Bankson 1977). It was designed to be a broad-based screening device. Of the 153 items on the test, 38 have been designated for "quick screen" purposes. Five general areas are assessed within the Bankson test: semantic knowledge, morphological rules, syntactic rules, visual perception, and auditory perception. Part I, semantic knowledge, includes vocabulary-type items such as nouns, verbs, prepositions, quantitative opposites (e.g., big–small, easy–hard) and pictured objects to be identified by function. This part comprises nearly half of the entire battery. Part II, morphological rules, includes pronouns, verb tenses, plurals, and comparatives. Part III, syntactic rules, includes subject–verb agreements, sentence-repetition tasks, and the child's judgment as to whether sentences read by the examiner are syntactically correct. Part IV, visual perception, includes matching, discrimination, association, and sequencing tasks. Part V, auditory perception, includes short-term memory and discrimination tasks.

It is a test for expressive-language function in the sense that the child's task is to supply the word for the action or picture identified by the examiner or to complete an elliptical sentence begun by the examiner. Bankson also suggests, in the instructional manual, that seven of the eight semantic-knowledge tests can be tested receptively. If an item is erred expressively but the correct response is identified receptively, the item is still scored as an error for comparative purposes, but the examiner has some more information on which to plan a remedial program.

Comparisons for the child's test performance are available as means, standard deviations, and percentile rankings for the total raw score according to half-year age separations from 4–1 to 8–0 years. Validity is expressed in terms of correlations with the *Peabody Picture Vocabulary Test* (Dunn 1965), the *Test for Auditory Comprehension of Language* (Carrow 1973), and the *Boehm Test of Basic Concepts* (Boehm 1971). The correlations are moderate at best, ranging from 0.54 to 0.64.

Bankson's (1977) interpretation of the test results is that

> children who score at the 30th percentile and below need further language assessment. Those at the 15th percentile and below are those who are most certain to be enrolled for clinical language instruction, while those from the 16th through 30th percentile are those for whom a classroom enrichment approach, directed to specific linguistic weaknesses, may be appropriate. (p. 4)

Illinois Test of Psycholinguistic Abilities (ITPA)

The *Illinois Test of Psycholinguistic Abilities* was published as an experimental edition in 1961 (McCarthy and Kirk) and in a revised edition in 1968 (Kirk, McCarthy, and Kirk). The ITPA is based on the Osgood (1957) theoretical behavior model. The Osgood two-stage ($S-r_m-s_m-R$) model is similar to language models for aphasia, which utilize decoding, association, and encoding components. Aphasia tests such as the *Language Modalities Test of Aphasia* (Wepman and Jones 1961) would fit in this category. Aphasia tests will be discussed in chapter 10.

The ITPA was designed to be a diagnostic tool in the sense that it identifies areas of relative strength and weakness. Paraskevopoulos and Kirk (1969) described the ITPA as a "diagnostic psychoeducational test . . . that assesses specific abilities and achievements of a child in such a way that remediation of defects can logically follow" (p. 4). For this purpose, the ITPA subtests (see Figure 5–4) represent the following:

1. Four channels of communication
   a. auditory reception
   b. visual reception
   c. verbal expression
   d. manual (gestural) expression
2. Two levels (hierarchy) of organization
   a. representational
   b. automatic (called automatic-sequential in the 1961 edition)
3. Three psycholinguistic processes
   a. receptive processes
   b. organizing processes (formerly called association)
   c. expressive processes

Norms are provided for children 2 through 10 years of age, and the test takes approximately 30 to 45 minutes to administer. The titles are generally descriptive of the content of those subtests, but the degree to which they are actually separable functions is a theoretical question. Because this test is unique and model specific, a short description of the subtests will be given.

Test 1. *Auditory Reception.* This is a yes–no type test with simple, short questions. It is actually a controlled vocabulary test with questions such as "Do dogs eat?," "Do airplanes fly?," "Do sidewalks sprinkle?"

Test 2. *Visual Reception.* The child is first presented with a stimulus picture (for about 3 seconds) and is then asked to find a similar picture from a choice of four pictures. The correct choice is semantically similar but not physically identical. For example, a picture of a boy running is to be matched with a choice of four pictures of girls: one reading, one standing, one writing, and one running.

FIGURE 5–4   Three-dimensional clinical model of the *Illinois Test of Psycholinguistic Abilities* (ITPA) showing two input and two output channels, two levels, and three psycholinguistic processes. The numbers included with the subtest names indicate the order in which the subtests are administered.

(Adapted from S. A. Kirk, J. J. McCarthy, and W. D. Kirk, *Illinois Test of Psycholinguistic Abilities.* Urbana: University of Illinois Press, 1968. Used by permission.)

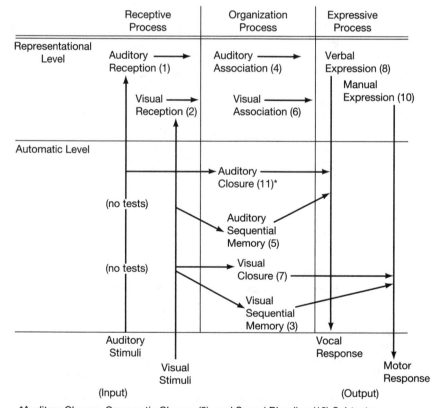

*Auditory Closure, Grammatic Closure (9), and Sound Blending (12) Subtests.

In other words, the child must identify the *meaning* of the picture, not just the object pictured.

Test 3. *Visual Sequential Memory.* A series of from 1 to 8 chips with geometric designs is illustrated in the test manual. A test pattern is shown to the child and then removed after about 5 seconds. The child is asked to reproduce the illustrated order of the chips from the available 17 chips.

Test 4. *Auditory Association.* This is an analogy-type test in which the child is asked to complete sequences such as "Daddy is big, baby is ____," "Smoke goes up, rain comes ____," and "A bee has a hive, a man has a ____."

Test 5. *Auditory Sequential Memory.* This is a digit-span test that differs from most other digit-span tests (such as in the Binet or Wechsler tests) in that the digits are presented at half-second intervals.

Test 6. *Visual Association.* In this test, the child is asked to associate one centrally located picture with one of four pictures located peripherally on the page. For example, a picture of a bone is to be matched with a choice of a pencil, a baby's rattle, a pipe, and a dog.

Test 7. *Visual Closure.* In this subtest, the child is shown picture strips with dogs, fish, bottles, and the like. He is first shown the sample picture of the object to be identified and is then asked to find as many of those as he can in the picture strip in 30 seconds.

Test 8. *Verbal Expression.* Five common objects are shown (separately) to the child: nail, ball, block, envelope, and button. His task is to describe the object as completely as he can. The response is credited with points for labels (it is a nail), for descriptions (the nail has a point), and for functions (carpenters use it).

Test 9. *Grammatic Closure.* What the ITPA categorizes as grammatic closure, we earlier discussed as a test of morphology. The difference is that the ITPA uses real words with responses that require past tense, plurality, possessive, comparative, and some derived adjective forms.

Test 10. *Manual Expression.* Pictured objects are shown to the child, and his task is to demonstrate the appropriate actions. For example, objects pictured include a hammer, a telephone, and a toothbrush.

Test 11. *Auditory Closure.* Words with sounds omitted are auditorily presented to the child, and his task is to supply the completed word. For example, a da—y is daddy, and bo—le is bottle.

Test 12. *Sound Blending.* This subtest is approximately the reverse process from what is tested in Auditory Closure. In one of the three sections, the child has a plate of pictures as a guide, and the examiner divides the words into two or three parts: d-og, f-oot. The second section divides words with two to seven sounds, which the child is to identify without picture cues. The third section divides nonsense words into three to six sounds for the child's identification.

The subtests all have standardized instructions and specific guidelines for probes to be used in eliciting responses. Some of the subtests have specific basal and ceiling levels depending on the age of the child and the accuracy of his performance.

Scoring the ITPA. Each of the 12 subtests will generate a raw score, and tables in the manual convert these scores to psycholinguistic-age scores and scaled scores for interpretation. For purposes of scoring, the Auditory Closure and the Sound Blending subtests are considered supplementary tests. A conversion chart is also included in the manual to convert the total raw score to a psycholinguistic-age score. A comparison of the child's psycholinguistic-age score (PLA) and his chronological age (CA) will yield a psycholinguistic quotient (PLQ) which the ITPA authors suggest (1968, p. 64) has close correspondence with overall intellectual level. The primary diagnostic purpose of the test, however, is accomplished by use of the scaled scores (SSs). These SSs are charted as a profile of abilities for the subtests, and from this profile should come the information as to whether or not the child has important discrepancies in her abilities. The point of reference for comparison is the mean scaled score (the sum of the basic scaled scores divided by 10). A median rather than a mean SS is used when profile discrepancies are all unidimensional, that is, when discrepancies are either all high or all low. Differences of ±6 SSs are considered within the average range of variability; ±7, ±8, ±9 are considered borderline discrepancies; and differences of ±10 are considered "substantial" discrepancies. In other words, these would indicate significant strengths or weaknesses in the child's psycholinguistic profile according to the ITPA. The suggested remediation procedure would be to utilize the areas of strength in an attempt to improve areas of weakness.

Reliability and Validity.   The ITPA was standardized on approximately 1,000 "average" children from 2 to 10 years of age. That is, the children were selected to be of average intellectual functioning, school achievement, personal-social adjustment, and sensory-motor integrity and were from predominantly English-speaking families (Paraskevopoulos and Kirk 1969). Because the test was designed for the primary purpose of identifying educational deficiencies, the choice of "average" children as a standardizing population seems highly logical. Weiner and Hoock (1973) have expressed some concern about the socioeconomic levels represented and the geographical location of the sample population. They have stated: "The published ITPA norms are most adequate for white children who live in small cities in the midwestern U.S." (p. 622). Paraskevopoulos and Kirk (1969) have recognized the geographical restriction and have called for the development of normative data for more diverse socioeconomic and geographical groups.

Reliability in terms of both internal consistency of test items and stability (test-retest) is relatively high for all subtests. "Statistical significance" and "psychological significance" are two different constructs, however. The validity of the ITPA would concern its psychological significance. Comparisons have been made primarily with intelligence test results. Data published by Paraskevopoulos and Kirk (1969, p. 162) revealed highly significant ($p = 0.01$) correlations between all 12 subtest scores and chronological age of the subjects in the standardization sample, but these data do not necessarily mean that the subtests or the complete ITPA profile measures language skill as it is usually defined in the clinic.

In a review of the ITPA, Carroll (1972) spoke to this point. He believed that the term "psycholinguistic abilities" was a misnomer and suggested instead "[it] might less misleadingly have been named something like the 'Illinois Diagnostic Test of Cognitive Functioning'" (p. 819). Later in the same review, he summarized his *cognitive* rather than *linguistic* complaint in these words:

> To a degree then, the ITPA may be regarded as just another test of a limited number of intellectual abilities—verbal comprehension and general information, immediate

memory span, and perhaps special capacities in the visual and auditory perceptual domains, as well as a special kind of expressive verbal fluency. (p. 821)

In reply to a number of similar reactions, Kirk and Kirk (1978) have responded that the major dissatisfactions expressed have been the result of the misuse of the ITPA rather than uses intended for the test. For example, they stress that the major intent of the instrument was to determine differential abilities and disabilities (intraindividual differences) rather than an overall level of functioning:

> Using the overall score to evaluate a child to compare him with other children rather than to compare his own subtest scores with each other are common misconceptions of the use of the test. (p. 61)

and further:

> . . . its main function is to help assess discrepancies in cognitive and perceptual functioning, and in some aspects of language and memory performance. (p. 70)

We have paid considerable attention to the ITPA in terms of detailed description. It has been a frequently used—and frequently abused and misused—instrument in the evaluation of language-remediation programs. Therefore, it seems appropriate to repeat that the ITPA was designed primarily as an educational psychometric tool for assessment of intraindividual variations. The ITPA score does maintain a high correlation with intelligence test results, but language skills, at least in the normal range of intelligence, are not usually in high agreement with intelligence.

Sequenced Inventory of Communication Development (SICD)

The SICD (Hedrick, Prather, and Tobin 1975) is a revision of the *Sequenced Inventory of Language Development* (Hedrick and Prather 1970). It was designed to assess children's growth in communication skills from 4 to 48 months of age. Items for the SICD were adapted from the *REP Scale* (D'asaro and John 1961), the *Denver Development Scale* (Frankenberg and Dodds 1967), the ITPA (Kirk, McCarthy, and Kirk 1968), plus some additional items and procedures generated by the authors. It is a receptive and an expressive instrument and contains subtest areas not frequently included in language tests. Figure 5–5 illustrates the test model.

The receptive scale subtests include awareness, discrimination, and understanding. Levels within these subtests are concerned with both sounds (localization) and words (discrimination and understanding). Some items are scored by a behavioral response; others are scored from parental report. The test items are sequenced according to the chronological age at which 75 percent of the standardization sample exhibited these behaviors.

Expressive-scale subtests include both expressive behaviors and expressive measurements. Expressive behaviors are categorized as imitating, initiating, and responding. These three are further subdivided as motor response, vocal response, and verbal response. "Motor" in this sense refers to pointing, gesturing, or manipulating responses; "vocal" indicates a sound not classifiable linguistically; and "verbal" refers to words or linguistically classifiable sounds. Initiating behaviors are scored primarily from parental report, since test situations usually generate responding behaviors. The expressive measurements included are verbal output and articulation. The quantitative portion of verbal output is obtained from MLR and SCS scores for 50 responses; the descriptive portion includes information on emergence of parts of speech, such as prepositional phrases, adverbs, third-person pronouns, and so on and is also obtained from the MLR protocol. Articulation is assessed for children two years and older with items selected from the *Photo Articulation Test* (Pendergast and others 1969). Fifty consonant productions in initial and final word positions and 18 vowels are included.

The standardization test sample included 252 children, 21 at each of 12 discrete age levels at four-month intervals from 4 to 48 months. All children were from the greater Seattle, Washington, area; white; equally divided at each age level into high, middle, and low socioeconomic groups; approximately equally divided between boys and girls; and judged to be normally developing. Testing time was reported to be from 30 minutes for infants to 75 minutes for children 24 months and older.

FIGURE 5–4   Test model of the *Sequenced Inventory of Communication Development.*
(Adapted from Hedrick, Prather, and Tobin [1975].)

Receptive Scale						
Awareness		Discrimination		Understanding		
Sound	Speech	Sound	Speech	Words+	Words	4 months Age levels 48 months

Expressive Scale										
Expressive Behaviors									Expressive Measurements	
Imitating			Initiating			Responding			Verbal Output	Articulation
Motor	Vocal	Verbal	Motor	Vocal	Verbal	Motor	Vocal	Verbal	Quant.	Descrip.

Scoring of SICD. Two primary age scores are computed: receptive communication age (RCA) and expressive communication age (ECA). Item numbers are listed in chronological order on the score sheet under the appropriate areas. The examiner circles the item numbers crediting receptive and expressive behaviors to a child and computes the percentages of items credited at each age level. Generally, the child is assigned an RCA or an ECA at the older of two consecutive levels on which he has successfully completed more than 75 percent of the items. More detailed descriptions for scoring and interpretation can be found in the manual (1975).

Reliability and Validity. Reliability was reported primarily in terms of stability (test-retest) and is appropriately high. Validity, or the degree to which a test actually samples behaviors it purports to measure, is always a function of the comparator instrument or judgments. The verbal output portion of the SICD was compared with MLR and SCS data. None of these measures purports to test exactly the same attributes, but the correlation ranged from 0.75 to 0.80. The highest correlation was between RCA and ECA ($r = 0.95$), which would indicate an overall consistency of the tests. A possibly more important supporting estimate of validity was high agreement among RCA, ECA, and chronological age in the test subjects. We have already discussed the difficulty in interpreting MLR and SCS data, but those measures would appear to be more corroborative than essential to the SICD profile.

Preschool Language Scale–3

The *Preschool Language Scale–3* (Zimmerman, Steiner, and Pond 1992) is, as noted, the third version of the PLS originally published in 1969. (Zimmerman, Steiner, and Evatt 1979). The authors reported that the need for modification from earlier versions was partly because of greater family involvement in both the description of problems and their remediation.

The PLS–3 has four receptive and four expressive language tasks for each six-month interval from birth to 4–11 and four receptive and four expressive tasks for each 12-month interval for five and six years. Administration time is 15 to 30 minutes depending on the child's age. Raw scores convert to standard scores and percentile ranks. Normative data were derived from a relatively small national sample (451 children—37 at each age level, none of whom were identified as needing language remediation, and described as approximately representative of sex and race/ethnicity according to the 1980 U.S. census).

What the earlier tests termed "Verbal Ability" was changed in the PLS–3 to "Expressive Communication" to include some prelinguistic and nonverbal communication skills. For example, some early comprehension items may be termed attentional behaviors. There was some modification and replacement of items to better reflect developmental progression. Memory tasks were revised to replace digit span with sentence repetition—which would more specifically be language behavior.

Standard scores are age based. Basal levels (three consecutive tasks credited, suggested beginning one year below CA) and ceiling levels (five consecutive no credit items) are specified. Raw scores for Expressive Communication and Auditory Comprehension can be converted to standard scores, confidence bands (SEM), percentile ranks, and confidence bands for ages. "Normal" range is defined as one standard deviation. Age-equivalent scores can also be derived from subscale raw scores. The sum of Expressive and Comprehension raw scores also can be used to derive a standard score and percentile rank.

Reliability (test-retest and interrater) ranged from 0.89 to 0.94. Validity statements were defined as the number of children identified by the PLS–3 as compared to the states' (schools') identification of the same children. Three-year-olds were correctly identified, according to criteria for their state, 66 percent of the time, four-year-olds 80 percent of the time, and five-year-olds 70 percent of the time. Most of the incorrect identifications (misses) were in failing to identify as language delayed (according to PLS–3) a child who had previously been identified as such.

From the data displayed in the examiners' manual, there was much less likelihood of classification by the PLS–3 of a language disorder when outside criteria— whatever they were—said that the child was normal than when the child had been identified as delayed or deviant. An obvious variable in this statistic is the test protocol used by the various states/schools to decide that the child is language delayed.

McCarthy Scales of Children's Abilities (MSCA)

The *McCarthy Scales of Children's Abilities* (McCarthy 1972) is also more generally developmental than specific to language in children. It is included here, in spite of some redundancy with tests already discussed, and in spite of its relative age, because it has some uniqueness and precision in description. The MSCA contains six scales: Verbal, Perceptual-Performance, Quantitative, General Cognitive, Memory, and Motor. The tests involve language, numerical concepts, motor coordination, and other skills to reflect cognitive and motor ability. The six scales are composed of 18 separate tests but with considerable overlap on some subtests for the areas to which they contribute. The five verbal tests, seven perceptual-performance tests, and three quantitative scales do not overlap in abilities tested, and these three areas make up the General Cognitive Tests. Memory (four tests) and motor (five tests) are overlapping with other scales. All of the memory tests are included on the General Cognitive scale. Three of the five motor tests are independent of General Cognitive (do not overlap with other tests), and two overlap with perceptual-performance items.

Test scores are assigned weighed values. Weighted raw scores are derived by multiplying the child's raw score by the test's assigned weight. A composite raw score for a scale equals the sum of the child's weighted raw scores on all of the tests comprising that scale. Scaled scores are provided according to chronological age of the child tested, as well as percentile ranking for General Cognitive Index and the MSCA indices. These scaled scores, therefore, provide a profile of the child's abilities on the six scales included. Comparisons would then be possible with other children of the same age, as well as within the child for relative ability within the areas tested.

The test was designed for children ranging from 2½ to 8½ years of age. There are standardized instructions for administering the scale, and test-retest reliability data reported are high. Validity was not reported in the manual. In terms of comparison with other general developmental scales, the MSCA would at least appear to have high face validity.

COGNITIVE/SEMANTIC OR CONCEPT TESTS

Language Assessment Tasks (LAT)

Earlier in this chapter, we commented that there were no available standard measures of semantics. To the degree that semantics is represented by language-function and language-content judgments, the *Language Assessment Tasks* (Kellman, Flood, and Yoder 1977) are an exception to that statement, although the LAT is not standardized. The LAT is unique in one other respect—it was designed primarily to provide a description of language function for the child from 9 to 14 years of age. The bulk of the language descriptions available are for younger children. We know of no other measure that provides a similar breadth of language description for this age range.

The LAT is divided into sections to provide measures of comprehension, production, language content, and a judgment of communicative function. Subtest results are plotted as a function of age scores to develop a profile of abilities for comparison with Piaget's cognitive levels.[2] According to Kellman, Flood, and Yoder (1977):

> If the level of language development is approximately equal to the cognitive level, it suggests that there is not a language delay, even though the language development level may be below chronological age. If the language development level is below the cognitive level, it suggests there is a delay in language development. The degree of language delay is determined by the gap between the cognitive level and the language development level. (p. xi)

Subtests include functional tests of syntax and semantics for both comprehension and production areas. For example, in the comprehension-of-syntax section, the child is asked to demonstrate, by her actions, an understanding of *before* and *after* ("Clap your hands after you sit down"). Comprehension of semantics includes the child's expressed understanding of the meaning of idioms ("What does 'feeling blue' mean?") and her explanation of riddles. Also included in the comprehension section is a subtest entitled "Paralinguistics" (identified as intonation, stress, and junction) in which, for example, the child must distinguish between *green house* and *greenhouse*.

In the production section, syntax judgments are made from elicited oral (and written) language samples. Semantics includes vocabulary, word definitions, and the use of *wh*-questions in eliciting information. Language-content items incorporate both labels and concepts expressed in subtest areas identified as temporal (e.g., order and duration), spatial (e.g., right-left), classification (e.g., "A radish, lemon, beets, carrots. Which one doesn't belong? Why?" and "What do they have in common?"), and causality ("What causes day and night?"). The communicative function area is a judgment of how well the child uses language to gain or give information, to express beliefs or feelings, to entertain, to interact—in short, how well can she use language to solve problems?

---

[2]The Piaget divisions or stages of cognitive development used by the LAT include Sensorimotor period, birth to 2 yrs.; Preoperational period, 2–7 yrs.; Early Preoperational period, 2–4 yrs.; Late Preoperational period, 4–7 yrs.; Concrete Operations period, 7–11 or 12 yrs.; Formal Operations, 12 yrs.–adulthood.

Year and month norms are provided for some of the subtest areas; other sub-test results are interpreted by the Piaget cognitive divisions with an age spread of two to three years. In the LAT authors' introductory statement, they agree that "the LAT is not a polished tool. It is still rough, and may continue to be so for a long time." They have, however, collected a number of language tasks from available literature and have created a few more for the purpose of the test profile; some of these have been normed, and some have not. The validity of the composite has not been determined, but there does appear to be considerable language-function description available from this protocol for the age range at which it is directed, and we know of no other test like it.

Basic Language Concepts Test (BLCT)

The *Basic Language Concepts Test* (Engelmann, Ross, and Bingham 1982) is a revision of the 1966 *Basic Concept Inventory* authored by Engelmann. The 1966 version was a criterion-referenced test for kindergarten and first-grade children designed to test skills that children would need to be successful in second grade. The revised test is broader in age range, maintains the same type of coverage, and is shorter in time of administration (nondiscriminatory items were removed), but essentially the same concept underlies both versions. What is being tested are basic language concepts considered necessary for initial school learning. The BLCT is designed for children from four to six-and-one-half years; norms are expressed as mean number of errors for ages (six-month divisions) by test sections. A total error score of 30 is considered inadequate language concept for a kindergarten-aged child. That is, 30 or more errors indicates that the child has "few of the skills neces-sary for basic academic instruction" (p. 4).

For normative comparisons across all age ranges, selected percentile ranks are shown for number of correct responses (by age) for sections of the test. The more important numbers for clinical or academic decisions would be the particular items erred as marked on a "circle chart" of the test results where item numbers are grouped to indicate errors in plurality, verb tense, negation, and so on.

The test was designed to identify specific types of problems with language. The first section has a set of picture stimuli, but the child's task is not merely to point to the picture named but to identify concepts such as plurality, negation, and size. For example, a picture of a table, a boy, a man, and a dog is presented. The instructions are to "find the ones that are not a dog," "find the ones that talk," "find the ones that are not the biggest." The second section has a set of sentences to be repeated and questions to be answered. For example, "A boy is not walking when he is running" (to be repeated) and then "When is a boy not walking?" The third part is a set of pattern-recognition tasks. For example, the examiner slaps the table and claps her hands three times in the same sequence. Then, after the fourth time, the child is to judge whether that fourth production was the "right" way or the "wrong" way. Or, the examiner says the numbers 7-7-7 and 4-4-4 and asks the child to repeat them. This item would not be a test of digit-span short-term memory but a test of pattern recognition. Those examples seem more appropriate to a pat-tern-recognition task than this next example of what is also termed pattern recogni-tion in the BLCT. In this next example, the child is asked to listen to the examiner say broken words such as m—ilk and ta—ble, and the child is asked to tell the intended word. The ITPA, discussed earlier, termed that task as "sound blending," and some other tests on the market have called it "auditory closure." It is not a pattern-recognition task per se but requires a knowledge of the *words* of the language rather than recognition of pattern.

Glaser (1963) defines a criterion-referenced measure as one that indicates *why* a child failed a particular task that is expected of him and that is required in order to move to the next academic level. In that sense, validity of the test seems adequately demonstrated with a reported 86 percent agreement between BLCT scores and teacher judgments on a sample of approximately 200 children.

Test of Language Development—Primary (TOLD–P)
Test of Language Development—Intermediate
(TOLD–I)

The *Test of Language Development–Primary* (Newcomer and Hammill 1982) was designed to test children from four to nine years of age. Similar in content to many other tests for this age range, it includes receptive and expressive tasks (termed listening and speaking systems) that are used to assess vocabulary (semantics), syntax, and phonology. Receptive-syntactic abilities (grammatic understanding) are tested by picture identification; expressive syntax is assessed by sentence imitation and a "grammatic completion" subtest that calls for the child to supply morphological endings relative to verb tenses, plurals, possessives, and so forth. Phonology is tested by same-different word–discrimination judgments for the receptive part and by means of a work-articulation test for the expressive portion.

The test makers state that the abilities tested are assumed to be cognitively influenced. They make a stronger case for that argument in the intermediate than in the primary version.

The *Test of Language Development–Intermediate* (Hammill and Newcomer 1982) is designed for older children (8–6 to 12–11) and by content appears more likely to test cognitive or language-usage abilities. There are five subtests of the TOLD–I. On the first subtest, the child is asked to form a compound or complex sentence from two or more simple sentences that are provided. Judgments of truth or falsity (e.g., "all trees are oaks," "all oaks are trees") based on general knowledge of relationships and categories are included on the second subtest. On the third subtest, the child is asked to rearrange four to seven words to make a sentence; and on the fourth subtest, the child is asked to state how three items (igloo, tepee, and palace) are alike. The fifth subtest of the TOLD–I is termed a test of grammatic comprehension, but "grammar" in this case is a judgment of prescriptive grammar ("Is this sentence correct?: 'Them girls stole the cake.'") rather than of generative grammar. A generative grammar is the relationship of sound to meaning. Prescriptive grammar is the "correct" way—what your fifth-grade English teacher tried to teach you. We may assume the clinician is also interested in "grammatically correct" utterances—but you may question whether this sort of item indicates an inappropriate sound-to-meaning relationship.

Test scores are converted to standard scores and percentile ranks for subtest areas and for combinations of areas for both the TOLD–P and the TOLD–I. The purpose of the standard scores and the percentile ranks for the subtests is to determine a profile of strength and weakness areas within the child's overall performance. How well these subtest areas, or the total score, represent diagnostic proficiencies or deficiencies for the planning of a language-intervention program is not addressed.

Clinical Evaluation of Language Fundamentals–Revised

Clinical Evaluation of Language Fundamentals–Revised (Semel, Wiig, and Secord 1987) is a revision and modification of the earlier *Clinical Evaluation of Language Functions* (Semel and Wiig 1980) partly, according to the authors, as a recognition that the 1980 version tested more of language form than of language use (function). Standard score comparisons, standard error ranges, and confidence levels are available by year separations from 5–0 to 16–11 years.

There are some minor revisions, for example, changes in subtest titles without an important change in content, what the authors term as major revisions with change in content of subtests, plus some deletions and additions to content. One of the more important differences is that the standard score comparisons are now age-referenced rather than grade- and age-referenced, which removes some confusion as to how to treat the results of a child who may not be at the expected grade for his age. The CELF–R dropped the screening version (receptive only) used earlier. The previous age separation included kindergarten through fifth grade as an "elementary group," but the CELF–R has one set of subtests for five- to seven-year-old children and a slightly different set of subtests for eight- through sixteen-year-old children.

The CELF-R has eleven subtests: three receptive and three expressive plus five supplementary subtests. In general, the tests are designed to measure memory, morphology, syntax, and semantics. Standard score comparisons may be made for each of the subtests separately, and for the sums of the three receptive and three expressive scores. What may be more descriptive for intervention planning is an item analysis summary included with each of the subtests. For example, in the Linguistic Concepts subtest for five- to seven-year-olds, the child is asked to demonstrate an understanding of concepts such as inclusion/exclusion ("Point to all of the the red lines and all but one of the yellow lines") and of condition ("Point to a blue line if you see a red line"). Item numbers representing the tested concepts are included for your summary analyses.

Reliability, internal consistency, and standardization sample appear to be adequately established. The CELF–R Technical Manual reports that approximately 90 percent of the children classified by the school system as language-learning delayed (LLD) were similarly classified by the CELF–R when using only the Receptive and Expressive Language subtest standard scores. When using the total language scores, approximately 85 percent were classified in common. We do not, however, know what specific criteria were used to select or identify the children who were identified by the school systems as LLD.

One other comparison study the CELF–R authors used to establish validity was a comparison between scores for the CELF–R and the *Peabody Picture Vocabulary Test–Revised*, which we discussed earlier. The moderate correlations obtained ($rs = 0.44$ with receptive scores, 0.46 for expressive scores and 0.52 for total scores) suggest a relatively low loading of the CELF–R on vocabulary. Comparisons of CELF–R and the *Wechsler Intelligence Scale for Children–Revised*

(WISC-R) show correlations generally in the 20s to low 40s. Both of these comparisons are included here to reiterate that language form and function, vocabulary recognition, and intelligence are different constructs. One does not well predict the other. Correlations between the CELF–R and the *Test of Language Development–Intermediate* (TOLD-I) were somewhat higher ($r = 0.49$ for receptive, 0.73 for expressive, and 0.68 for total language) but still indicate more difference than commonality in content.

Language Form Versus Language Function

What is important about tests such as the TOLD and the CELF–R is the attempt to determine language function rather than just mastery of the forms of language. As we just discussed, the CELF was modified, according to its authors, to reflect the testing of form rather than function. However, the essence of many of the original items was maintained.

Spekman and Roth (1984) and Muma (1984) criticized the earlier CELF in relation to construct validity and size and definition of normative sample. Much of this criticism appears to be answered in the CELF–R. One other example of test format for older children (beyond language form) and especially those subtest items that attempt to assess reasoning with language, is the *Screening Test of Adolescent Language* (STAL) (Prather, Breecher, Stafford, and Wallace 1980).

The *Screening Test of Adolescent Language* is a brief, simple screening test with much less detail, and it is less well standardized than the other tests. It includes a vocabulary section in which the child must provide a word synonymous with a word supplied by the examiner, a sentence-imitation task (the CELF–R has similar subtests), and a less usual section—a language-processing task in which the child is to indicate what is wrong with a sentence and why ("I went with my sister to the shoe store to buy a pair of combat boots to wear to the junior prom"), and an explanation of three common proverbs.

This test has no norms, but some criterion levels for grades 6 through 12 are provided. No rationale is given for why these particular elements are included as screening elements. However, the type of vocabulary items, the exercise in logic—reasoning with language, and the translation of proverbs are appropriate examples of language use (pragmatics).

The *Test of Problem Solving* (TOPS) (Zachman, Jorgensen, Huisingh, and Barrett 1984) is another example of an attempt to measure reasoning with language. It is a norm-referenced test for 6- to 12-year-old children. The child is shown a picture indicating a problem (e.g., a bicycle with a flat tire) and asked how that may have happened and then why that is a problem ("Why shouldn't he ride his bike with a flat tire?"). Answers are scored as "2," "1," or "0" depending on appropriateness, completeness, and grammatical correctness. Examples are given as guidelines for each of these three, but therein lies a problem.

Bernhardt (1990) selected a group of clinicians experienced in speech-language testing but unfamiliar with the TOPS to test the validity of the protocol. Each of her judges was provided with protocol responses from the test and asked to assign 0, 1, or 2 values according to the test instructions. Bernhardt's concern was the validity of the ratings (not whether the judges could be trained to make ratings similar to the test authors). Her results showed less than 50 percent agreement between these judges' values and the intended TOPS values, which challenges the content validity of the TOPS.

Skarakis-Doyle and Mallet (1991) reported an investigation of the test-retest reliability of the TOPS and also found it to be inadequate. They reported testing and retesting eight weeks later a group of children from 6–2 to 11–8 years. In addition, 20 percent of the tape-recorded answers were scored by a second examiner. The intrajudge reliability on an item-by-item comparison indicated a reliability score of 82 percent. A comparison of total test scores for the two administrations of the test yielded a correlation of $r = 0.28$, which is to say that test-retest reliability falls short of the 0.90 reliability coefficient recommended as the minimum standard for a diagnostic test (Salvia and Ysseldyke 1988), especially for the between-examiner (interjudge) reliability.

No single test is expected to provide all of the definition that we would like as diagnosticians. Test formats have been constructed to represent the test authors' different purposes and different constructs. Just as you would be more concerned with descriptions of test performance than with test scores in planning your remediation, you would be advised to use a variety of formats and contents for your description of what needs remediation. Earlier we discussed structured and nonstructured observations. You would probably want to use both. One style is more likely to demonstrate what the child can do and the other is more likely to give you a version of what the child does do.

Lahey (1990), in a paper concerned with "who should be called language disordered," discusses such caveats as "the goal of identification must be clearly distinguished from other goals of assessment" and "language performance must be sampled in more than one context, including, for purposes of identification, contexts that stress the language system."

REVIEW AND OVERVIEW

In earlier chapters we discussed tests of social and general development as part of our diagnostic concern. Articulation and speech perception also have been covered. This chapter concerned itself with children's language. Motor development, motor proficiency, and structural disorders (physical restrictions) will be discussed later as will be aphasia, closed head injuries, and other primarily adult communication problems. This "sectioned-for-convenience" coverage requires an occasional reminder that our primary concern is not with speech and language per se, but with communication.

Language is a symbol system. Units of speech are signs—as signs acquire meaning they become symbols. The stop sign at the corner is only a sign. When that distinctive octogonally shaped sign is interpreted to mean "stop," then it has become a symbol and has communicative value. "Language is a symbol system children use to represent their learning about people, objects, events, and relationships in their world" (van Kleeck and Richardson 1990). Our concern with speech and language skill concerns social, educational, and economic functioning. As a 1993 *Asha* publication describes the clinical indications for spoken language assessment, "individuals of all ages are assessed as needed, requested, or mandated, or when they have communication, educational, vocational, social, and health needs due to their language."

We are concerned with language use as an index of cognitive function and cognitive function as a base for language. We are concerned with speech and language as related to social and family interaction. These interactions may be part of the problem as well as a large part of the remediation. In that 1990 chapter on speech and language assessment, van Kleeck and Richardson discuss a variety of parameters to be assessed and spend considerable time discussing the assessment of the "cognitive domain" for a number of reasons and from a number of theoretical viewpoints. Their point also is that our primary concern is not for language per se, but the use of language in family, social, educational, and vocational actions and interactions. Our diagnostic description is for guidance in the direction of intervention. Our intervention concern is for the most efficient function of the individual in her family, society, and world.

When Sir Henry Head published his text on *Aphasia and Kindred Disorders of Speech* (1926), he entitled the chapter on aphasia language testing "Chaos." The same could be said for testing the various aspects of language development almost three-quarters of a century later. The chaos that Head referred to, and the chaos in language testing, is apparent from the parade of language scales we have discussed (see Table 5–3), is due to an awkward blending of divergent theories and empirical biases. Some of the tests reviewed have been based on specific theoretical viewpoints and some on what their authors believed was helpful information for planning an intervention program. For some, it is difficult to discern what the theoretical base was, and for others, there is disagreement on whether the test is an adequate reflection of the theory proposed as the base. Finally, examples are included for which both base models and theories and lack of models and theories have been criticized.

Language-delayed children are an extremely heterogeneous group. There may or may not be a difference between children categorized as language delayed and language disordered, or even language-learning disordered, which may also depend on your theoretical or philosophical biases. No one test, or group of tests, is most appropriate for a population with a diversity of etiologies and linguistic behaviors. There is some hint of a Chinese menu in this listing. You are invited to choose one from column A, two from column B, and so forth until you have (temporarily, at least) satiated your epistemological appetite. To recall a comment made in Chapter 1, you must still know what information you are seeking and what descriptions will be most adequate to your purposes before you can choose from among the available test styles, formats, and contents.

It is appropriate to reiterate that these are primarily tests of performance in controlled-circumstance situations. They may more fully indicate what a child can do rather than what a child does do. In other words, you may need to expand your diagnostic endeavors beyond these example formats to get a more complete description of the child's behavior.

In the listings in Table 5–3, the first assessment procedures may be categorized as quantitative measures of the child's conversation (usually from a child–adult "interview"). The next set focuses on vocabulary and on language form, including single words, word combinations, and sentences. These include both

TABLE 5–3   Summary of language tests

Name	Ages	Type of Norms	Skills Tested (Scoring)
Mean Length of Response (MLR)	1½–4½ yrs. (McCarthy) 3–8 yrs. (Templin)	Means and standard deviations	Expression—words per response
Mean Length of Utterance	—	—	Expression—morphemes per response
Structural Complexity Score (SCS)	3–8 yrs.	Means and standard deviations	Expression—weighted score for complexity of utterance in simple to compound, etc., terms
Developmental Sentence Scoring (DSS)	2–7 yrs.	Percentile rankings	Expression—values for words and types of words
Developmental Sentence Types (DST)	—	—	Expression—relative description but no scores
Length-Complexity Index (LCI)	—	—	Expression—values for linguistic complexity of phrases
Peabody Picture Vocabulary Test–Revised (PPVT-R)	2–40 yrs.	Standard scores, percentile ranks	Receptive vocabulary
Vocabulary Comprehension Scale (VCS)	2–6 yrs.	Mean ages for individual words sampled	Vocabulary comprehension—receptive
Test of Word finding (TWF)	6½–13 yrs.	Standard scores, percentile ranks, ages, and grades	Word retrieval, speed, and accuracy
Morphology (Berko or Berry-Talbot)	—	—	Expressive—regular morphologic past tense, plural, possessive, progressive, and comparative endings
Northwestern Syntax Screening Test (NSST)	3–8 yrs.	Percentile rankings	Expressive and Receptive
Carrow Elicited Language Inventory (CELI)	3–8 yrs.	Means, percentile ranks, standard scores for total and subgroup scores	Expressive
Assessment of Children's Language Comprehension (ACLC)	3–6½ yrs.	Mean percentage for subparts of test	Receptive (vocabulary only for items used in other three sections)

(continued)

TABLE 5–3 Summary of language tests (continued)

Name	Ages	Type of Norms	Skills Tested (Scoring)
Test for Auditory Comprehension of Language–Revised (TACL–R)	3–10 yrs.	Percentile ranks, age-equivalent, standard scores for age and grade	Receptive—total and subtests
Bankson Language Screening Test (BLST)	4–8 yrs.	Means and standard deviations plus percentile ranks	Expressive
Illinois Test of Psycholinguistic Abilities (ITPA)	2–10 yrs.	Language age by category subtest and total	Receptive and expressive
Sequenced Inventory of Communication Development (SICD)	4–48 mos.	Age scores	Receptive and expressive
Preschool Language Scale–3 (PLS–3)	0–6 yrs.	Age score—standard score	Receptive and expressive
McCarthy Scale of Children's Abilities (MSCA)	2½–8½ yrs.	Standard score, weighted scaled	General development with subtest profile
Language Assessment Tasks (LAT)	9–12 yrs. (gr 4–8)	Age scores	Profile of receptive and expressive communicative function
Basic Language Concepts Test (BLCT)	1st grade	Criterion referenced	General development school prediction
Test of Language Development–Primary (TOLD–P)	4–9 yrs.	Standard scores, percentile ranks	Receptive and expressive
Test of Language Development–Intermediate (TOLD–I)	8–13 yrs.	Standard scores, percentile ranks	Receptive and expressive
Clinical Evaluation of Language Fundamentals–Revised (CELF–R)	6–12 yrs.	Standard scores, percentile ranks	Receptive and expressive
Screening Test of Adolescent Language (STAL)	Grades 6–12	No norms—passing criteria	Expressive (language reasoning)
Test of Problem Solving (TOPS)	6–12 yrs.	Norm referenced	Expressive (language reasoning)

receptive and expressive tasks utilizing picture-identification and sentence-repetition formats. The basic assumption in repetition-of-form tasks is that the child should not reliably repeat constructions that are not in his productive repertoire. For the most part, the upper-age boundary on tests of this sort is seven to eight years. Most of the tests that go beyond this age range were designed to be measures of language function. This distinction is in harmony with the Piagetian concept of 7-

to-12 years as the Concrete Operations period and beyond 12 years as the Formal Operations period. It is not necessary to accept Piagetian theory to believe that language in 7-plus or 12-plus-year-old children reflects more complex propositions than that of children under the age of seven.

The "pragmatic revolution" of the seventies and eighties has generated a new series of test formats and, in some aficionados, an aversion to formal test formats that they believe restrict the ability to measure the efficiency of functional communication. Be that as it may, as a diagnostician, your description cannot be complete without attention to both the form and the function of language, and your description of adequacies and inadequacies should include judgments of both formal (restricted or controlled) and informal situational efficiency and effectiveness.

The tests we have presented are examples of the kinds of information that can be obtained. Age ranges for which the tests were designed, types of normative comparisons available (mean score for age, age scores, percentile ranks), and types of skills tested (expressive, receptive) are listed. This listing does not make a qualitative judgment for a clinician in search of the "best test." It is not intended to. Nor is it intended to include popular versus unpopular or commonly used versus uncommonly available tests and procedures. The descriptions are intended to provide some basis for the clinician's judgment in choosing among them. No one test will provide all of the necessary information for a remediation regimen if a problem has been diagnosed. The age, the area of concern, and the capability of the child in question are all important factors in your test selection. The primary misuse of the diagnostician's responsibility would be in the assumption that one test is "all good" and another is "all bad."

This presentation has assumed that a judgment of "language disorder" must be based on an understanding, in both form and function, of what is to be expected with chronological age. The description available, from an appropriate combination of test results, should give an indication of the child's abilities and disabilities within his language system.

REFERENCES

ADLER, S., Assessment of language proficiency of limited English proficient speakers: Implications for the speech-language-specialist. *Lang. Speech Hearing Serv. Schools,* 22, 12–18 (1991).

AMERICAN SPEECH-LANGUAGE-HEARING ASSOCIATION, Preferred practice patterns for the professions of speech-language pathology and audiology. *Asha* 35, No. 3 (Supp. No. 11) 57 (1993).

ARNDT, W. B., A psychometric evaluation of the Northwestern Syntax Screening Test. *J. Speech Hearing Dis.,* 42, 316–319 (1977).

BANGS, T. E., *Vocabulary Comprehension Scale.* Lamar, Tex.: Learning Concepts (1975)

BANKSON, N. W., *Bankson Language Screening Test.* Baltimore: University Park Press (1977).

BATES, E., *Language and Context: The Acquisition of Pragmatics.* New York: Academic Press (1976).

BERKO, J., The child's learning of English morphology. *Word,* 14, 150–177 (1958).

BERNHARDT, B., A test of the *Test of Problem Solving* (TOPS). *Lang. Speech Hearing Serv. Schools,* 21, 98–101 (1990).

BERRY, M. F., AND R. TALBOT, *Exploratory Test for Grammar.* Rockford, Ill.: Berry and Talbot, 4322 Pine Crest Road (1966).

BLOOM, L., Talking, understanding, and thinking. In *Language Perspectives—Acquisition, Retardation, and Intervention,* eds. R. L. Schiefelbusch and L. L. Lloyd. Baltimore: University Park Press (1974).

BOEHM, A. E., *Boehm Test of Basic Concepts* (Manual). New York: Psychological Corporation (1971).

BROWN, R., *A First Language: The Early Stages.* Cambridge, Mass.: Harvard University Press (1973).

BROWN, R., AND C. FRASER, The acquisition of syntax. In *Verbal Behavior and Learning*, eds. C. N. Cofer and B. S. Musgrave. New York: McGraw-Hill (1963).

BURNS, E., Psychometric deficiencies of the short-form version of the Northwestern Syntax Screening Test. *J. Speech Hearing Dis.*, 47, 331–333 (1982).

CARROLL, J. B., Review of Illinois Test of Psycholinguistic Abilities: Revised Edition. In *The Seventh Mental Measurements Yearbook*, ed. O. K. Buros. Highland Park, N.J.: Gryphon Press (1972).

CARROW, E., *Test for Auditory Comprehension of Language*. Lamar, Tex.: Learning Concepts (1973).

CARROW, E., *Carrow Elicited Language Inventory Manual*. Lamar, Tex.: Learning Concepts (1974).

CARROW, E., AND J. LYNCH, Comparison of semantic versus syntactic comprehension in three groups of linguistically deviant children. Unpublished manuscript cited in E. Carrow, *Test for Auditory Comprehension of Language*. Lamar, Tex.: Learning Concepts (1973).

CARROW, M. A., The development of auditory comprehension of language structure in children. *J. Speech Hearing Dis.*, 33, 99–111 (1968).

CARROW-WOOLFOLK, E., *Test for Auditory Comprehension of Language–Revised*. Allen, Tex.: DLM Teaching Resources (1985).

CHOMSKY, N., *Aspects of the Theory of Syntax*. Cambridge, Mass.: M.I.T. Press (1965).

CHOONG, J., AND J. MCMAHON, Comparison of scores obtained on the PPVT and the PPVT-R. *J. Speech Hearing Dis.*, 48, 40–43 (1983).

DARLEY, F. L., AND K. L. MOLL, Reliability of language measures and size of language sample. *J. Speech Hearing Res.*, 3, 166–173 (1960).

D'ASARO, M. J., AND V. JOHN, A rating for evaluation of receptive, expressive, and phonetic language development of the young child. *Cerebral Pal. Rev.*, 22, No. 5 (1961).

DEVER, R. B., A comparison of the results of a revised version of Berko's test of morphology with the free speech of mentally retarded children. *J. Speech Hearing Res.*, 15, 169–178 (1972).

DOLL, E. A., *The Vineland Social Maturity Scale*. Minneapolis: American Guidance Service, Inc. (1946).

DUCHAN, J. F., Language assessment: The pragmatics revolution. In *Language Science*, ed. R. Naremore, San Diego: College-Hill Press (1984).

DUNN, L. M., *Expanded Manual for The Peabody Picture Vocabulary Test*. Circle Pines, Minn.: American Guidance Service, Inc. (1965).

DUNN, L. M., AND L. M. DUNN, *Peabody Picture Vocabulary Test–Revised*. Circle Pines, Minn.: American Guidance Service, Inc. (1981).

ENGELMANN, S., D. ROSS, AND V. BINGHAM, *Basic Language Concepts Test*. Tigard, Oreg.: C. C. Publications, Inc. (1982).

FEY, M. C., Understanding and narrowing the gap between treatment research and clinical practice with language impaired children. In *The "Future of Science and Services" Seminar*, ed. C. M. Shewan. *Asha Reports* No. 20 (1990).

FILLENBAUM, S., *Syntactic Factors in Memory*. The Hague: Mouton (1973).

FILLMORE, C. J., The case for case. In *Universals in Linguistic Theory*, eds. E. Bach and R. T. Harms. New York: Holt, Rinehart and Winston (1968).

FOSTER, R., J. J. GIDDAN, AND J. STARK, *Assessment of Children's Language Comprehension, Manual*. Palo Alto, Calif.: Consulting Psychologists Press, Inc. (1973).

FRANKENBERG, W. K., AND J. B. DOBBS, *Denver Developmental Screening Test. J. Pediatrics*, 71, 181–191 (1967).

FRASER, C., U. BELLUGI, AND R. BROWN, Control of grammar in imitation, comprehension, and production. *J. Verb. Learn. Verb. Behav.*, 2, 121–135 (1963).

GERMAN, D. J., *Test of Word Finding*. Allen, Tex.: DLM Teaching Resources (1986).

GERMAN, D. J., *Test of Adolescent/Adult Word Finding*. Allen, Tex.: DLM Teaching Resources (1990).

GLASER, R., Instructional technology and the measurement of learning outcomes: Some questions. *Amer. Psychol.*, 18, 519–521 (1963).

HAHN, E., Analyses of the content and form of the speech of first-grade children. *Q. J. Speech*, 34, 361–366 (1948).

HAMMILL, D. D., AND P. L. NEWCOMER, *Test of Language Development–Intermediate*. Austin, Tex.: Pro-Ed (1982).

HEAD, H., *Aphasia and Kindred Disorders of Speech, Vol. I*. London: Cambridge University Press (1926).

HEDRICK, D. L., AND E. M. PRATHER, *Sequenced Inventory of Language Development (SILD), Experi-*

mental Edition. Seattle: Child Development and Mental Retardation Center, University of Washington (1970).

HEDRICK, D. L., E. M. PRATHER, AND A. R. TOBIN, *Sequenced Inventory of Communication Development Examiner's Manual*. Seattle: University of Washington Press (1975).

KELLMAN, M., C. FLOOD, AND D. YODER, *Language Assessment Tasks*. Copyright by Kellman, Flood, Yoder (1977).

KIRK, S. A., AND W. D. KIRK, Uses and abuses of the ITPA. *J. Speech Hearing Dis.*, 43, 58–75 (1978).

KIRK, S. A., J. J. MCCARTHY, AND W. D. KIRK, *Illinois Test of Psycholinguistic Abilities (Examiner's Manual)*. Urbana: University of Illinois Press (1968).

KLEE, T. M., AND D. L. RATUSNIK, On the utility of the NSST short form: A reply to Burns. *J. Speech Hearing Dis.*, 47, 333–334 (1982).

LAHEY, M., Who shall be called language disordered? Some reflections and one perspective. *J. Speech Hearing Dis.* 55, 612–620 (1990).

LASS, N., J. NORTHERN, L., MCREYNOLDS, AND D. YODER, eds. *Handbook of Speech-Language Pathology and Audiology*. Toronto: B. C. Decker (1988).

LAWRENCE, C. W., Assessing the use of age-equivalent scores in clinical management. *Lang. Speech Hearing Serv. Schools*, 23, 6–8 (1992).

LEE, L. L., Developmental sentence types: A method for comparing normal and deviant syntactic development. *J. Speech Hearing Dis.*, 31, 311–330 (1966).

LEE L. L., *Northwestern Syntax Screening Test*. Evanston, Ill.: Northwestern University Press (1969, 1971).

LEE, L. L., *Developmental Sentence Analysis*. Evanston, Ill.: Northwestern University Press (1974).

LEE, L. L., Reply to Arndt and Byrne. *J. Speech Hearing Dis.*, 42, 323–327 (1977).

LEE, L. L., AND S. M. CANTER, Developmental sentence scoring. *J. Speech Hearing Dis.*, 36, 315–340 (1971).

MARQUARDT, T. P., AND J. H. SAXMAN, Language comprehension and auditory discrimination in articulation-deficient kindergarten children. *J. Speech Hearing Res.*, 15, 382–389 (1972).

MCCARTHY, D., *The language development of the preschool child*. Institute of Child Welfare Monograph Series. No. 4. Minneapolis: University of Minnesota Press (1930).

MCCARTHY, D., Language development in children. In *Manual of Child Psychology*, ed. L. Carmichael. New York: John Wiley (1954).

MCCARTHY, D., *McCarthy Scales of Children's Abilities*. New York: Psychological Corporation (1972).

MCCARTHY, J. J., AND S. A. KIRK, *The Illinois Test of Psycholinguistic Abilities, Examiner's Manual*. Urbana: University of Illinois Press (1961).

MCDADE, H. L., M. A. SIMPSON, AND D. E. LAMB, The use of elicited imitation as a measure of expressive grammar: A question of validity. *J. Speech Hearing Dis.*, 47, 19–24 (1982).

MESSER, S., Implicit phonology in children. *J. Verb. Learn. Verb. Behav.*, 6, 609–613 (1967).

MINER, L., Scoring procedures for the Length-Complexity Index: A preliminary report. *J. Commun. Dis.*, 2, 224–240 (1969).

MINIFIE, F., F. L. DARLEY, AND D. SHERMAN. Temporal reliability of seven language measures. *J. Speech Hearing Res.*, 6, 149–156 (1963).

MUMA, J. R., SEMEL AND WIIG'S CELF: Construct validity? *J. Speech Hearing Dis.*, 49, 101–104 (1984).

NEWCOMER, P. L., AND D. D. HAMMILL, *Test of Language Development–Primary*. Austin, Tex.: Pro. Ed. (1982).

NEWFIELD, M. U., AND B. B. SCHLANGER, The acquisition of English morphology by normal and educable mentally retarded children. *J. Speech Hearing Res.*, 11, 693–706 (1968).

NICE, M. N., Length of sentences as a criterion of a child's progress in speech. *J. Ed. Psych.*, 16, 370–379 (1925).

NIPPOLD, M. A., Evaluating and enhancing idiom comprehension in language-disordered students. *Lang. Speech Hearing Serv. Schools*, 22, 100–106 (1991).

NIPPOLD, M. A., AND S. T. MARTIN, Idiom interpretation in isolation versus context: A developmental study with adolescents. *J. Speech Hearing Res.*, 32, 59–66 (1989).

OLSWANG, L. B., AND A. L. CARPENTER, Elicitor effects on the language obtained from young language-impaired children. *J. Speech Hearing Dis.*, 43, 76–88 (1978).

OSGOOD, C. E., A behavioral analysis of perception and language as cognitive phenomena. In *Contemporary Approaches to Cognition*, ed. J. S. Bruner. Cambridge, Mass.: Harvard University Press (1957).

OWENS, R. E., JR., *Language Development. An Introduction*. Columbus, Ohio: Chas. E. Merrill (1984).

PARASKEVOPOULOS, J. N., AND S. A. KIRK, *The Development and Psychometric Characteristics of the Revised Illinois Test of Psycholinguistic Abilities.* Urbana: University of Illinois Press (1969).

PAUL, R., AND P. JENNINGS, Phonological behavior in toddlers with slow expressive language development. *J. Speech Hearing Res.*, 35, 99–107 (1992).

PENDERGAST, K., AND OTHERS, *Photo Articulation Test.* Danville, Ill.: Interstate Printers & Publishers (1969).

PIAGET, J., AND B. INHELDER, *The Psychology of the Child.* New York: Basic Books (1969).

PRATHER, E. M., S. V. BREECHER, M. L. STAFFORD, AND E. M. WALLACE, *Screening Test of Adolescent Language.* Seattle: University of Washington Press (1980).

PRUTTING, C. A., T. M. GALLAGHER, AND A. MULAC, The expressive portion of the NSST compared to a spontaneous language sample. *J. Speech Hearing Dis.*, 40, 40–48 (1975).

RAMER, A. L. H., AND N. S. REES, Selected aspects of the development of English morphology in black American children of low socioeconomic background. *J. Speech Hearing Res.*, 16, 569–577 (1973).

RATUSNICK, D. L., AND R. A. KOENIGSKNECT, Internal consistency of the Northwestern Syntax Screening Test. *J. Speech Hearing Dis.*, 40, 59–69 (1975).

RATUSNIK, D. L., T. M. KLEE, AND C. M. RATUSNIK, *Northwestern Syntax Screening Test*: A short form. *J. Speech Hearing Dis.*, 45, 200–208 (1980).

RESCORLA, L., The language development survey: A screening for delayed language in toddlers. *J. Speech Hearing Dis.*, 54, 587–599 (1989).

SALVIA, J., AND J. K. YSSELDYKE *Assessment in special and remedial education*, 4th ed. Boston: Houghton Mifflin (1988).

SANDER, E. K., When are speech sounds learned? *J. Speech Hearing Dis.* 37, 55–63 (1972).

SCHLESINGER, L. M., Production of utterances and language acquisition. In *Ontogenesis of Grammar*, ed. D. L. Slobin. New York: Academic Press (1971).

SCHLESINGER, I. M., Learning grammar: From pivot to realization rule. In *Language Acquisition: Models and Methods*, eds. R. Huxley and E. Ingram. New York: Academic Press (1971).

SCHLESINGER, I. M., Relational concepts underlying language. In *Language Acquisition and Intervention*, eds. R. L. Schiefelbusch and L. L. Lloyd. Baltimore: University Park Press (1974).

SCHLESINGER, I. M., The role of cognitive development and linguistic input in language acquisition. *J. Child Language*, 4, 153–169 (1977).

SCOTT, C. M., AND A. E. TAYLOR, A comparison of home- and clinic-gathered language samples. *J. Speech Hearing Dis.*, 43, 482–495 (1978).

SEARLE, J. R., *Speech Acts Theory.* New York: Cambridge University Press (1969).

SEMEL, E. M., AND E. H. WIIG, *Clinical Evaluation of Language Function.* Columbus, Ohio: Chas. E. Merrill (1980).

SEMEL, E., E. H. WIIG, AND W. SECORD, *Clinical Evaluation of Language Fundamentals–Revised: Technical Manual.* San Antonio, Tex.: Psychological Corporation (1987).

SEMEL, E., E, WIIG, AND W. SECORD, *Clinical Evaluation of Language Fundamentals–Revised.* San Antonio, Tex.: Psychological Corporation (1988).

SHRINER, T. H., A review of mean length of response as a measure of expressive language development in children. *J. Speech Hearing Dis.*, 34, 61–68 (1969).

SHRINER, T. H., AND D. SHERMAN, An equation for assessing language development *J. Speech Hearing Res.*, 10, 41–48 (1967).

SIEGEL, G. M., AND P. A. BROEN, Language assessment. In *Communication Assessment and Intervention Strategies*, ed. L. L. Lloyd. Baltimore: University Park Press (1976).

SKARAKIS-DOYLE, E., AND C. A. MALLET, Test-retest reliability: Another evaluation of the *Test of Problem Solving. Lang. Speech Hearing Serv. Schools*, 22, 278 (1991).

SLOBIN, D. I., Imitation and grammatical development in children. In *Contemporary Issues in Developmental Psychology*, eds. N. S. Endler, L. R. Boulter, and H. Osser. New York: Holt, Rinehart and Winston (1968).

SLOBIN, D. I., Cognitive prerequisites for the development of language. In *Studies of Child Language Development*, eds. C. Ferguson and D. I. Slobin. New York: Holt, Rinehart and Winston (1973).

SLOBIN, D. I., *Psycholinguistics*, 2nd ed. Glenview, Ill.: Scott, Foresman (1979).

SLOBIN, D. I., AND C. A. WELSH, Elicited imitation as a research tool in developmental psycholinguistics. In *Studies of Child Language Development*, eds. C. A. Ferguson and D. I. Slobin. New York: Holt, Rinehart and Winston (1973).

SMITH, C., An experimental approach to children's linguistic competence. In *Studies of Child Language*

Development, eds. C. A. Ferguson and D. I. Slobin. New York: Holt, Rinehart and Winston (1973).

SNYDER, L. S., Cognition and language development. In *Language Science*, ed. R. C. Naremore. San Diego: College-Hill Press (1984).

SPEKMAN, N. J., AND F. P. ROTH, Clinical Evaluation of Language Function (CELF) diagnostic battery: An analysis and critique. *J. Speech Hearing Dis.*, 49, 97–100 (1984).

TEMPLIN, M. C., *Certain Language Skills in Children*, Institute of Child Welfare Monograph Series, No. 26, Minneapolis: University of Minnesota Press (1957).

TEMPLIN, M. C., The study of articulation and language development during the early school years. In *The Genesis of Language*, eds. F. Smith and G. A. Miller. Cambridge, Mass.: M.I.T. Press (1966).

THORUM, A. R., *The Fullerton Language Test for Adolescents*, 2nd ed. Palo Alto, Calif.: Consulting Psychologists Press (1986).

UNDERWOOD, B. J., The language repertoire and some problems in verbal learning. In *Directions in Psycholinguistics*, ed. S. Rosenberg. New York: Macmillan (1966).

VAN KLEECK, A., AND A. RICHARDSON, Assessment of speech and language development. In *Developmental Assessment in Clinical Child Psychology: A Handbook*, eds. J. H. Johnson and J. Goldman. Elmsford, N.Y.: Pergamon Press (1990).

WECHSLER, D., *The Measurement and Appraisal of Adult Intelligence*. Baltimore: Williams and Wilkins (1958).

WEINER, P. S., The perceptual level functioning of dysphasic children: A follow-up study. *J. Speech Hearing Res.*, 15, 423–438 (1972).

WEINER, P. S., AND W. C. HOOCK, The standardization of tests: Criteria and criticisms. *J. Speech Hearing Res.*, 16, 616–626 (1973).

WEPMAN, J. M., AND L. V. JONES, *The Language Modalities Test for Aphasia*. Chicago: University of Chicago Education-Industry Service (1961).

WHITACRE, J. D., H. L. LUPER, AND H. R. POLLIO, General language deficits in children with articulation problems. *Lang. Speech*, 13, 231–239 (1970).

WHORF, B. L., *Language, Thought and Reality: Selected Writings*. Cambridge, Mass.: Technology Press (1956).

WIIG, E. H., AND W. SECORD, *Test of Language Competence–Expanded (TLC-E)*. New York: The Psychological Corporation, Harcourt Brace Jovanovich (1989).

WILLIAMS, H. M., An analytical study of language achievement in preschool children, Part 1, (and) An analytical scale of language achievement. In *Development of Language and Vocabulary in Young Children. University of Iowa Studies in Child Welfare*, 13, 9–18 and 49–77 (1937).

WINITZ, H., Language skills of male and female kindergarten children. *J. Speech Hearing Res.*, 2, 377–386 (1959).

ZACHMAN, L., C. JORGENSEN, H. HUISINGH, AND M. BARRETT, *The Test of Problem Solving*. Moline, Ill.: LinguiSystems (1984).

ZIMMERMAN, I. L., V. G. STEINER, AND R. L. EVATT, *Preschool Language Manual*. Columbus, Ohio: Chas. E. Merrill (1969, 1979).

ZIMMERMAN, I. L., V. G. STEINER, AND R. E. POND, *Preschool Language Scale–3*. San Antonio, Tex.: The Psychological Corporation, Harcourt Brace Jovanovich (1992).

6

Evaluation of Uncertainty: Developmental Skills, Motor Skills, and Nonverbal Intelligence

*"The time has come," the Walrus said, "to talk of many things: Of shoes—
and ships—and sealing wax—of cabbages—and kings—. . ."*

Lewis Carroll
Through the Looking Glass

INTRODUCTION

The evaluation of communication skills is a process akin to a research project. It involves the asking of answerable questions in such a way that our results are meaningful. In order to know when and where and how the results of our research project (or diagnostic endeavors) provide predictions and descriptions of behavior, we must be able to define the variables that are expected to affect the outcome. A number of these variables, such as motor skills or proficiencies, visual-motor perceptual skills, and nonverbal intelligence abilities, do not directly involve communication processes but are importantly related to an understanding of the growth and development of the child and of the developmental scaffolding from which communication evolves.

We review a relatively small number of these tests as exemplars. Our purpose is not to review tests in a wide number of areas in order to paint an appraisal mosaic but rather to isolate areas of assessment that should lead to a greater understanding of why the child communicates (or doesn't communicate) as she does. Depending on the general populations or individuals the clinician is concerned with, this short listing may be considered either as an example of test formats to be mastered as part of the diagnostic armamentaria or as test protocols to request from a source (psychologist, occupational therapist) to whom the child or adult is referred.

DEVELOPMENTAL SKILLS

In many ways, language maturation parallels motor and physical maturation. For more than half a century (Abt, Adler, and Bartelme 1929), it has been recognized that early language development could be used as a predictive yardstick[1] for the child's general and intellectual potential (Gesell and Amatruda 1941). This is not to say that a causal relationship exists between motor and speech development, but in the absence of specific etiologies that may affect skills differentially, there is a pattern of consistency in normal behavioral evolution (Gesell and Amatruda 1947; Lenneberg 1966; McGraw 1963). Growth and maturation proceed at characteristic rates for each developmental aspect (Lenneberg 1966). Our consideration of developmental skills in this chapter is an outgrowth of the recognition that motor and perceptual functioning and nonverbal intelligence as well as verbal language skills provide information on neurological integrity and maturation.

Gesell Motor and Adaptive Scales

Gesell and his associates (1934, 1940, 1941, 1948) were concerned with four fields of developmental behavior: motor, adaptive, language, and personal-social. The *Gesell Motor and Adaptive Scales* are an empirically based product of their 20-year study of normal children aimed at generating a system of developmental diagnosis for infants and children. The scales assume that motor, adaptive, language, and social behaviors are all a function of mental growth and require progressively more coordinated patterning of behavior based on neurological integrity and maturation. In other words, "We cannot or need not separate or distinguish physical patterns and behavior patterns. The child is a unitary organism and from the very beginning is growing as a single unit" (Gesell and Ilg 1947, p. 16).

Since we have previously discussed language and personal social behaviors, our primary focus insofar as the Gesell scales are concerned will be on motor and adaptive behaviors. The *Gesell Motor and Adaptive Scales* are not measures of intelligence, and the age-scale items of the instrument are not to be taken as specific rules of thumb. Rather, the scales are designed to yield a very general picture of the child's growth in adaptive behaviors primarily during the first five years of life.

---

[1]For a more complete review of perceptual-motor programs and test instruments, what predictions can be made, and what predictions cannot be made, see Cratty (1970).

Both the motor and adaptive scales span the ages from 18 to 72 months at 6-month divisions, but Gesell considered 5 to be the "nodal" age (Gesell and Ilg 1947, p. 251). Items on the scale are listed as age norms but were designed to be used for general orientation and interpretation rather than as standards of behavior that the child must meet.

The Motor Scale consists largely of walking and balance activities; for example, the child runs without falling at 24 months; alternates feet going up stairs at 36 months; walks downstairs with the last few treads one foot to a tread at 48 months. The Adaptive Scale has a number of eye–hand coordination tasks, especially at the earlier age divisions. For example, a tower of 6 or 7 blocks is to be built at 24 months, 8 blocks at 30 months, and 9 blocks at 36 months. Many drawing and counting tasks are also included, such as copying geometric figures, draw-a-man, and counting objects. These are age-related tests, which means that the total number of correct responses credits the child with a year–month age score for motor age level or adaptive age level.

There is also a *Preliminary Behavior Inventory* (Gesell and Amatruda 1947), which is a screening test of observations for motor, adaptive, language, and personal-social behaviors. This abbreviated scale with one or two items per age designation at intervals from four weeks to six years is not to be used as a diagnostic inventory. Suggested use of the instrument is for the examiner to check the most advanced behaviors in each field. Gross deviations or disparities indicate the need for a diagnostic behavior examination.

The *Denver Developmental Screening Test* (Frankenburg and Dodds 1967) is essentially a display of the Gesell test items in a different form. A few of the test items, however, are placed at slightly different age levels than on the Gesell scales. For example, building a tower of 8 cubes is shown on the Gesell Adaptive Scale at the 30-month level. According to the Denver chart, 25 percent of children 21 months of age can build a tower of 8 cubes, 75 percent can perform the task at between 24 and 30 months, and 90 percent have accomplished this feat at approximately 39 months.

Behaviors to be evaluated on the test are segmented into four categories: gross motor, language, fine-motor adaptive, and personal-social. Items are arranged on an age scale with one-month separations from one to 24 months and by half-year divisions from 2–6 to 6 years. For convenience in deriving an approximate developmental age for each of the four categories, the Denver response sheet is marked with ages along the horizontal axis. Developmental item skills are shown horizontally on bar graphs beginning in line with the age-scale markers where 25 percent of the standardization population of 1,036 children had mastered the skill. The bar graph becomes shaded at the point where 75 percent of the tested children performed the test item and terminates where 90 percent of the children satisfied the criterion item. Many of the items are directly tested, but some items, especially at the earlier age levels, are keyed to allow credit by parental report. Items passed are marked with "P," refused items by "R," failed items by "F," and no opportunity by "N.O." Failure or delay is defined as failure to successfully perform an item at an age level at which 90 percent of comparably aged children passed. Normal children are expected to show a scattering of successes and failures on items within an area and between categories. The manner in which the items are displayed on the response sheet allows the examiner to more easily make informed judgments of the overall developmental picture presented by the child. Test-retest and interexaminer reliability have been established at 0.95 and 0.90 respectively.

The *Inventory of Early Development* (Brigance 1978) is another broad-based tool for early assessment. The measure, designed for children from birth to seven years, has several purposes: (1) as an assessment tool to evaluate performance or developmental level, to identify strengths and weaknesses, to determine instructional objectives in keeping with the child's developmental level, and to serve as a basis for referral; (2) as an instructional guide; (3) as a record-keeping system that is ongoing and specific; (4) as a tool for structuring individual educational programs; and (5) as a resource for parent and professional training. The inventory includes 98 skill sequences up to the developmental age of six years. Areas assessed include psychomotor, self-help, speech and language, general knowledge and comprehension, and early academic skills.

The Brigance scale is not intended to be administered in its entirety. The clinician chooses the areas to be assessed based on his reasons for testing (assessing development, instructional planning, etc.). Within each sequence, the level to begin is determined by the approximate developmental level of the child. The tester can then test to higher or lower levels. Assessment procedures are flexible and may include parental interview or various types of formal and informal procedures and observations. The scale is derivative. That is, items and sequences are based on previous studies of child development with the age of acquisition predicated on a consensus of published age norms. For each sequence, references are cited that were the source for establishing and validating the sequences and developmental ages.

Assessment of gross motor skills may serve as an example. Suggested methods for gathering information include interviewing the parent or guardian, individual assessment, game playing with the child, and observation during a play period or during class activities, all depending on the age of the child and the ability investigated. The tester may demonstrate the skill to be assessed if the child does not perform because of lack of understanding of instructions. Gross motor skill sequences include standing; walking; stairs climbing; running; jumping; hopping; kicking; balance board walking; catching, rolling, throwing and bouncing a ball, and using rhythm and wheel toys. The expected level of performance for *standing*, for example, includes standing with broad stance at one year, standing on one foot for one second at three years, and standing heel to toe at seven years. Each sequence is continued until the child fails two or three consecutive items or until the skill level is determined at the discretion of the tester. Similarly, sequences for *self—help* skills include feeding/eating, undressing, unfastening and fastening, toileting, grooming, bathing, and knowing front and back and inside compared to outside of clothing. Expected performance in feeding sequences ranges from suckling reflex observable at birth, to holding a glass with one hand to drink at two years, to preparing a sandwich at seven years. The sequence is continued until failure on two consecutive items.

The *Inventory of Early Development* is an assessment protocol rather than a test. It is criterion-referenced based upon norms derived from earlier studies of development within a broad spectrum of behaviors from gross-motor skills to academic performance and speech and language. The inventory should be viewed as a descriptive picture of developmental behaviors without specific suggestions about diagnostic distinctions relative to delayed or abnormal performance.

TESTS OF MOTOR SKILL

The *Oseretsky Test of Motor Proficiency* was originally published in Russian in 1923. It was adapted into Portuguese and later translated into English (Doll 1946). It was designed for children from 4 to 16 years of age and was described as "a year-scale of tests of motor maturation for measuring genetic levels of motor proficiency [and] . . . affords a standard means for the clinical evaluation of behavioral development." The test was designed to evaluate manual abilities, motor skills, and motor equilibrium—that is, to show the value of children's motor reactions and their causes so that children could be trained to control and coordinate movements. The test is composed of 85 items divided into six groups for each age level: (1) tests for general static coordination (balance), (2) tests for dynamic coordination of the hands, (3) tests for general dynamic coordination, (4) tests for motor speech, (5) tests for simultaneous voluntary movement, and (6) tests for synkinesia (associated involuntary movements). The original Oseretsky test suffered from significant procedural shortcomings. For example, Doll (1946) noted that:

> It is not clear from most of the test directions to what extent the examiner may assist the child by supplementing the verbal directions with demonstration. Since many of the test directions presumably would not be clearly understood without demonstration, the lack of which increases the intellectual requirements of the tests, it may be assumed that demonstrating the tasks is not only permissible but desirable or even imperative. . . . the tests are not free from a rather marked intellectual loading since the problem of comprehending the task and to some degree responding to it is inherent in the testing. (p. 2)

These procedural shortcomings have led to two notable adaptations of the test.

Sloan (1955) modified and adapted the Oseretsky scale, and his experimental results were published as the *Lincoln-Oseretsky Motor Development Scale*. A total of 380 boys and 369 girls between the ages of 6 and 14 were tested on the 85 original Oseretsky items. The number of subjects at the various age levels ranged from 39 to 46. All subjects were obtained from the public schools in small towns in central Illinois and were from moderate to "low-moderate" socioeconomic-level families. They were selected on the basis of age and grade placement alone. None were reported to have a marked intellectual deficiency, but individual intelligence tests were not administered.

On the basis of statistical analyses of the performance of the children on the Oseretsky scale, test items that did not contribute to the total score were eliminated, and the format of the test was changed. The six types of items used by Oseretsky were maintained, but the 36 items retained are structured as a single order of difficulty rather than represented at each age level. As with the original Oseretsky scale, varying amounts of credit are given for speed of performance, dominant and non-dominant hand performances are weighted differently, and boys and girls are scored separately. An example of an item from the test is the act of throwing a ball. Equipment necessary includes a ball and a 10-inch square target placed 8 feet in front of the child at chest height. With both right hand and left hand separately, the subject is asked to bring her hand to the shoulder (as in a shot put) and throw the ball at the target. Scoring is based on the number of times the target is hit. An improper throw (overhand or underhand, for example) is not counted. If the child hits the target four times (out of five), she is given three points; three hits or two hits, two points; one hit, one point; and no hits, no points. Consequently, scoring is determined by how many points are credited to the child on the item and not whether she passed or did not pass.

The directions for the Lincoln-Oseretsky scale are concise, the amount of credit per item is explicitly stated, and the total number of points for the child's age and sex can be interpreted according to means, standard deviations, and percentile scores provided for children 6 to 14 years of age. As a validity statement, Sloan reported that the test correlated well with chronological age and was capable of discriminating between children of different ages. Split-half reliability ranged from a low of 0.59 (for 14-year-old girls) to a high of 0.94. For the 9 age groups on which data were collected, reliability coefficients were 0.80 and above, except for the 13 and 14-year-old boys (0.72 and 0.78 respectively) and the 14-year-old girls.

The *Bruininks-Oseretsky Test of Motor Proficiency* (Bruininks 1978) is an expansion as well as an adaptation of the Oseretsky scale. The test is designed to assess the motor skills of children from 4–6 to 14–6 years of age. The battery includes eight subtests comprised of 46 items to provide an index of motor proficiency for both gross and fine motor skills. The short form contains 14 items and serves as a survey of general motor proficiency.

Four subtests of the battery (running speed and agility, balance, bilateral coordination, and strength) assess gross motor skills; three subtests (upper limb coordination, response speed, and visual-motor control) measure fine-motor skills, and one subtest (speed and upper-limb dexterity) tests both gross and fine motor skills. Approximately 40 percent of the items are revised tasks from the *Oseretsky Test of Motor Proficiency*, and the test includes three subtests not included in the original Oseretsky version.

Performance on each item is scored according to the time required to complete the task, the number of units completed per unit time, the number of errors observed during performance of the task, or as pass or fail based upon established criteria. The raw scores are converted to scale values that can then be totaled. The test was standardized on 765 subjects between 4–6 and 14–6 years of age. The sample included approximately an equal number of boys and girls, and racial and community size representation were considered in the subject selection.

The raw scores are converted to point scores, and point scores are converted to derived scores based on chronological age. Norms are expressed as four types of derived scores: subtest standard scores at six-month intervals from 4–6 years to 14–5 years, percentile ranks, stanines, and age equivalents. By comparing the derived scores with the scores of subjects from the standardization, the subjects' performance can be compared to the reference group. The complete battery yields three estimates of motor proficiency: a gross motor composite score, a fine motor composite score, and a battery composite score. The performance on each composite is expressed as a standard score with a mean of 50 and a standard deviation of 10 for each age level. The test appears to have adequate construct validity. Test-retest reliability based upon results from 63 second graders and 63 sixth graders was found to be 0.77 for the gross motor composite, 0.88 for the fine motor composite, and 0.89 for the battery composite.

The *Motor Problems Inventory* (Riley 1972) is primarily an empirically based test. It consists of 15 items that are described as included in "traditional examination procedures used by speech and language pathologists, traditional psychological observations, and the traditional neurological examination." The items are categorized as small muscle coordination, laterality, gross motor coordination, and general observations. No special equipment is required except for a stopwatch and a room sufficiently large to allow gross muscle activities, such as hopping, skipping, and running.

Small muscle coordination includes items such as finger snapping and diadochokinetic movements of the tongue and lips. Laterality items include lateral alternating movements of the tongue, slapping the thighs with the hands bilaterally, and hand-eye-foot preferences. Gross motor coordination is observed in hopping, balancing, walking, and running activities. General observations are concerned with hyperactivity, perseveration, distractibility, and legibility of handwriting.

Each of the 15 items is scored as "no problem," "some problem," or "much problem" according to criteria shown with each of the items. These three terms are given weights of 0, 1, and 2 respectively. The range of scores for the 15 items is, therefore, 0 to 30. Normative comparisons are based on the range of scores for children of preschool, kindergarten, and first through fifth grade. The standardization population consisted of 209 children with from 30 to 60 children at each of the grade levels except that there were no children included at the second- and fourth-grade levels. The normal-range, significant-problem, and severe-problem designations for these two ages were judged by interpolations of the curves.

Validity and reliability data are based on comparison of the instrument to "soft" neurological signs and test-retest consistency. The test is reported to be of value for screening special education classes, selecting children to be referred for neurological examination, and as a measurement of the motor component in speech, language, and education disorders. However, no statistics are cited for the agreement of the test scores with speech and language disorders.

The motor development-proficiency scales we have discussed have one assumption in common: Coordination skills and patterns of behavior reflect the integrity of the neurological system. Children on the low end of the coordination continuum will tend to be classified differently according to the theoretical biases favored in the academic or clinical environment in which the clinician finds herself. These children have been variously categorized with terms ranging from aphasoid to clumsy. To explore the rationale for the variety of terms used would require more of a defense of the theoretical biases than a listing of diagnostic criteria. Our purpose is not to argue whether one term is better than another for describing a syndrome but rather to provide a rationale for appraisal instruments that aid in establishing a more complete description of the patient and the problem referred. For the same reason, we will include several examples of scales that provide measurements of visual perception.

TESTS OF VISUAL PERCEPTION

Tests of visual-perceptual skills are expected to have diagnostic relevance to children with learning disabilities, especially those problems related to reading and assigning meaning to visual symbols. The *Developmental Test of Visual Perception* (Frostig and others 1966; Maslow and others 1964) has five major components: eye–hand coordination; figure–ground perception; form constancy; position in space; and spatial relationship.

Tests of eye–hand coordination require the child to draw straight and curved lines between narrow boundaries or to draw straight lines to a target. Figure–ground tasks require the child to discriminate between intersecting shapes and to find hidden figures. Form constancy requires a discrimination of circles and squares in different sizes, positions, and shading among other figures on the page. Position in space is a test of directionality. The differentiation required is to separate figures in a like position from those that are reversed or rotated. In the spatial relationship subtest, the task is to copy patterns by linking dots.

The 1963 standardization (Maslow and others 1964) is based on the performance of over 2,100 unselected nursery school and public school children from three to nine years of age. The five subtest areas are considered relatively distinct. Each can be converted to a perceptual age equivalent, and a total perceptual age and quotient can be derived. Maslow and others reported that the perceptual quotient was more informative than the perceptual age. Means, standard deviations, and upper and lower quartile rankings are provided at half-year levels between five and eight years of age.

Validity has been expressed in terms of agreement with Goodenough (1955) intelligence test results and with beginning reading scores in early elementary classrooms. The correlations ranged from 0.31 to 0.50. Measures of reliability were generally higher.

The *Developmental Test of Visual Motor Integration* (Beery 1967) was devised as a measure of visual-perceptual and motor-behavior integration in young children. It is geared toward academic assessment rather than clinical diagnosis, and its primary users are elementary school teachers. The test is composed of 24 geometric forms to be copied with pencil and paper. The forms are arranged in the order of increasing difficulty and can be administered to children from 2 to 15 years of age, individually or by group administration. The recommended procedure is to evaluate the child's reproduction of a form according to a series of criteria provided using illustrations to aid in doubtful cases. At the corner of each scoring-criteria page are notations of age norms for a particular form. For example, male 5–6 means that 50 percent or more of the boys from the standardization population succeeded on the form at approximately five years and six months of age. Testing is discontinued after the child has failed on three consecutive forms although he may be allowed to attempt more difficult items. Age equivalents from raw scores are provided for boys and for girls from 2–10 to 15–9 years.

A validity estimate was derived from correlations between the test scores and age. The correlation between chronological age and test scores was 0.89 and was higher for mental age. Correlations were found to be higher in first-grade children than in older children. Test-retest reliability from a sample of 171 subjects was 0.83 and 0.87 for boys and girls respectively.

The *Motor-Free Visual Perception Test* (Colarusso and Hammill 1972) purports to test visual perception without confounding by motor activity. The test is composed of 37 items selected to assess spatial relationships, visual discrimination, figure–ground, visual closure, and visual memory. The items are individually administered and are multiple choice. The only response required from the child is that she point to the one of four alternatives that she thinks is the correct response. The child is not allowed to trace any figures and is generally given 15 seconds to make a selection although it is not a timed test.

The test was standardized on an unselected sample of 881 normal children who were four to eight years old and who resided in 22 states. Included were children from all races, economic levels, and residential areas. Perceptual-age estimates for each possible raw score are provided and include upper and lower ages based on the standard error of measurement for the entire test. Therefore, if a child's raw score is 22, it is likely that his true raw score is between 20 and 24, his perceptual age is between 5–8 and 6–5, and the best estimate is 6–0. A perceptual quotient is derived in a similar manner. Perceptual quotients are provided for children at a one-year interval between 4–0 and 4–11 and at six-month intervals from 5–0 to 8–11. The perceptual age and the perceptual quotient, then, should not be interpreted without considering the standard error of measurement for the raw scores.

Test-retest reliability was found to range from 0.77 to 0.82, split-half from 0.81 to 0.84, and Kuder-Richardson from 0.71 to 0.82. Construct validity was evaluated by means of age differentiation, correlations with similar tests, and internal consistency. The test correlated higher with other measures of visual perception (0.49) than it did with tests of intelligence (0.31) or school performance (0.38). The authors indicated that these findings support the validity of the measure because it would be expected to correlate higher with visual perception devices than with measures of intelligence and school performance.

Our discussion of developmental tests would not be complete unless we considered the *Bender Visual Motor Gestalt Test* (Bender 1938). The test is composed of nine designs selected by Bender from figures used by Wertheimer (1923) to study visual perception. The patient's task is to reproduce the nine figures that are then scored for imperfections. A separate set of instructions for the test was published along with the figures by Bender in 1946. Since its inception, the test has received intensive study and has proven useful for investigating adults (e.g. Pascal and Suttell 1951) and children (e.g., Clawson 1962) with disorders ranging from psychiatric disturbances to mental retardation and brain damage. Koppitz (1963, 1975) has devoted two volumes to reviews of the accumulated work with the test.

Since our concern is with visual-motor integration as a developmental skill, we will not consider the use of the test as an indicator of brain damage or emotional disturbance. Similarly, we will not review the several scoring systems for the test or the relationship of test results to intelligence, school achievement, mental age, or learning ability. Our focus will be on the scoring system developed by Koppitz (1963, 1975) and the results of the test as estimators of visual-motor maturity.

The Developmental Bender Test Scoring System (Koppitz 1963, 1975) contains 30 items that are used to quantify the imperfections in the reproductions of the nine gestalt designs. The total score is based on the distortion of shape, rotation, failure to integrate design parts, and perseveration in the copying of the figures. Theoretically, the score can range from 0 to 30 although scores of more than 20 are unusual. It is important to point out that the score is indicative of negative aspects of the copied designs; that is, with improved copying accuracy, the score will decrease rather than increase.

Koppitz (1975) has noted that by the age of nine the average child will make few if any errors and that below the age of five the designs are difficult to score. Consequently, the age range of the test is approximately five to nine years, although it may be of use for children above nine if they are markedly immature or have significant visual-motor integration problems.

The 1974 standardization of the test on 975 children yielded means and standard deviations at half-year intervals from 5 to 12 years; age equivalents from less than 4 to 12 years; and percentiles as function of chronological-age levels. For example, if a 7-year-old child received a score of 12, he would be functioning at the 10th percentile for children of his age, which is equivalent to the visual-motor integration of a child 5 years and 2 months of age. The score of 12 falls more than one standard deviation below the mean for his age, and he would be considered to have "extremely poor" visual-motor integration.

The Bender gestalt test appears to have adequate although not high test-retest reliability. Koppitz (1975) reviewed nine studies that found reliability coefficients from 0.53 to 0.87, although additional instability would be expected in brain-damaged and emotionally disturbed children. Correlations between the Bender and the *Frostig Developmental Test of Visual Perception* are not high (0.39 to 0.52), although the test results do correlate more positively (0.82) with the *Beery Developmental Test of Visual-Motor Integration* (Krauft and Krauft 1972).

TESTS OF INTELLIGENCE

Intelligence is a general ability composed of a large number of interrelated functions. Intelligence is not a thing—it is a construct defined by behavioral responses to a variety of specific factors or functions. Factors include verbal skills, numerical facility, reasoning, memory, spatial relations, and visual perception. Tests of intelligence are geared toward testing one or more of these factors to assess the intellectual ability or capability of the child or adult.

Typically, tests of intelligence are divided into performance and verbal scales. Nunnally (1970) noted, however, that:

> It has been the custom to call instruments "performance" tests if they deemphasize language requirements, employ three-dimensional materials, and require manipulative responses. Because of these components, the performance tests usually measure motor coordination, speed, perceptual factors and spatial factors. Instruments are usually referred to as "verbal" tests if they are printed forms, emphasize verbal comprehension, and require symbolic responses. Because of the ease with which certain kinds of test materials can be placed on printed forms, the verbal tests tend to measure verbal comprehension, numerical computation, and the reasoning factors. There is no clear-cut separation between the factors found in verbal and performance tests, but there is a tendency for different factors to arise in the two kinds of materials. (p. 281)

As noted earlier, our descriptions here will be restricted primarily to performance or "nonverbal" scales.

MEASURES OF INTELLECTUAL POTENTIAL: PERFORMANCE SCALES

Performance tests require an overt nonverbal manipulative response. Judgments of intelligence are made based upon what the child can demonstrate with her hands, point to, arrange, insert, or put together (Horrocks 1964). They were developed because many individuals demonstrate deficits in hearing, language, and/or speech and, consequently, will be handicapped on test instruments that are verbally demanding. Performance scales, therefore, are particularly important in the evaluation of communicatively handicapped patients. These scales may not be completely nonverbal in that the patient may engage in verbal behavior during the course of completing manipulative tasks. However, the instructions and the tasks require no overt verbalizations to the extent that instructions are pantomimed or acted out.

Performance tests serve the important function of helping to rule out mental retardation in a patient with limited verbal abilities since these measures estimate the patient's nonverbal cognitive abilities. They are also important because they provide information on the content of language. Bloom and Lahey (1978) note that tests of this type fit into a content-of-language category:

> . . . (1) the test gives information about the child's capacities for representational thought and ability to act on represented information (in the mind) as opposed to empirical information (in the context); (2) the test does not require that the child respond to much verbal instruction nor that the child interact verbally with the examiner in order to complete the task; and (3) completion of the tasks does not require that the child verbalize the answers, but instead, the scoring reflects nonverbal solutions. If most of these tasks are successfully completed by the child, then it is possible to conclude that the child is able mentally to represent aspects of the world that are not perceptually present in the situation, and to perform actions that are contingent on these mental representations. Although the tasks in such tests are not direct measures of the content coded by language, age appropriate scores with these measures can suggest that the child's concepts of the world, and the ideas that are coded by language are most likely intact.

We will review several performance tests with the purpose of providing information on their format, design, standardization, and information obtained.

The *Merrill-Palmer Scale of Mental Tests* (Stutsman 1948) is primarily a performance test but also contains several verbal items. The test was designed for children 24 to 48 months of age and is composed of 93 items arranged in ascending order of difficulty with 3 to 14 items at each 3-month interval. The speed and accuracy with which the tasks are completed determines the age level credited to the child on many of the items. Timed items include pegboards, a form board, picture puzzles, tower building, picture matching, buttoning, and pyramid building with cubes. Nontimed items are the verbal and copying tasks. Language tests include repetition of words and phrases, answering questions, and an action-agent test with items such as "What cries?" and "What runs?" The copying tasks include reproduction of a circle, a cross, and an asterisk.

A child is tested to a base level where all items are passed and upward to a level where more than one-half of the test items are failed. The test was standardized on 300 boys and 311 girls from 18 to 77 months at 6-month intervals with 41 to 81 children at each level. The raw score is used to determine a mental age, a percentile, and a standard score. Computation of an intelligence quotient is not recommended since the I.Q. deviations are not the same size at various age levels. The reliability of the test has not been determined, but Stutsman (1948) reported that the test differentiates between bright and dull children, and a correlation of 0.92 between chronological age and the total score on the test has been reported (Horrocks 1964).

The Merrill-Palmer scale is frequently the test of choice with the reluctant low-verbal two- to four-year-old child. Its colorful, age-graded, toylike items appeal to most children. Verbal instructions used with the performance items are simple and are usually accompanied by pantomime. The test affords a unique opportunity for observing personal behavior that may be clinically significant, such as the child's persistence, frustration level, and dependency. However, it tends to overestimate the intellectual capacity of the language-impaired child and underestimates the ability of the awkward child due to the many timed items.

The *Leiter International Performance Scale* (Leiter 1969) is a nonverbal mental-age scale for assessing the intelligence of patients between 2 and 18 years of age. Its primary use is with children with speech, hearing, and language disorders. Materials include blocks with pictures, colors, or designs that the child places in slots of an adjustable frame containing a stimulus card. The child is given three months of credit for each of the 54 tasks passed after the establishment of a basal age. Basal age is defined as correct completion of all four tests at an age level. Above 10 years, 6 months of credit is provided for each correct completion of a task. The test is terminated when all items are failed for two consecutive age levels.

The total score on the test is converted to a mental age that can be used to establish an intelligence quotient. The first or Hawaiian standardization of the scale was later found to overestimate the mental age of the child by approximately 18 months. A second standardization of the scale was completed to alleviate this problem but was found to underestimate the performance of the child by approximately 6 months. Therefore, the intelligence quotient is corrected by the addition of five points to the derived score. The mean at each age level with the quotient correction is 100 with a standard deviation of 16.

The *Arthur Adaptation of the Leiter International Performance Scale* (Arthur 1952) is a restandardization and not a revision of the *Leiter International Performance Scale*. It was restandardized because the norms of the first standardization by Leiter were too high. The test was reorganized to remove tasks demanding acquired skills such as telling time and to eliminate the timing of any of the test items to facilitate use of the instrument with motor-impaired patients. Some of the items at the upper age levels were omitted.

The test is designed for children from three to eight years of age and for other patients whose intellectual capacity would be expected to fall within this range. The lowest items on the test are determiners of the patient's ability to learn rather than tests of acquired knowledge or skill. The child is given credit if she is able to successfully complete the task without demonstration or help during a trial, no matter how many previous opportunities were given. There are 4 items at each 12-month age level for which the child can receive 3 months of credit. The exception is the 4-year level where the child receives 2.25 months of credit per item.

The test was standardized on 289 children from 3 to 7.99 years of age with 58 to 64 children at each age level. The mean intelligence quotient is 100 at each age level, and although not reported by Arthur, the standard deviation is estimated to be 16 (Leiter 1969).

The major asset of the test is in ruling out mental retardation and identifying the child with superior or above-average intelligence. If the nonverbal child scores above her chronological age on the test, it is recommended that teaching be through the visual modality.

The *Hiskey-Nebraska Test of Learning Aptitude* (Hiskey 1966) is a unique performance scale in that separate instructions and norms are provided for deaf and normal-hearing children from 3 to 17 years of age. The scale is composed of 163 items of increasing difficulty on 12 subtests. For children 3 to 10 years old, 8 subtests are presented. Instructions are pantomimed for the deaf and presented orally for the normal-hearing child. Four of the subtests—bead patterns, memory for color, visual attention span, and paper folding—evaluate memory. For example, the bead-patterns subtest requires the child to copy a design at the earlier age levels, while at older age levels he must reproduce the design from memory following a short exposure. Similarly, on the memory-for-color subtest, the child must match colored sticks following a short exposure by the examiner. Tasks not having a memory component are picture association, pictorial identification, block patterns, and completion of drawings. In general, these four subtests tap concept formation, spatial relationships, reasoning ability, and visual closure and attention.

Seven subtests are administered to children from 11 to 16 years of age. Visual attention span, block patterns, and completion of drawings are identical to those administered to younger children. The tests specific to this age group include memory for digits, puzzle books, pictorial analogies, and spatial reasoning. The memory-for-digits test requires the child to remember numbers on a card and to reproduce them from a set of digits provided by the examiner. Puzzle blocks are a set of eight colored blocks cut into parts. Each must be combined to make a cube. Pictorial analogies require the child to select a correct picture from a series of choices to complete the analogy. Spatial reasoning contains 10 geometric designs presented one at a time followed by the presentation of a set of four fragmented geometric designs from which the child must choose the correct form that could be assembled from the original design.

An age score is derived from each subtest. A learning age for deaf children and a mental age for hearing children is determined from the median of the subtests. A learning age, rather than a mental age, is used with deaf children to reduce the possibility of comparing the two groups. A learning age of five years, for example, is interpreted to mean that the child is able to do those tasks that an average deaf child of five can perform. A learning quotient can be determined for the hearing-impaired child by dividing the learning age by the chronological age. However, age improvement gradually reduces from 12 to 16 years, and learning ages and learning quotients have less significance at older than at younger age levels. One out of every four months of chronological age is dropped out above 12 years, and a constant chronological age is used for computations above 16 years. For the normal-hearing child, an intelligence quotient is determined by dividing mental age by chronological age. The intelligence quotients have been set with a mean of 100 and an arbitrary standard deviation of 16 at each age level.

The test was standardized on 1,079 deaf children and 1,074 hearing children from 2–6 years to 17–5 years at one-year intervals. Children from 2–6 years to 3–5 years were grouped as three-year-olds, children from 3–6 years to 4–5 years were considered in the four-year group, and so forth. The three-year group was very limited in size, and the norms for the upper limits are based on extrapolations. Therefore, the extremes of age must be considered reduced in reliability. The test has adequate concurrent validity as revealed by correlations with the Stanford-Binet (L–M) for normal-hearing children. Moreover, reliability is high as judged by coefficients from 0.947 to 0.904 on split-half and Spearman-Brown statistical procedures.

The Hiskey-Nebraska offers a wide array of untimed performance tasks but is somewhat arduous for the young child. A deaf child must be at least four years of age before test administration is not difficult. It is also problematical as to which instructions (verbal or nonverbal) and which norms (hearing or deaf) to use with the hard-of-hearing child who is administered verbal instructions accompanied by demonstration.

The *Raven Progressive Matrices* (1960, 1963, 1965) are nonverbal and determine intellectual functioning by means of a single factor, visual perception. They are a

> test of the ability to apprehend meaningless figures presented for observation, see the relations between them, conceive the nature of the figure completing each system of relations presented, and by doing so, develop a systematic method of reasoning. (Raven 1960, p. 2)

The *Standard Progressive Matrices* (1960) are composed of 60 items divided into 5 sets (A, B, C, D, E) of 12 each. On each set, the problems become more difficult. Stimuli are black and white drawings from which a part has been removed, and there are six possible choices to complete the design. The patient chooses the one that successfully completes the design. The test is typically untimed and can be individually or group administered. The individual administration format was designed for children from 6 to 13½ years of age, although the test may be administered at any age; the same items are administered no matter what the age of the patient.

The test was standardized on subjects from 6 to 65 years of age. The total score is the number right, which can be compared to the percentiles of the normative population that included 735 children from 6 to 13½ years of age, 1,407 children from 8 to 14 years, and 5,857 adults. By definition, the test requires intact visual perceptual skills for successful completion.

The *Coloured Progressive Matrices* (Raven 1963) were designed for children from 5 to 11, for old people; and for communication-impaired, intellectually subnormal, and intellectually deteriorated patients. It is composed of 3 sets of 12 items. Sets A and B are identical to the first two sets of the Standard Matrices except they are colored. Test Ab is a new set. The score is the total number correct, which can be compared to percentile norms for children from 5 to 11½ years of age or to norms for healthy old people from 65 to 85 years of age. If the Coloured Matrices are found to be too easy, sets C, D, and E are administered, the results of Set Ab are discarded, and the total score is compared to norms for the Standard Matrices.

The *Advanced Progressive Matrices* (1965) were derived from the *Standard*

Progressive Matrices and were designed for people of more than average intellectual ability. Set I is composed of 12 problems that tap the same intellectual processes encompassed in the Standard Matrices and is used to introduce the method of working. Set II contains 48 items similar to sets C, D, and E of the Standard Matrices. Percentile norms are provided for children from 11½ to 14 years of age at half-year intervals and for adults from 20 to 40 years old at decades.

The matrices are most useful for identifying mental retardation in low-verbal and nonverbal adults and older children. The test is unique in that the Coloured Matrices have percentile norms for the normally aged and appears to be an appealing instrument for evaluating the patient with senile dementia.

However, the test will not typically be used as the sole estimate of intellectual functioning, and its reliability is in doubt for young children and the severely retarded.

The *Test of Nonverbal Intelligence* (Brown, Sherbenou, and Dollar 1982) is similar in format to the Ravens Matrices and is based on problem solving. The test items require the child to identify relationships among abstract figures. Each item is composed of a group of figures with one or more figures missing, and the task is to choose the correct foil to complete the series from four or six options. The symbols depicted include one or more "characteristics of shape, position, direction or rotation, contiguity, shading size or length, movement, and pattern within the figure" (p. 4). The child must examine the differences and similarities among the figures in the set and the alternatives available in the response, establish the rule that binds the test items and foils, and then select a correct option based on the rule. Rules used in the construction of the test involve simple and more complex matching, addition, subtraction, alteration, progressions, classification, and intersections.

The test was constructed for use with individuals who are difficult to test on more traditional measures, such as those who are deaf, language delayed, mentally retarded, or learning disabled, since intelligence tests that rely on reading, writing, speaking, and listening are not appropriate for these populations. Brown and others (1982) also note that the test is less biased on the basis of cultural factors such as ethnicity and socioeconomic status because it is untimed; instructions are pantomimed; preliminary practice items are incorporated in the test; the content involves problem solving rather than pictures or writing; performance rather than paper-and-pencil tasks are used; and novel problems that avoid the confounding effect of previously learned information are to be solved.

The test is composed of two forms each with 50 items and may be administered by competently trained professionals (teachers, psychologists, speech-language pathologists, etc.) who adhere to the standards governing the administration and interpretation of educational tests. The age range is from 5 years to 85 years and 11 months. Suggested starting points for age ranges are provided. The basal is five consecutive items correct and the examiner may need to work backward from the starting point to establish the basal. The ceiling is three of five items incorrect. A total score is determined by computing the total items correct below the ceiling. The score then can be converted to a scaled score with a mean of 100 and a standard deviation of 15 and to a percentile rank.

The test was standardized on 1,929 subjects from 5–0 to 85–11 years and included no subjects with suspected intellectual deficits. Demographic characteristics of the sample appeared to approximate proportions of the 1980 U.S. census, suggesting that the standardization group was representative in terms of ethnicity, age, gender, geographic location, and so forth. Interpretive derived scores (TONI quotients) and percentiles are provided for each form of the test at varying intervals that range from 1 year at 5 to 6–11 years, 18 months from 7–0 to 8–5, 2½ years at 12–5 to 14–11, and larger intervals in adulthood (e.g., 25 to 49–11 years). Compared to other measures of intelligence, the age intervals appear quite large, particularly for the developmental period from 5 to 15 years.

In summary, performance scales are specifically designed for patients with speech, hearing, and language deficits who would typically be penalized on tests requiring communicative abilities. The scales offer an estimate of intellectual potential without confounding by language impairment.

Screening Tests of Intelligence

An important need in assessment of communicative disorders is a brief measurement instrument to provide an estimate of intellectual functioning when a trained psychologist is not available or when the time available for assessment is limited. The *Kaufman Brief Intelligence Test* (KBIT) (Kaufman and Kaufman 1990), a recent addition to instruments available to assess intellectual functioning, appears to fulfill this need. The test is a measure of verbal (vocabulary—including word knowledge and verbal concept formation) and nonverbal (matrices—ability to determine relationships and problem solve) intelligence and therefore appears to be broader in scope than the *Test of Nonverbal intelligence* and the Ravens Matrices. The test requires only 15 to 30 minutes to administer and can be given by paraprofessionals or technicians if adequately trained. The test is to be administered individually. The age range is 4 to 90 years. The measure is intended for screening purposes and not for diagnosis or neuropsychological interpretation.

Subtest 1 is an 82-item measure of vocabulary that includes two parts: Expressive vocabulary (45 items) administered to all testees, which requires the individual to name a pictured object and Definitions (37 items) administered to individuals eight years of age or older, which requires the person to provide a word based on two clues (phrase description and partial spelling). The Matrices subtest (Subtest 2) is composed of 48 items that deal with meaningful (people, objects) and nonmeaningful (symbols, designs) visual stimuli. The items are multiple choice with five, six, or eight choices available in the response field, depending on the difficulty of the item. Teaching of the task is allowed on sample items and the first two scored items of the vocabulary and matrices subtests. The intent of the teaching is to help ensure that the child knows exactly what kind of response is expected.

Suggested starting points are provided for each subtest and items are grouped in units of four or five items. The ceiling is incorrect responses to all items within a unit, and, with one exception, the total score is the ceiling item minus errors. Four interpretive procedures are completed for the vocabulary and matrices scores: (1) conversion to scaled scores; (2) determination of the standard score error of measurement band; (3) conversion of the scaled score to percentiles and assignment to descriptive categories; and (4) determination of the significance of scale score differences on the verbal and nonverbal measures.

The KBIT was standardized on a sample of 2,022 subjects from 4 to 90 years

TABLE 6–1   Summary of developmental and related measures

Tests	Ages
Developmental Scales	
Gesell Motor and Adaptive Scales	1–72 months
Denver Developmental Screening Test	1–72 months
Inventory of Early Development	0–7 years
Motor Skills Tests	
Oseretsky Test of Motor Proficiency	4–16 years
Lincoln-Oseretsky Motor Development Scale	6–14 years
Bruininks-Oseretsky Test of Motor Proficiency	4–5—14–5 years
Motor Problems Inventory	Preschool–5th grade
Visual-Motor Perception Tests	
Developmental Test of Visual Perception	3–9 years
Developmental Test of Visual-Motor Integration	2–15 years
Motor-Free Visual Perception Test	4–8 years
Bender Visual-Motor Gestalt Test	5–9 years
Performance (nonverbal) Intelligence	
Merrill-Palmer Scale of Mental Tests	24–48 months
Leiter International Performance Scale	2–18 years
Arthur Adaptation of the Leiter International Performance Scale	3–8 years
Hiskey-Nebraska Test of Learning Aptitude	2–5—17–5 years
Raven Progressive Matrices	6–65 years
Test of Nonverbal Intelligence	5—85–11 years
Screening Intelligence Test	
Kaufman Brief Intelligence Test	4–90 years

of age stratified on the basis of gender, geographic region, socioeconomic status, and race or ethnic group. Standard scores for vocabulary and matrices subtests are provided at 3-month intervals from 4 to 13 years, at 6-month intervals from 13 to 16 years, and at 1-year intervals from 16 to 18 years, with larger intervals for adults ranging from 5 to 10 years. Tables also are provided for determining the confidence intervals for the two subtests and the composite (two subtest scaled scores combined) with larger age groupings at older ages, as well as percentiles, descriptive categories, and stanine values derived from standard scores.

Split-half and test-retest reliability for the vocabulary, matrices, and composite scores generally is high. The average split-half reliability for vocabulary was 0.92; for matrices 0.87 and for the composite 0.93. Test-retest reliability coefficients were similar to the split-half coefficients. Based on increased scores with increases in chronological age and KBIT vocabulary and matrices correlations (0.69 and 0.59, respectively) with the WISC–R and the WAIS–R full-scale intelligence quotients, the measure appears to have good construct validity. Concurrent validity is supported by correlations of the KBIT composite score with the *Slosson Intelligence Test* (Slosson 1981) and the *Test of Nonverbal Intelligence* (Brown and others 1982) results, which ranged from 0.23 to 0.76.

SUMMARY

In this chapter, we lumped a potpourri of test formats (see Table 6–1), which, at least by their titles, would appear to have little in common. From the rationales of these separate test areas, however, the common theme that emerges is that coordinated motor development, visual-motor perception, and intelligence are all functions of integrated neurological development. Results from tests of this type have an important bearing on the understanding of communication abilities because they provide information about the general development of the child.

REFERENCES

ABT, I. A., H. M. ADLER, AND P. BARTELME, The relationship between the onset of speech and intelligence. *J. Amer. Med. Assoc.*, 93, 1351 (1929).

ARTHUR, G., *The Arthur Adaptation of the Leiter International Performance Scale*. Washington, D.C.: Psychological Service Center Press (1952).

BAYLEY, N. A., The development of motor ability during the first three years. *Monogr. Soc. Res. Child Develop.*, 1, 1–26 (1935).

BEERY, K. E., *Developmental Test of Visual Motor Integration: Administration and Scoring Manual*. Chicago: Follett Publishing Co. (1967).

BENDER, L., A visual motor Gestalt test and its clinical use. *Amer. Orthopsychiat. Assoc. Res. Monogr.*, No. 3 (1938).

BENDER, L., *Bender Motor Gestalt Test: Cards and Manual of Instructions*. New York: American Orthopsychiatry Association (1946).

BLOOM, L., AND M. LAHEY, *Language Development and Language Disorders*. New York: John Wiley (1978).

BRIGANCE, A. H., *Inventory of Early Development*. North Billerica, Mass.: Curriculum Associates (1978).

BROWN, L., R. SHERBENOU, AND S. DOLLAR, *Manual for the Test of Nonverbal Intelligence*. Austin, Tex.: Pro-Ed (1982).

BRUININKS, R. H., *Bruininks-Oseretsky Test of Motor Proficiency: Examiner's Manual*. Circle Pines, Minn.: American Guidance Service, Inc. (1978).

CLAWSON, A., *The Bender Visual Motor Gestalt for Children: A Manual*. Beverly Hills, Calif.: Western Psychological Services (1962).

COLARUSSO, R., AND D. HAMMILL, *Motor-Free Visual Perception Test*. San Rafael, Calif.: Academic Therapy Publications (1972).

CRATTY, B. J., *Perceptual and Motor Development in Infants and Children*. New York: Macmillan (1970).

DOLL, E. A., *The Oseretsky Tests of Motor Proficiency: A Translation from the Portuguese Adaptation*. Minneapolis: Educational Test Bureau (1946).

FRANKENBURG, W. K., AND J. B. DODDS, *The Denver Developmental Screening Test*. Denver: University of Colorado Medical Center (1967).

FROSTIG, M., W. LEFEVER, AND J. WHITTLESEY, *Developmental Test of Visual Perception: Administration and Scoring Manual*. Palo Alto, Calif.: Consulting Psychologists Press (1966).

GESELL, A., *The First Five Years of Life*. New York: Harper & Row (1940).

GESELL, A., *Studies in Child Development*. New York: Harper & Row (1948).

GESELL, A., H. THOMPSON, AND C. AMATRUDA, *Infant Behavior: Its Genesis and Growth*. New York: McGraw-Hill (1934).

GESELL, A., AND C. S. AMATRUDA, *Developmental Diagnosis*. New York: Hoeber (1941).

GESELL, A., AND C. S. AMATRUDA, Developmental diagnosis: Normal and abnormal child development. In *Clinical Methods and Pediatric Applications*, 2nd ed. New York: Hoeber (1947).

GESELL, A., AND F. L. ILG, *Infant and Child in the Culture of Today*. New York: Harper & Row (1947).

GOODENOUGH, F. L., *Measurement of Intelligence by Drawings*. New York: Harcourt Brace Jovanovich (1955).

HISKEY, M., *Manual: Hiskey-Nebraska Test of Learning Aptitude.* Lincoln Nebr.: Union College Press (1966).

HORROCKS, J., *Assessment of Behavior.* Columbus, Ohio: Chas. E. Merrill (1964).

JOHNSON, D., AND H. MYKLEBUST, *Learning Disabilities: Educational Principles and Practices.* New York: Grune & Stratton (1967).

KAUFMAN, A., AND N. KAUFMAN, *Kaufman Brief Intelligence Test.* Circle Pines, Minn.: American Guidance Service, Inc. (1990).

KOPPITZ, E., *The Bender Gestalt Test for Young Children.* New York: Grune & Stratton (1963).

KOPPITZ, E., *The Bender Gestalt Test for Young Children. Vol. II: Research and Application, 1963–1973.* New York: Grune & Stratton (1975).

KRAUFT, V., AND G. KRAUFT, Structured vs. unstructured visual-motor tests for educable retarded children. *Percep. Motor Skills,* 34, 691–694 (1972).

LEITER, R., *General Instructions for the International Performance Scale.* Chicago: Stoelting Company (1969).

LENNEBERG, E. H., The natural history of language. In *The Genesis of Language,* eds. F. Smith and G. A. Miller, Cambridge, Mass.: M.I.T. Press (1966).

MASLOW, P., AND OTHERS, The Marianne Frostig Developmental Test of Visual Perception. 1963 Standardization. *Percep. Motor Skills,* 19, 463–499 (1964).

MCGRAW, M. D., *The Neuromuscular Maturation of the Human Infant.* New York: Hafner (1963).

NUNNALLY, J., *Introduction to Psychological Measurement.* New York: McGraw-Hill (1970).

PASCAL, G., AND B. SUTTELL, *The Bender-Gestalt Test: Quantification and Validity for Adults.* New York: Grune & Stratton (1951).

RAVEN, J., *Guide to the Standard Progressive Matrices: Sets A, B, C, D, E.* London: H. K. Lewis (1960).

RAVEN, J., *Guide to Using the Coloured Progressive Matrices, Sets A, B, Ab.* London: H. K. Lewis (1963).

RAVEN, J., *Advanced Progressive Matrices: Sets I and II.* London: H. K. Lewis (1965).

RILEY, G. D., *Motor Problems Inventory: Manual.* Los Angeles: Western Psychological Services (1972).

SLOAN, W., The Lincoln-Oseretsky Motor Development Scale. *Genetic Psych. Monogr.,* 51, 183–252 (1955).

SLOSSON, R., *Slosson Intelligence Test for Children and Adults–Revised.* New York: Slosson Educational Publications (1981).

STUTSMAN, R., *Guide for Administering the Merrill-Palmer Scale of Mental Tests.* New York: Harcourt Brace Jovanovich (1948).

WERTHEIMER, W., Studies in the theory of Gestalt psychology. *Psychol. Forsch.,* 4 (1923).

7

Examination of the Speech-Production Mechanism

Physiology without anatomy is unfounded, anatomy without physiology is useless.

Franz Joseph Gall

The examination of the speech-production mechanism is very much a descriptive task. There are observations to be made and behaviors to be quantified, but there are no psychometrically based tests to aid in these tasks. Similarly, the data obtained typically do not allow a determination of adequacy from computation of a derived score that can be compared to normative data because the reference for adequacy lies within the experience of the examiner and not within the numbers tables. It is of paramount importance, then, that the examiner makes his observations systematically and with an understanding of why the patient is asked to perform each task.

Two evaluations are made as part of the examination. The first entails a determination of structural integrity. This involves a careful description of the size, shape, and relationship of the speech-production structures. Functional integrity, the second consideration, involves determining the adequacy of the system for producing speech-related movements. Structure and function are not separable, but we have divided the evaluation into these two parts because some of the observations are made of skeletal, dental, and muscular structures at rest, and others are made while the structures are executing speech-related movements.

Few aspects of the appraisal of speech disorders are treated in such a cursory and perfunctory manner as the speech-mechanism examination. This relatively superficial treatment of an integral part of the appraisal has resulted because clinicians frequently do not have a clear understanding of what they are looking for and the inferences they are to draw from what they find. The examination does not take long to complete, is not unusually difficult, and is as important and should be as routine as the audiological evaluation.

The idea that the oral-peripheral examination of the patient is as integral a part of patient assessment as auditory testing brings up an important point. Audiological procedures are geared toward determining the anatomic and functional integrity of the hearing mechanism. An otoscopic examination and tympanometry are carried out to determine the status of the tympanic membrane–ossicular chain system, and test batteries are used to assess the integrity of the auditory nerve and higher neural functions of audition. The audiological examination, then, is essentially an evaluation of a set of structures and the neural mechanisms that subserve them. Likewise, an examination of the speech-production mechanism is an evaluation of structures and the neural mechanisms responsible for their innervation.

Perusal of any standard neurology text (Alpers and Mancall 1971; Brain and Walton 1969; DeJong 1958) quickly reveals the close similarity between procedures used by the speech pathologist during the course of the oral-peripheral examination and the cranial nerve examination of the neurologist. The two examinations have similarities, but they are by no means identical. The cranial nerve examination involves testing the sensory and/or motor functions of each of the highly specialized cranial nerves for evidence of peripheral or central nervous system damage. The oral-peripheral examination entails the evaluation of only some of the nerves. It is abbreviated to the extent that some motor functions, such as eye movements, and some sensory processes, such as olfaction and taste, are omitted or only screened while highly integrated execution of speech movements is evaluated in detail. It is an extension of the cranial nerve examination as well because respiratory muscles, whose innervation is by means of the spinal nerves, are also examined. A listing of the cranial nerves and an abbreviated description of their functions are provided in Table 7–1.

Before considering the procedures of the oral examination, several aspects of speech production need to be examined. Speech is an overlaid function, since the primary role of the respiratory, laryngeal, and articulatory systems is the maintenance of life-support systems by means of vegetative breathing and feeding. Consequently, it is readily apparent that the speech mechanism is capable of producing muscular forces and structural displacements, velocities and accelerations considerably greater than are normally necessary for speech production. Two examples may suffice to demonstrate this point. We have all seen the circus performer who hangs by her teeth from the high trapeze. She is capable of developing enough force between her teeth to support her weight. Speech activities, in comparison, never approximate these maximal abilities of the masticatory musculature. Similarly, if we examined the average subglottal pressure needed for speech production, we

TABLE 7-1   The cranial nerves and their functions (abbreviated)

Cranial Nerve	Function
I. Olfactory	Sense of smell
II. Optic	Vision
III. Oculomotor	Eye movement
IV. Trochlear	
V. Abducens	
VI. Trigeminal	Jaw movements
	Sensation for face
VII. Facial	Facial movements
	Taste for anterior two-thirds of tongue
VIII. Auditory	Hearing
	Maintenance of equilibrium
IX. Glossopharyngeal	Pharyngeal movements
	Sensation to soft palate and pharynx
	Taste to posterior third of tongue
X. Vagus	Sensation for pharynx, larynx
	Thoracic and abdominal viscera
	Pharyngeal and laryngeal movements
XI. Spinal Accessory	Shoulder girdle movements
XII. Hypoglossal	Tongue movements

would find it to be approximately 5 to 10 cm H_2O while the respiratory unit is capable of producing pressures in excess of 50 cm H_2O, such as during heavy lifting. We must be aware then that the tasks we ask the patient to perform are well within the physiological capabilities of a normal adult or child.

In light of the significant differences between typical and maximal performance, it is not surprising that the speech-production apparatus is capable of substantial compensations for structural or functional inadequacies. Examples are readily available for both speech-impaired and normal speakers. Children with repaired cleft lip who have reduced lip tissue and scarring continue to produce bilabial plosives. In fact, bilabial plosives are one of the least frequent types of errors for repaired-cleft speakers. Similarly, speakers with partial or complete glossectomy (partial or complete resection of the tongue) may produce speech that is only minimally reduced in intelligibility.

The functional compensatory abilities of normal speakers have also been demonstrated. Lindblom and Sundberg (1971) and Lindblom, Lubker, and Gay (1979) have shown that normal speakers can produce formant frequencies with bite blocks between their teeth, at the first glottal pulse of a vowel, that approximate those of an unimpeded condition. This suggests that the speech-production mechanism is capable of substantial and immediate reorganizational abilities. Moreover, Hixon, Mead, and Goldman (1976) observed that subjects maintained a relatively constant subglottal pressure during speech, using widely varying patterns of muscular forces while standing and sitting, positions in which the force of gravity would have considerably different effects. More informal examples are the ability to produce speech while eating or with a pipe between the teeth without a significant reduction in intelligibility. The point to be made is that the speech-production mechanism is capable of significant compensation for typical or novel constraints imposed on its activity.

When maximal compensation has been reached, it appears that any additional psychological or physiological loading has the effect of deteriorating performance. Indirect evidence is readily available for aphasic patients who demonstrate reduced performance when fatigued or under emotional stress and for stutterers who typically have a greater number of disfluencies when in situations of great communicative demand. Knowledge of the patient's condition at the time of testing is, therefore, important to making inferences regarding the integrity of the speech-production apparatus and may offer information on probable prognosis as well.

Articulatory structures are variable even in a "normal" group of speakers. If dental configurations were used as an example, it would be found that less than half the population has what could be described as "normal" dentition. Likewise, there are variations in tongue size, palatal vault height, and size of the mandible. More than for almost any other group of judgments to be made, the variations on normal will have to be considered in determining the anatomic integrity of the patient being examined, as well as the significance of the deviations in relation to the speech presented.

Finally, the entire examination should be completed even if only a part of the speech-production apparatus is involved. If you have a medical examination, the physician will evaluate a number of systems: neurological, cardiovascular, genitourinary, and so on, whether you have an ulcer or head trauma, which points out the fact that no system of an organism is functionally independent. The examination should be completed in its entirety, whether the source of the problem is limited, such as an acquired quadriplegia due to an upper spinal cord lesion, or involves the entire speech-production system, such as in Parkinson's disease.

We present some procedures for evaluating the speech-production mechanism, including the voice evaluation and oral-peripheral examination. The descriptions should not be considered exhaustive but rather representative. Other descriptions of these examinations are provided by Darley, Aronson, and Brown (1975), Dworkin (1978), Mason (1969), and Mason and Simon (1977). We also discuss how instrumentation may be used to enhance and extend these clinical observations.

Before we begin, a few comments about maximal performance measures are in order. Traditionally, maximal performance has been an integral part of the assessment of the speech-production apparatus. Recently, Kent, Kent, and Rosenbek (1987) reviewed this body of literature. They noted that maximum duration of phonation, maximum fricative duration, maximum phonation volume, maximum expiratory pressure, fundamental frequency range, maximum sound pressure level, maximum occluding force of the articulators and diadochokinetic rate are comparable to tests of strength, range of motion, and speed in the neurological examination. They concluded that these measures provide useful information on phonatory and articulatory performance, constitute a potential test battery for speech assessment, and show that the demands of typical speech production are within these maximum performance levels but are inadequate because they contain high intrasubject and intersubject variability, are not necessarily independently interpretable, and are lacking in several respects such as in differences in expected performance across the life span. Based on this review, the maximum performance measures cited as part of the following assessment paradigm must be viewed cautiously. Until a new generation of measures and standardization is complete, however, they are included as the best available tools for determining important information about the capabilities of the speech-production apparatus.

EVALUATION OF RESPIRATORY
AND LARYNGEAL SYSTEMS

The respiratory system is relatively resistant to disease processes and traumatic lesions that would affect the development of air pressures and air flows necessary for speech production. This is perhaps related to the crucial role of respiration for the maintenance of an oxygen supply to the cells of the body. Witness to this is the patient with a traumatic lesion to the spinal cord at the fifth cervical vertebra. Although the effects of this type of lesion are to produce a quadriplegia with paralysis of some of the respiratory muscles, the patient continues to be able to produce speech with only a minimal impairment since intelligible speech does not require more than tidal volume. Respiratory deficits that affect phonation and articulation relate more to the inability to coordinate respiratory activities with laryngeal and upper-airway functions. Consider the patient with congenital cerebral palsy of an athetoid type who begins expiration and then suddenly stops due to involuntary movement resulting from contraction of the inspiratory musculature. This patient has sufficient respiratory activity to maintain life and to generate pressures and flows but cannot adequately control the input and output of the respiratory unit for speech production. Since the respiratory and laryngeal processes are so closely related, they are typically examined together as part of the evaluation of the speech-production mechanism.

Individuals with voice problems may be identified from screening or be referred. Screening of children in the schools may be problematic, since colds, allergies, and vocal abuse may result in temporary hoarseness where direct intervention is warranted. Case (1991) suggests that the child be questioned to determine whether the hoarseness is temporary, notes that the classroom teacher should also be contacted, and recommends a follow-up screening two weeks later if a problem is noted. Interestingly, Davis and Harris (1992) found that classroom teachers can consistently identify children with voice problems and therefore are a good source of information when screening elementary school children. With referral from a physician, it is expected that information regarding duration, severity, and possible etiology of disorder has been explored. A detailed history and evaluation may be necessary for individuals who are self-referred with a history of voice problems.

Evaluation of voice disorders can be divided into two broad categories: history of the problem and examination of the respiratory-phonatory system. It is assumed that a general history has been obtained by interview so that this portion of the history will relate specifically to the voice disorder itself. It also is assumed that patients will be evaluated for other than respiratory and laryngeal dysfunction. An example of a voice evaluation form is included in Figure 7–1.

```
                         VOICE EVALUATION

A. HISTORY OF SPEECH DISORDER

   1. Patient's description of the problem
      Severity _____
      Effect on communication _____
      Etiology _____
   2. Development of the Problem
      Onset _____
      Progression _____
      Consistency _____
      Duration _____
   3. Previous Voice Evaluation or Therapy
      _____
   4. Vocal Habits
      Occupation _____
      Vocal Abuse _____
   5. Additional Significant History
      Familial _____
      Medical _____
      Social _____
      Emotional (concern for problem) _____
      _____


B. RESPIRATORY AND LARYNGEAL EXAMINATION

   1. Respiratory Efficiency

      Observations of breathing:  Clavicular _____
      Abdominal _____Thoracic_____
      Shortness of breath _____
      Audible breathing _____

      Breath Control:
      Counts on one breath _____
      Sustain a, i, or u: Trials ____ ____ ____
      Prolong voiceless fricative /s/ ____ ____ ____
      Prolong voiced fricative /z/ ____ ____ ____

      Muscular tension of the chest and neck that appears to be
      related to breath supply and control? _____
      _____


   2. Laryngeal Observations

      Tension _____
      Muscular contractions exhibited during phonation that are similar
      to those exhibited during swallowing _____
      _____

      Indirect Laryngoscopy _____
      _____
```

FIGURE 7–1 Example voice evaluation form.

C. PHONATION

1. Pitch
   Subjective appropriateness _____
   Habitual Pitch _____
   Pitch Range (# of notes) _____
   Optimum Pitch _____

   Pitch Control
   Discrimination _____
   Imitation of high, medium, and low pitches _____
   _____
   Production of a tone _____
   Imitation of upward and downward inflectional patterns _____
   _____
   Ability to maintain steady pitch _____
   _____

2. Loudness
   Subjective appropriateness for situations

   Ability to alter loudness:
   Imitate soft, medium, and loud sounds _____
   _____
   Glide from loud to soft during production of vowels _____
   _____
   Discrimination of loudness _____

3. Quality
   Type of Disorder
   Breathy _____Harsh_____Hoarse _____
   Denasal _____Nasal_____Aphonia _____
   Severity _____
   Changes in Quality during: Reading   Prolonging Vowels
     Vary Pitch   _____   _____
     Vary Loudness   _____   _____
     Vary Rate   _____   _____
   During Physical Exertion   _____   _____
   During Exaggeration of
     Articulatory Movements   _____   _____

4. Related Observations
   Pitch Breaks_____ Phonation Breaks _____
   Hard Glottal Attack_____ Glottal Fry _____
   Spastic Dysphonia_____ Other _____
   _____

D. Oral Peripheral Examination

E. Hearing Screening

FIGURE 7–1   Example Voice Evaluation Form (continued)

History of the Problem.   The case history information we discussed in Chapter 2 was general in purpose. Voice and a number of other problems require further specific background. A voice history will entail a self-description of the problem by the patient and a general history of the problem as deduced from the patient's history and collateral information, such as results of medical examinations, vocational and family history, and so on.

The self-description of the voice problem should include questions regarding the nature of the problem—what does the voice problem sound like and feel like; the severity of the problem—how significantly does it affect the communication process; the effect of the problem—how "bad" is the problem, and how "different" does the voice sound; and the etiology of the problem according to the patient. The purpose of this portion of the history taking is to evaluate the patient's view of the nature, severity, etiology, and effect of the voice problem.

The general history of the voice problem will explore other aspects of its development. When did it begin? Was there a sudden or gradual onset? Has the problem become progressively worse, or has the course of the problem been characterized by plateaus and intermittent remissions? Has the problem been previously evaluated and treated? If so, by whom? Is the problem consistent, or does it appear to be affected by voice usage, time of day, and so forth? The patient's voice usage habits should be explored in detail if there appears to be hyperfunction. The results of medical examinations, previous therapy, general medical history, and social familial history should be explored with care. The important thing for you to remember is that you want to gain all the information possible about the patient and her disorder before, during, and following its onset. The importance of this exploration of the problem cannot be underestimated because of the host of metabolic, traumatic, neurologic, and emotional factors that produce voice disorders.

The interview process also allows the examiner to note important aspects of the voice disorder that will require further exploration. For example, is habitual pitch appropriate to the patient's age and sex? Is loudness suitable to the situation? Is the patient breathy, hoarse, harsh? What are voice usage patterns?

Physical Examination.   The examiner should carefully observe respiratory and laryngeal characteristics. The type of vegetative and speech respiratory patterns should be noted. Normally, the only respiratory pattern of particular concern is the use of clavicular breathing. Clavicular breathing involves upward movement of the clavicles to increase the size of the respiratory unit. It is of concern because it is less efficient than thoracic-abdominal breathing patterns and because it may bring about tension in extrinsic laryngeal muscles. Any shortness of breath and struggle to breathe should be noted. The tension in the accessory (extrinsic) muscles of the larynx should be observed because vocal hyperfunction is frequently evidenced by an increase in extrinsic laryngeal muscle tension. The tension can be noted by palpation of the neck musculature during phonation of vowels, counting, and conversational speech.

Considerable controversy exists regarding the role of the speech pathologist in the indirect examination of the larynx. Needless to say, every individual with a voice problem whom you are asked to examine should be evaluated by a laryngologist before proceeding with therapy since it is the physician's task to differentially diagnose the disorder and to provide surgical and drug therapy if these are deemed necessary. Boone (1983) noted that:

> . . . the diagnostic examination of the vocal folds belongs to the laryngologist. After the laryngologist has made a diagnosis, the speech-language pathologist trained in laryngoscopy may occasionally use mirror laryngoscopy to view the cords indirectly; this will facilitate the treatment of the patient by allowing him or her to make judgments about vocal cord adequacy. (p. 79)

What then is the speech pathologist's role in indirect observation of laryngeal structure and function? We agree with the statement of Moore (1957):

> The [indirect laryngoscopy] examination technique can and should be learned by the voice pathologist, since it is a help to be able to observe laryngeal conditions and to follow changes which occur in the course of therapy. It should be emphasized, however, that the diagnosing of laryngeal diseases and disorders is the province and responsibility of the laryngologist. (p. 686)

The physical examination, therefore, should involve a careful observation of respiratory patterns, laryngeal extrinsic musculature tension, and indirect laryngoscopy. Indirect laryngoscopy is utilized to note the status of the larynx and to follow the course of laryngeal changes resulting from therapy but is never utilized to make differential diagnoses, which are clearly the province of the physician. Indirect laryngoscopy requires a minimum of time, a limited number of inexpensive instruments, and an average degree of dexterity. The patient is seated with knees together, head tilted slightly forward, and chin up. The examiner is seated on a stool approximately level with the patient's knees and directly in front. A light is positioned behind and slightly to the right of the patient's head. A head mirror is worn by the examiner and is used to focus a beam of light onto a laryngeal mirror introduced into the oral cavity. With the tongue firmly held with a piece of gauze by the examiner and with the back of the mirror lifting the soft palate, a slight rotation of the mirror will allow visualization of the laryngeal structures. Structures should be examined in a serial order. A detailed discussion of these procedures is provided by Netter (1964). The student should practice these procedures with careful attention to detail and under the direct supervision of a physician or speech pathologist trained in these techniques before attempting to utilize them in the course of therapy or diagnosis.

Determining Respiratory Efficiency.   Several tasks may be utilized to provide information about the efficiency with which the patient utilizes the respiratory system for phonation. One method is to ask the patient to count as far as possible on one breath after being provided with a rate-of-count model of approximately three digits per second (Boone 1977). The length of time she is able to count and the number of digits produced is recorded. Additionally, information regarding total performance is noted, such as how the patient maximally inspires and how well she sustains exhalation. A similar task is to ask the patient to prolong a vowel such as /a/, /i/, or /u/ as long as possible at a comfortable pitch and loudness level. The average of three productions can then be compared to norms available regarding maximal performance (Ptacek and Sander 1963; Yanagihara and Koike 1967;

Yanagihara and others 1966). For example, Ptacek and Sander found maximum phonation time for vowels averaged 25 seconds for men and 17 seconds for women. The presence of voice tremor, intermittent arrests of the voice, and intermittent waxing and waning of loudness is noted. Another method of determining the ability to sustain expiration is to ask the patient to read as many words as possible from a selected passage without renewing her air supply. A related task is to ask the patient to prolong the voiceless fricative /s/ as long as possible. This provides information on how well the patient can maintain expiration without phonation. The patient is then asked to produce the voiced cognate /z/ as long as possible. Typically, the patient without vocal pathology will be able to maintain each of the fricatives the same length of time, while the patient with vocal-fold pathology will be unable to maintain the voiced fricative as long as the voiceless due to reduced phonatory efficiency, assuming that velopharyngeal functioning is within normal limits. Eckel and Boone (1981) found that 95 percent of patients with glottal margin pathologies (e.g., nodules) have /s–z/ ratios higher than 1.4, indicating marked reduction in voiced durations. It should be noted, however, that maximum durations are age dependent (e.g., Tait, Michel, and Carpenter 1980) and are expected to vary depending on intensity, pitch, number of trials, feedback, and the vowel produced (Schmidt, Klingholz, and Martin 1988; Stone 1983). Sorenson and Parker (1992) found no significant difference in maximum /s/ duration between 11 children with vocal pathology and matched normal-speaking children. However, /z/ durations and /s–z/ ratios were significantly different, lending support to the use of the ratio as a tool in evaluating glottal efficiency. Moreover, Fendler and Shearer (1988) have demonstrated that the ratio appears to have good test-retest reliability.

Several types of information can be obtained from these procedures. First, the ability of the patient to sustain a controlled exhalation with and without phonation can be described. Second, the relative efficiency of phonation can be determined by comparing the duration of sustained productions of voiced and voiceless fricatives. Third, reductions in maximal performance can be noted for sustained vowels. Although this information may be of some value, remember that normal speech production typically does not require a maximal effort on the part of the patient.

Evaluation of Aspects of Phonation.   Several important aspects of the phonatory process are typically examined as part of the voice evaluation. These include pitch, loudness, and quality. Each of these parameters of voice production will be considered individually although these processes are intricately related. Some of the information you will obtain is subjective and based on observations and ratings, other data (fundamental frequency, intensity, duration) might best be characterized as objective and obtained from instrumental analysis. We first consider clinical procedures and rating scales; we then return to instrumental analyses later in this chapter.

Pitch.   Earlier in our discussion, we noted that you should make some judgment during the initial interview as to whether the pitch of the patient's voice is "too high" or "too low" in relation to the patient's age and sex. Additionally, you will want to obtain information regarding the patient's habitual pitch, optimal pitch, and pitch range.

Habitual pitch is the central tendency of pitches used by an individual (Fairbanks 1960). As such, it represents a range that may be influenced by situational variables and the emotional status of the patient. Several methods may be utilized to determine habitual pitch. One suggested by Boone (1983) as the easiest and most valid involves the recording of conversational speech and oral reading from the patient during the first visit to the clinic. The speech sample is then analyzed by stopping the tape recorder at selected points and attempting to match the patient's habitual pitch by means of a pitch pipe. This is accomplished by starting at approximately the mean fundamental frequency of male or female speakers (128 Hz or C_3, for adult males, 213 Hz or A_3, for adult females, 256 Hz or C_4 for prepubertal child) and then moving by gradations (sharps and flats) until the habitual pitch is approximated (the distribution of fundamental frequency for males and females is presented in Figure 7–2). This procedure should be repeated seven or eight times or more during the course of analyzing the speech sample. The modal pitch (most frequently occurring) is determined and designated as the patient's habitual pitch. Boone suggests that utilizing modal rather than mean pitch offers a more valid estimate of habitual pitch.

Another model of determining habitual pitch has been suggested by Fairbanks (1960). A reading sample of approximately 180 words is selected. The selection is divided into three 60-word segments. During the reading of the first 60 words, normal inflectional patterns are utilized by the patient. During the reading of the second 60 words, the patient is asked to compress the range until by the end of this section he is chanting in a monotone. He should then complete the reading utilizing this monotone and finish with a humming or singing of notes equal to his habitual pitch. A pitch pipe or piano can then be utilized to identify the habitual

FIGURE 7–2   Distribution of fundamental frequency for males and females.

(From W. Zemlin. *Speech and Hearing Science*. Englewood Cliffs. N.J.: Prentice Hall, 1968. Used by permission.)

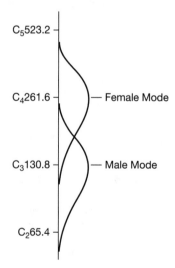

pitch. The whole procedure may be repeated to determine the accuracy of the estimate. Other procedures utilized to determine habitual pitch include asking the patient to sing a tone without a model and then attempting to match the produced tone on a pitch pipe or piano. Similarly, the patient can be asked to count to 10 and then to prolong a vowel, the pitch of the vowel being determined with a pitch pipe. Repetition of these procedures will allow a determination of modal habitual pitch.

The total pitch range can be determined by asking the patient to sing up and down the scale. Boone (1983) suggested that this be accomplished by providing the patient with three-second models of the tones to be produced (recorded by a male, female, or child). The patient is asked to match each tone and to take a breath between each production. The patient is first asked to match notes to the lowest tone, then to go up the scale to the highest notes he can produce including the falsetto, matching tones back down to the lowest note and then back up to the highest note again. This procedure provides an estimate of the total pitch range of the patient. The total number of tones is recorded. The examiner should be aware, however, that patients will not be equally skilled in matching tones.

Optimum pitch is the perceptual correlate of the maximal efficiency of vibration of the vocal folds. This suggests that the vocal folds have an optimal rate of vibration determined by their length, mass, and natural elasticity. A number of methods have been suggested for estimating the optimal frequency of vibration.

1. Determine the total pitch range including falsetto. Optimum pitch is located one-fourth of the way from the bottom of the pitch range. For adult females, it may be one to two notes below the one-fourth level (Fairbanks 1960).
2. Determine the total pitch range excluding falsetto. One-third of the distance from the bottom of the pitch range will be the optimum pitch.
3. Ask patient to take a deep breath and intone "ah" on expiration (Murphy 1964).
4. Ask patient to grunt "ah" or "oh," gradually prolonging the utterances until a passage is chanted at the original grunt pitch level (Murphy 1964).
5. Ask patient to stop up his ears and sing "ah" or hum "m" up and down the scale until the pitch level at which the tone swells or is louder is identified (Murphy 1964).
6. Cough sonorously on an /i/ sound (Murphy 1964).
7. Yawn and sigh should produce optimum pitch (Boone 1983).
8. Say "uh'huh" and note pitch (Boone 1983).

After an optimal pitch level has been determined, the patient may be asked to produce several vowels and words to help substantiate the determined pitch. These procedures will reveal approximately the same optimal pitch level. Fisher (1966) suggests that the optimal pitch in normal speakers fulfills several requirements: (1) It is within the pitch range where maximal vocal fold efficiency of vibration is located; (2) there are at least four notes below the modal optimum pitch for downward intonations; and (3) there is at least an octave above modal optimum pitch for upward intonations. She suggested further that the habitual (modal) pitch should be changed if it is less than four notes above the lowest note that can be phonated clearly or if the modal pitch is as much as two notes from optimum pitch. Finally, she suggested that 10 notes is the minimal range of intonation required for production of "factual" speech. This range will include three notes below the modal pitch and six notes above the optimal modal pitch. Moreover, she suggests that an increase in the upper range interval (from modal optimal pitch to the highest pitch) will increase the effectiveness of speech more surely than any other one device. Wilson (1987) has provided composite tables of mean fundamental frequency and acceptable fundamental frequency limits for males and females between 1 and 18 years of age that the examiner may find of value in determining the appropriateness of habitual pitch levels.

Pitch-control skills are also evaluated if the habitual pitch of the patient is to be changed to optimal pitch. Van Riper (1978) recommended that the following pitch skills be examined: (1) ability to discriminate between two pitches that differ in a single note (these can be sung or played on a piano or pitch pipe); (2) ability to hum at high, medium, and low pitches after they are presented by the examiner; (3) ability to produce a tune alone or in conjunction with the examiner; and (4) ability to follow upward and downward inflectional patterns. Finally, the ability to maintain a steady pitch for a specified period of time should be examined.

Loudness.   Loudness can be defined as the perceptual correlate of acoustic energy produced by the speech mechanism. Two aspects of the loudness parameter are considered in the voice evaluation: (1) its suitability to the conversational setting, and (2) the ability of the patient to volitionally alter it. Appropriateness of the loudness level used by the patient can be assessed by requesting that he produce levels consistent with situations. For example, the examiner should gradually move away from the patient and ask him to produce speech consistent with the distance from the examiner. Ability to control loudness can be assessed by asking the patient to sustain tones at soft, medium, and high intensity levels, to imitate loudness of sustained sounds and words presented by the examiner, and to glide from loud to soft during production of vowels. Finally, the ability to discriminate different loudness levels can be determined by presenting two tones of differing loudness and asking the patient to judge which of the two is louder. This procedure is facilitated by having pairs of words or vowels tape-recorded and ready for use. Reduced variation in loudness during conversational speech is also noted. Typically, loudness problems are indicative of psychological or organic problems. The examiner should also remember that there is no optimal loudness level for an individual, loudness depends upon the situation in which the patient finds himself.

Quality.   A wide variety of terms have been utilized to describe voice-quality problems. We utilize only four: breathiness, harshness, hoarseness, and nasality. Breathiness is voice quality characterized by an audible escape of air. Harshness is typified by aperiodicity of vocal-fold vibration and is usually accompanied by hard glottal attacks and low pitch. Hoarseness is defined as a combination of breathiness and harshness with both audible escape of air and aperiodicity of vocal-fold vibration.

Two types of abnormal nasal resonance are typically identified as part of the voice evaluation. Hypernasality is a voice-quality disorder due to abnormal coupling of the oral and nasal cavities and is characterized acoustically by antiresonances and reduced formant frequencies. Denasality is produced by abnormal reduction in the amount of coupling typically utilized for production of nasalized consonants such as /m/ and /n/. Insofar as voice-quality disorders are due to problems at the level of the larynx, hyper- and hyponasality are not voice problems but articulation problems. That is, the phonemes are inappropriately articulated—either as nasal resonance where oral resonance is expected or as a lack of nasality on intended nasal phonemes. Fairbanks's (1940) definition, for example, was:

> The test of the existence of a voice quality disorder is whether or not the quality that is heard is independent of phonemes, or, in other words, whether or not the phenomenon heard can be superimposed upon a good example of a voiced sound. (p. 202)

By that definition, hyper- and hyponasality are *not* voice-quality disorders. From a remediation standpoint, the therapeutic regime for abnormalities of nasal resonance will usually have some features common to articulation therapy and some procedures similar to voice therapy.

Several procedures should be utilized to estimate voice-quality disturbances. By this time in the evaluation, you will have collected and taped a number of speech samples from the patient and should be able to describe and estimate the severity of the disorder from these samples. If these samples are insufficient, you may wish to obtain a sample of connected speech, oral reading, and isolated production of vowels and voiced continuants. From careful listening, an estimate of the disorder can be obtained and recorded on a rating scale that considers breathiness, hoarseness, and harshness.

Also, the effects of varying pitch, loudness, and rate on voice quality should be evaluated. Ask the patient to read a speech sample and prolong vowels at lower and higher than habitual pitch levels, at higher and lower than habitual loudness levels, and at faster and slower than habitual rates. Examine the effects of physical exertion and relaxation on voice quality by requesting that the patient produce words or an extended vowel during pushing or pulling activities and during relaxation. Finally, note whether voice quality is improved when articulatory movement is exaggerated during the reading of a passage. Pay careful attention to the presence of laryngeal extrinsic musculature tension during these activities. Also, carefully note the presence and frequency of hard glottal attacks during production of conversational speech and reading. Wilson (1979) provides rating scales for estimating the amount of vocal abuse produced by a patient. The scales include vocal abuse categories of shouting, screaming, cheering, excessive talking, strained vocalizations, reverse phonation, explosive release of vocalizations, abrupt glottal attack, throat clearing, coughing, talking in noise, and other factors. Each category is rated in amount (0 = none; 1 = little; 2 = frequent; 3 = excessive) and degree (1 = mild; 2 = moderate; 3 = severe). Although these ratings can be completed as part of the voice evaluation, other persons acquainted with the patient such as teachers, friends, and relatives may also need to be interviewed.

Wilson (1979) has devised a voice profile for efficiently recording the results of observations from the evaluation. A scale of severity is included which ranges from 1 for a minimal problem to 7 which reflects significant interference with communication. A second "cross" scale is used to rate the relative "openness" of the vocal folds during phonation and ranges from –4 (totally open = aphonia) to +3 (hyperadduction = inability to maintain phonation) on the ordinate and pitch deviance from +3 (high) to –3 (low) on the abscissa with the juncture of the two lines (a rating of 1) indicating normal function. Nasality is rated from +4 (nasality on all voiced sounds) to –2 (lack of nasal resonance). Similarly, there are ratings for rate (slow/fast), intensity (soft/loud), and vocal range (monotone/variable pitch) from –2 to +2. Space is also provided to note whether the problem is constant or variable.

Summary of Voice Evaluation.   These procedures should yield a large body of information regarding the patient's voice problem, including presenting complaint, history of the disorder, habitual pitch, pitch range, optimal pitch, habitual loudness level and ability to alter loudness, type of voice-quality disturbance, and the effects of rate, loudness, and pitch on overall quality, respiratory and laryngeal efficiency, and the types of abusive vocal behavior utilized by the patient. For children, procedural guides developed by Boone (1980) and Wilson (1987) may aid in improving the efficiency of gathering this information. From the information gained, a prognosis should be made and appropriate therapy instituted, if warranted.

Prognosis in Voice Disorders.   Prognosis will depend on many factors including the etiology of the disorder, the duration of the problem, the severity of the disorder, and the motivation of the patient. Obviously, all medical, social, vocational, and speech and language evaluation results must be considered carefully in order to determine prognosis. A sample behavioral prognostic checklist for "functional" voice disorders has been developed by Murphy (1964). The checklist includes 11 vocal (e.g., severity and complexity of the voice disorders, loudness level, respiration, articulation), 5 auditory (hearing acuity, sound discrimination, ability to imitate vocal sounds, ability to carry a melody, auditory memory span), 14 psychosocial (e.g., general level of emotional adjustment, absence of associated symptoms, self-defensive behavior, general nonverbal spontaneity), and 3 miscellaneous criteria (intelligence, general physical condition, other) that are rated as inferior, below average, average, above average, or superior. The checklist also includes a rating of overall prognosis for improvement. Murphy indicated that the rating scale is for "discussion" purposes only. However, if it is coupled with other information about the patient and his problem, it may prove to be a valuable tool. An accurate prognosis can only be made by someone with "all the facts" and the clinical experience to evaluate them.

EXAMINATION OF THE ORAL-FACIAL SPEECH MECHANISM

The purpose of the examination of the speech mechanism is to describe the status and function of the articulatory and resonatory systems. As such, it is an important part of *any and all* speech and language evaluations and should be carried out systematically and efficiently. This section describes the procedures involved in conducting this portion of the examination. An example of an oral-peripheral examination form is included in Figure 7–3.

Positioning of the Client.   Mason (1969) has described how the patient should be positioned. She should be in a posture that most clearly approximates that which she uses during speaking. Typically, this involves positioning the client in an erect position in a chair, with eyes focused directly forward. Except when we

Name:_____Sex:_____Birthdate:_____Case No:_____
Referral reason:_____By:_____
Examiner:_____Date:_____

STRUCTURE (JUDGMENT)

L	T	Te	A	P

(L-Lips; T-Tongue; Te-Teeth; A-Dental Arch; P-Palate)

Normal Structure

Slight deviation—probably no adverse effect on speech

Moderate deviation—possible adverse effect on speech; remedial services may be required, particularly if other structures of speech are also deviant

Extreme deviation—sufficient to prevent normal production of speech; modification of structure required, either with or without clinical speech services

FUNCTION—Diadochokinesis

Average of three trials of 5-second duration each.

Single syllables: puh, tuh, kuh
Lip Approximation:
 (puh) ____, ____, ____, average per second ____
Tongue-tip-alveolar:
 (tuh) ____, ____, ____, average per second ____
Back-tongue-palate:
 (kuh) ____, ____, ____, average per second ____
 Combined syllables: (puh-tuh-kuh) ____, ____, ____
 average per second ____
 Gag reflex _____ (present or absent)

                    ****
If no significant deviations in structure or function, the form can be discontinued at this point. Continue with following page for more description, especially when deviations are noted.

FIGURE 7–3 Sample oral examination form.
(From W. Johnson, F. L. Darley, and D. C. Spriestersbach, *Diagnostic Methods in Speech Pathology.* New York: Harper & Row, 1963. By permission.)

(Indicate severity of deviation with description)
NOSE—structural deviations _____
        Function _____(structure, etc.) _____
Lips—structural deviations _____(repaired) _____
        cleft: Right___Left___Bilat.___Includes premaxilla _____
        corners retract: bilaterally_____symmetrically _____
                        Unilaterally: Right_____Left _____

MANDIBLE AND DENTAL STRUCTURES:
    Mandible: Normal____Prognathic____Retruded____
    Occlusion: Normal____Neutrocclusion____Distocclusion____
        Mesiocclusion____(relative to first molars)
    Lateral relationship: Normal____Crossbite R____L____
    Overbite: Normal____Open____Closed____
    Condition of teeth: _____

PALATE:
    Hard Palate: shape____arch____width____cleft____
    Soft palate: short____tight____blue____cleft____
        movement____ (gag____ "ha"____)
    Uvula: bifid____ absent____ normal____

TONSILS: absent____normal____enlarged____inflamed____infected____

ORO-PHARYNX: size____; movement: mesial____lateral____none evident____
TONGUE: Size____; tremor: (rest)____(protruded)____
        Function; curl____, point____
        move voluntary; up____down____right____left____
        sweep lips smoothly ____ move independently of mandible____
        tongue-thrust swallow ____

COMMENTS:

FIGURE 7–3   Sample oral examination form (continued).

are making structural evaluations of the palate, the client should not tilt her head backward for the intraoral examination. Studies (McWilliams, Musgrave, and Crozier 1968) have shown that modifications of a "natural" head posture can distort normal muscle relationships in the head and neck and produce physiologic differences that do not reflect normal function during speech production. Therefore, the patient should sit with her head in a natural upright position with her mouth aligned on a horizontal plane with the eye level of the examiner.

Facial Musculature.   The head and neck should be examined carefully. Any scars on the side of the head and neck should be noted. The symmetry of the face should be examined at rest. Drooping of the corner of the lip or ptosis (partial or complete closure of the eyelid) may indicate weakness. If upper-lip scarring is observed, the amount of upper-lip tissue, shape of the scar, and tightness of the upper lip should be recorded. Drooling, lack of forehead wrinking on one side, and incomplete labial closure are also indicative of muscle weakness.

Voluntary nonspeech movements should be tested. Ask the patient to smile, and note if the corners of the lips move equally on each side. Request she pucker her lips, and note if this activity is symmetrical. Reduced movement is suggestive of weakness. Ask her to blow out her cheeks and seal air in her mouth. Press gently on each cheek to determine if the labial seal is broken and air escapes. Reduced ability to maintain intraoral pressure is suggestive of weakness on that side of the face.

Mandibular Musculature.   At rest, the mandible is examined to determine if it droops on one side compared to the other. If the jaw deviates to one side or the other when it is maximally opened, it suggests weakness on the side toward which it deviates. The examiner should also test the strength of jaw depressors and elevators by requesting that the patient overcome the resistance offered by the examiner to jaw opening when it is elevated (occluded) or to jaw closing when it is depressed. Weakness is estimated by the difficulty the patient has in overcoming the resistance presented by the examiner. It should be remembered, however, that the jaw-closing muscles are capable of producing considerably more force than the jaw-opening muscles because of their role in mastication.

The Dentition and Alveolar Ridge.   To evaluate dental occlusal relationships, the clinician instructs the patient to bite down on her back teeth and to spread her lips. This procedure usually results in a normalized pattern of jaw closure rather than a thrusting forward of the mandible with contact of maxillary and mandibular incisors, which frequently occurs if the patient is simply asked to "bite down." With the teeth in contact, the examiner can observe the posterior and anterior occlusal relationship and the bony framework of the dental arch. The occlusal relationship should be described as well as the condition of the teeth, presence of misaligned and extraneous teeth, and edentulous space. A number of terms have been developed to aid in this descriptive process. These terms are based on variations from the normal occlusional pattern.

In normal adults, the maxillary arch has a slightly larger diameter than the mandibular arch. Therefore, the upper arch overlaps the lower arch such that the maxillary anterior teeth are labial (anterior) to the mandibular teeth. The teeth of the lower and upper arches are arranged so that each tooth is opposed by two teeth of the opposite arch except for the upper third molars and the lower central incisors (Zemlin 1968). The point of reference for describing malocclusions is the oppositional relationship of the first upper and first lower molars; that is, the first lower molar is one cusp anterior to the upper oppositional molar. *Neutrocclusion* is used to describe a malalignment of individual teeth when the anteroposterior (front–back) and lateral (side–side) relationship of the upper and lower dental arches is normal. *Distocclusion* is an abnormal retrusion of the mandible so that the lower dental arch is too far posterior in relation to the upper arch. *Mesiocclusion* refers to an excessive protrusion of the mandible in relation to the maxilla so that the lower arch overlaps the upper arch.

Several other terms may be of value in describing dental abnormalities. *Openbite* refers to the lack of contact between the upper and lower anterior teeth when the posterior teeth are in occlusion. Conversely, *closebite* refers to an excessive overlap of the lower teeth by the upper anterior teeth. *Crossbite* is used to describe a lateral overlap of the upper and lower arches, rather than the normal parallel alignment. In addition to describing the relative positions of the upper and lower arches, it is also useful to describe the relative position of individual teeth. *Labioversion* is a tilting of a tooth toward the lip, *buccoversion* is the deflection of the tooth toward the cheek; *linguaversion* is the tilting of the tooth toward the tongue. *Mesioversion* means that the tooth is medial to its normal position, and *distoversion* indicates that it is distal from normal position. *Edentulous* spaces refer to missing teeth, and *supernumerary* refers to extra or additional teeth. For a rather extensive discussion of dental malocclusions, the interested reader is referred to Bloomer (1971).

The Hard Palate.   When a patient is requested to open his mouth, he usually depresses the mandible maximally to allow the examiner a clear view of the oral cavity. This is only appropriate for a view of palatal or dental structure. It is not the recommended posture for a functional examination because when the mouth is opened as wide as possible, the musculature of the pharynx is immobilized due to the communication between oral and pharyngeal rings of musculature at the pterygomandibular joint (Mason 1969). The recommended mouth opening during the intraoral examination, according to Mason, is three-fourths of the maximal distance.

The hard palate is inspected with the patient's head tilted backward so that the entire hard palate is exposed at one time. This posture can be assumed for inspection of the hard palate because it is a rigid structure not distorted by head position. The primary features of the hard palate to be assessed as reviewed by Mason (1969) include midline coloration, location of its posterior border, and size and shape of the palatal vault. Normal midline colors are pink and white. A bluish coloration should raise suspicion about the adequacy of the bony framework of the palate, such as the possible presence of a submucous cleft. The posterior border of the hard palate can be located by drawing an imaginary line across the palate to join the posterior borders of the maxillae. This is approximately the posterior border of the palantine bone and is useful for evaluating the length of the hard palate and the point at which palpation for the posterior nasal spine should be performed in cases of suspected submucous clefts. The size and shape of the palatal vault should be carefully noted and recorded if it deviates significantly from "normal."

The Palatopharyngeal Musculature.   When examining this area, the examiner will want to assess the coloration of palatal and pharyngeal structures, the anatomic integrity of these structures, and the function of the palatopharyngeal musculature during voluntary and reflex activity. The normal coloration of the velum is similar to that of the hard palate. Any inflammation or marked redness of the velopharyngeal area should be referred to a physician for further examination. The size of the faucial tonsils should also be noted. Tonsillitis is evidenced by redness and engorgement of blood vessels of the tonsillar tissues.

The uvula at the posterior end of the soft palate is usually observable during the intraoral examination. It should be examined carefully since a bifid uvula may appear intact until it is separated with a tongue blade.

The soft palate should be carefully observed at rest. Unilateral weakness will be evidenced by one side of the palate resting at a lower level. Bilateral weakness is usually evidenced by both sides of the soft palate resting at a lower than normal level (near the dorsum of the tongue). Any signs of scars should be carefully recorded.

Only limited information can be obtained about the effectiveness of palatopharyngeal structures in gaining velopharyngeal closure because of the limited access of the examiner to a view of their size, shape, and function. The overall size and length of the soft palate are important, but these dimensions are difficult to ascertain because they depend upon the depth of the nasopharynx. A large nasopharynx can make a normal-sized soft palate appear small.

The effective length of the soft palate is a critical feature to be noted since that is the portion of the elevated velar tissue used to obturate the nasopharyngeal opening. Another way to define effective velar length is the amount of tissue filling the distance between the posterior border of the soft palate and the posterior pharyngeal wall on the horizontal plane of the soft palate (Mason 1969). Effective length is judged by asking the patient to say "ha" while the tongue is gently depressed. A judgment should be made by the examiner regarding the adequacy of velar movement for gaining obturation of the nasopharynx after she has observed the size of the nasopharynx and the effective length of the soft palate. The contribution of the faucial pillars to velopharyngeal closure should also be noted as the patient phonates. We will have more to say about evaluating velopharyngeal closure later in this chapter when we discuss instrumental approaches to diagnosis of speech disorders. Finally, a word of caution. The adequacy of the velopharyngeal mechanism should not be evaluated with the tongue protruded since the anatomic connection of the tongue and palate by means of the palatoglossus muscles will restrict soft-palate elevation during phonation. The symmetry of the soft-palate movement should be noted during phonation. If there is unilateral weakness, the uvula will tend to move toward the intact side. If there is bilateral weakness, production of a syllable such as "ha" results in a minimum of palatal movement.

The pharyngeal gag reflex is also elicited routinely as part of the examination. The reflex is typically elicited by gently placing pressure on the back of the tongue or by stroking the soft palate or pharyngeal wall with a tongue depressor. A normal response is a symmetrical posterior-superior movement of the soft palate and mesial movement of the faucial pillars. Asymmetrical movement or reduced movement of the palate or faucial pillars is suggestive of weakness. An inability to elicit a gag reflex is to be noted, but the examiner should be aware that a small percentage of normal subjects do not have a gag reflex. Significant differences in movement between the habitual movement associated with phonation of a vowel or syllable and movement noted during the gag reflex provide an estimate of potential for responding to speech therapy in cases of velopharyngeal insufficiency.

Tongue Musculature. The tongue is examined at rest and during voluntary activities. First, examine the tongue as it lies in the mouth. Note its size and whether it is shrunken or furrowed on one side. Also, look for the presence of involuntary contractions or twitchings of muscle fibers around the edges of the tongue, and inspect it for signs of involuntary movement. Muscle atrophy and fasciculations are suggestive of peripheral nervous system damage to the hypoglossal nerve. Next, ask the patient to protrude the tongue as far as possible. If there is unilateral weakness, the tongue will deviate toward the side of dysfunction; in bilateral weakness, the patient will be able to protrude the tongue little if at all. Lingual strength can be tested by asking the patient to resist the examiner's attempts to force the tongue to the left, right, or inward with a tongue depressor. Tongue strength (lateral) can also be tested by asking the patient to place his tongue against the inside of the check and then to resist attempts of the examiner to move it medially. Weakness is evidenced by greater ease in forcing the tongue medially on the side opposite the weakness. In cases of facial weakness, the lips should be manually retracted on the weakened side, and the examiner should evaluate lingual deviation by comparing the midline of the tongue with the middle of the jaw. Lingual range of motion is tested by asking the patient to touch the upper lip and alveolar ridge, corners of the mouth, and a point at the midline of the lower lip with the tip of his tongue. Finally, the patient is asked to move his tongue from side to side as quickly as possible. The rate and regularity of these movements are carefully observed and noted. The examiner may also be interested in the status of the lingual frenulum. The frenulum is considered adequate for speech production if the patient can touch the alveolar ridge with his tongue tip when the mouth is held half open. However, the anterior attachment of the frenulum to the under surface of the tongue and a "heart-shaped" appearance of the tongue upon protrusion may also reveal evidence of a restrictive frenulum.

Diadochokinesis. Diadochokinesis is the ability to make rapid alternating movements. Establishing the ability of the patient to produce rapid speech and nonspeech movements is frequently performed as part of the intraoral examination. For example, the examiner may ask the patient to move her tongue back and forth as quickly as possible or to repeat syllables at maximum rates. The important thing to remember is that reduced diadochokinetic rates in themselves are not important since we rarely produce syllables at the maximum rates physiologically allowable. Rather, the importance of diadochokinetic testing is to evaluate the ability of the patient to make consistent articulatory contacts without articulatory breakdowns and significant variations in rate. Typically, diadochokinetic rates are determined by asking the patient to produce the syllables /pa/, /ta/, and /ka/ and the syllable series /pataka/ as quickly as possible over three trials. The average of the three trials is then compared to established norms. The norms for boys and girls 9, 10, and 11 years old are presented in Table 7–2 (Bloomquist 1950). If a 9-year-old boy produced less than 3.8 repetitions per second (two standard deviations below the mean of 4.8), we might conservatively judge his performance to be "inadequate." Additional norms are available for children 3 to 5 (McKelvey 1976), 9 to 11 (Lundeen 1950), and 6 to 15 (Irwin and Becklund 1953). Kent, Kent and Rosenbek (1987) review additional databases.

Swallowing. Swallowing is also evaluated as part of the oral-peripheral examination. In a later chapter, we discuss dysphagia evaluation. In this section, we briefly review procedures for determining the presence of a reversed tongue-thrust swallow (tongue thrusting). Fletcher, Casteel, and Bradley (1961) suggest that this disorder be evaluated in the following manner: Tell the patient you want to observe how he swallows. Place fingers of both hands on the anterior portions of the masseter and over the hyoid bone so that muscle movement can be noted. At the same time, depress the lower lip with the thumbs to break the labial seal and to expose the tongue if it is protruded during swallowing. Ask the patient to swallow several times. Criteria for the tongue-thrusting pattern include absence of masseter action during swallowing, difficulty swallowing when the labial seal is broken, and tongue protrusion beyond the edges of the incisors. Although tongue thrusting may be examined, Mason and Proffit (1974) suggest that swallowing therapy is not indicated before puberty.

Several protocols have been developed that retain the most critical elements of the speech mechanism examination and provide interpretive comments relative to differential diagnosis. The *Dworkin-Culatta Oral Mechanism Examination* (Dworkin and Culatta 1980) contains 10 subtests to evaluate facial appearance, circumoral musculature, masticatory musculature, dentition and gingiva, hard palate, velopharyngeal mechanism, tongue, laryngeal mechanism, and oral and speech praxis. Following administration of the entire examination, abnormal signs are noted on a checklist. The signs are then compared to a tabled matrix of error profiles for 23 conditions varying from spastic dysphonia to oral apraxia, cleft lip, and macroglossia. Each of the 23 conditions is also described on the basis of site of neurological involvement (for example, extrapyramidal system, basal ganglia) or of anatomical abnormality (for example, velum, tongue) and the examinations and subcategories of tests that yielded the abnormal signs. The implications of the test

TABLE 7–2   Mean number of sounds repeated per second in three trials and standard deviation, subjects grouped according to age and sex

	AGE 9				AGE 10				AGE 11			
	Girls		*Boys*		*Girls*		*Boys*		*Girls*		*Boys*	
Sound	M	SD	M	SD	M	SD	M	SD	M	SD	M	SD
p	4.4	.47	4.8	.49	4.7	.76	4.9	.64	5.2	.52	5.5	.64
t	4.5	.65	4.6	.50	4.9	.82	5.0	.98	4.9	.47	5.5	.99
k	4.1	.53	4.2	.51	4.4	.53	4.6	.92	4.6	.55	4.9	.44
ptk	4.8	.72	4.3	.68	5.0	.47	5.0	.80	5.3	.58	5.0	.54

From Bloomquist (1950).

results are cited as an additional interpretive device relative to the abnormal signs from each of the tests. Also included are six sample reports from patients demonstrating spastic dysarthria, flaccid dysarthria, hyperkinetic dysarthria, mixed spastic-ataxic dysarthria, oral and speech apraxia, and phonological disorder with associated structural and physiological abnormalities. The formalized organization of the protocol adds structure to the assessment process, but its most important contribution is the interpretation of findings for the inexperienced clinician who has had little contact with patients demonstrating neurological or structural-based speech disorders.

The *Oral Speech Mechanism Screening Examination* (St. Louis and Ruscello 1981) is designed as a reliable screening examination of the speech-production mechanism and can be administered in 5 to 10 minutes by relatively inexperienced examiners. The measure is organized to make structural or functional judgments relative to the lips, tongue, jaw, teeth, hard palate, soft palate, pharynx, breathing, and diadochokinesis. Scoring is plus (+) for no deviation, minus (–) for deviation, not tested (NT), no response (NR), and incorrect execution (X) with arrows used to denote anatomical asymmetries. The examiner also makes notes or records observations of functional or structural adequacy for tasks dealing with speech movements. Three interpretations are possible for each of the structures or functions assessed: (1) normal, (2) abnormal with referral to another speciality for additional evaluation, and (3) further testing to verify and more fully describe the disorder. Also included in the manual is a detailed description of the importance of each structure to speech production, its appearance, and typical deviations. Mean agreement for two testers for each of four age groups administered the examination (excluding diadochokinesis) revealed intrajudge reliability of 95.5 to 98.4 percent and interjudge reliability of 95.1 percent. Given the small database, these agreement values should be viewed as preliminary estimates. The protocol is helpful in organizing the components of the oral-peripheral examination and in attempting to determine the reliability of the observations, but it includes a definite shortfall in the lack of tasks/observations that deal with respiratory/phonatory components of speech production.

To this point, the clinical procedures for evaluating the anatomic and structural integrity of the speech apparatus have been reviewed. These procedures are not to be used only in cases of obvious structural and functional dysfunction but rather as an integral part of the evaluation of patients regardless of the suspected speech and language problem. Clinical observations may be significantly enhanced through instrumental assessment, which may make up an important part of the examination if appropriate instrumentation is available. The purpose of the following review is to provide a rationale for instrumental assessment and some brief discussion of some available methodology. It is not intended to be exhaustive in terms of equipment and techniques since detailed discussions are available elsewhere (for example, Baken 1987).

INSTRUMENTAL APPROACHES TO THE EXAMINATION OF THE SPEECH MECHANISM

Instrumentation extends the senses of the observer and objectifies her observations. Its utilization for the diagnosis of speech disorders is in its infancy; its potential appears limited only by the creativity of the engineer and the interpretive powers of the diagnostician. Its usefulness lies in the ability of the diagnostician to gather detailed information directly from the abnormal speech apparatus rather than relying on perceptual information. This deductive shortcut might be likened to a mechanic's effort to diagnose the problem of a malfunctioning car motor. If he knows nothing about engines, it does not matter whether he listens to it, acoustically analyzes the noise of the troubled engine, or takes the motor apart; he will not be able to diagnose the problem even though evidence of its malfunctioning is available at each stage of his examination. If he knows how engines operate when in good repair, he may be able to diagnose the problem through listening or acoustical analysis, but he can make his best estimate of its dysfunction by taking it apart, examining each of the components, and inferring why the engine is not working properly.

Two features of this analogy from Netsell (1975) are important to instrumental approaches to the diagnosis of speech disorders. First, we must have some knowledge of normal processes in order to judge *if* the speech-production apparatus is disordered. This is an important point we made in our discussion of standardization of tests on "normal" subjects in order to make decisions about whether a communicative problem exists. The comparative process of determining normalcy is rendered considerably more difficult in instrumental analysis, however, by the lack of a large physiological database to aid in making our decisions. The process is complicated further by the variability demonstrated by normal speakers when electromyographic, structural movement, aerodynamic, and acoustical data are examined. The large variations in normal performance, coupled with the lack of a significant normative database, make diagnostic interpretations and decisions difficult based on instrumental data alone. Physiological data from disordered speech processes are an aid to diagnosis and appraisal; they are not the only information available and cannot be relied upon exclusively for making our decisions.

Second, collection of physiological data has the advantage of investigating the source of the disorder by allowing us to examine the problem more directly. If we wish to determine the physiological origin of a particular type of dysarthria from perceptual analysis, for example, we must make inferences across the levels of the speech-production process. We listen to the acoustic output from the patient, which is based on the resonant characteristics and sound-generation sources of the vocal tract; the sound sources are developed by changes in air pressure and flows within the vocal tract produced by alterations in structural movement. The movements, in turn, are produced by changes in muscular activity controlled by the nervous system. Given that the disorder has a neuromuscular origin, we are required to make inferences across several stages of the speech-production process. The inferential leap from perceptual information to the underlying neuromuscular pathology is no mean task for even the well-trained clinician; it is even more formidable because the movements of the articulatory structures cannot be separated from the constrictions that serve as sound sources or the movements that control vocal tract resonance (Abbs and Watkin, 1976). Even though the experienced diagnostician can make inferences from perceptual judgments of the acoustic waveform to the underlying neuromuscular pathology, she must, as we mentioned earlier, have a knowledge of normal functioning to determine the extent to which the patient's speech production differs from normal. The advantage of instrumental approaches is that we can get closer to the source of the problem and can quantify our observations in a highly detailed fashion; comparisons with normal performance then become more reliable and valid.

The ability to gather objective data closer to the source of the problem is not purchased without cost. As we seek to examine earlier stages of speech production, less and less of the process is available for measurement at one point in time. For example, spectographic analysis allows us to display most of the acoustic information available in the speech waveform at one time. A complete aerodynamic description requires that we monitor approximately seven relevant variables. Structural-movement data may be collected from 10 or more articulators, and muscle function, if we attempt to describe the entire speech activity, requires examining approximately 100 muscles. Since there are a finite number of parameters that can be recorded and interpreted at one time, as we move toward the origins of the speech-production process, we are able to monitor less and less of the total activity. This situation is comparable to a wedge-shaped piece of pie that gets tastier as we eat toward the point. We get a lot of pie at the periphery, but it does not taste very good. As we eat toward the point, it gets better and better, but we have less and less of it. The only wise course for the hungry person is to eat the entire piece, of course. Likewise, the diagnostician will want to use information from each stage of the speech-production process even if only a limited number of variables are available for study at each level.

The purpose of this section is to describe instrumentation useful for collecting information about disordered speech processes. It is understood that much of this instrumentation may not be readily available to the diagnostician; knowledge of its operation, however, may provide important insights for the student of differential diagnosis.

INSTRUMENTAL APPROACHES

The stages of the speech-production process along with some instrumental approaches to the study of each stage are presented in Figure 7–4. It should be obvious that the schematic diagram is a highly simplified graphic display of a very complex process and does not include feedback systems or interactive effects between the stages. Moreover, we have not attempted to list all possible investigative techniques but only a representative sample of those most commonly employed in speech research. Reviews of physiology instrumentation and their advantages and disadvantages are provided by Strong (1970), Abbs and Watkin (1976), Warren (1976), Hardy (1965), and Hixon (1972) and of speech acoustics instrumentation by Wakita (1976). Baken (1987) provides a detailed description of clinical measurement techniques for speech and voice.

MUSCLE ACTION POTENTIALS

We begin our discussion with electromyography because it allows examination of one of the earliest stages of the speech-production process. This is not to say that attempts have not been made to directly measure central or peripheral nervous system activity during speech production. Electromyography, however, is the first instrumental approach that can provide readily interpretable information.

Electromyography (EMG) is a method of displaying the time varying electri-

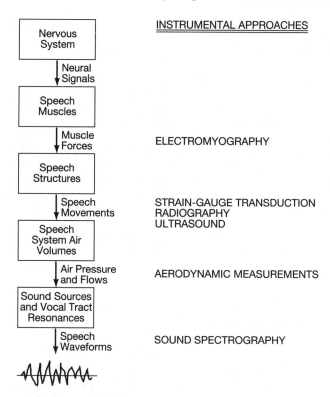

FIGURE 7–4   **Stages of the speech-production process and instrumental approaches to the study of each stage.**

(Adapted from J. Abbs and K. Watkin, Instrumentation for the study of speech physiology. In *Contemporary Issues in Experimental Phonetics*, ed. N. Lass. New York: Academic Press, 1976. Used by permission.)

cal activity associated with muscle contraction (Harris 1970). The source of the electrical activity is the resting potential of living mammalian cells—that is, the potential difference between the inside and the outside of an active cell.

Muscle fibers are functionally arranged such that a large number of fibers lie parallel, enclosed within a sheath. Groups of fibers within the muscle are connected to a single neuron and thereby comprise a motor unit. Each muscle is made up of a number of these motor units. When a suprathreshold stimulus is delivered to a motor unit, a wave of depolarization sweeps down the muscle fibers. The momentary changes in electrical activity can be recorded by use of electrodes or "probes" placed next to each other within or overlying the muscle.

Surface, needle, and hooked-wire electrodes are utilized for monitoring speech-muscle activity. No matter which are chosen, they must meet several requirements according to Abbs and Watkins (1976):

> . . . it is obvious that electrodes for measurement of speech muscle activity must (1) allow for placement in confined spaces (such as the oral cavity), (2) be light enough to

follow the movement of the muscle and yet remain in place (to minimize movement artifacts), and (3) be unobtrusive in relation to the speech movement activity that one is attempting to observe. (p. 97)

In general, each type of electrode has advantages and disadvantages. Surface electrodes are easy to apply and offer minimal discomfort to the patient but cannot be used to monitor activity from deep muscles or those muscles (such as the mentalis) that are small in comparison to the size of the electrode. Intramuscular electrodes (needles and hooked wires implanted into the muscle) can be used to monitor superficial and deep muscles as well as small muscles because they are lightweight and the recording area is small. There tends to be some discomfort associated with their implantation, but they are relatively painless once embedded. The hooked-wire electrode is superior to the needle electrode because it is smaller and more flexible. Consequently, it does not load the muscle as much while retaining the advantages normally gained from needle-electrode use—that is, easy implantation and measurement from a specific muscle area (Basmajian 1967).

Since the electrical activity recorded by the electrode is small, it must first be amplified. Following amplification, various types of signal manipulation may be used to maximize the ease with which the information can be interpreted when graphically displayed.

So what is the value of electromyographic data? In general, the absolute magnitude of the signal is of little value since it varies as a function of the electrode used, placement location, and tissue impedance. The magnitude of the signals from two muscles cannot be directly compared for the same reason. The value of electromyography lies in two areas. First, it is useful in examining the time relationship between muscle activity and associated speech gestures, and second, it provides information on the status of the neuromuscular system, such as the presence of hypertonicity or abnormal variations in the activation and inhibition of muscle activity.

STRUCTURAL MOVEMENT

Several techniques have been employed for the measurement of structural movement. Typically, the use of these procedures is mutually exclusive, and employment of more than one method at a time is rare. As with electromyography, there are advantages and disadvantages associated with the use of each technique.

Three primary instrumental approaches as reviewed by Moll (1965) and Bzoch (1970) are considered under the rubric of *radiography*, including "still" X-ray, laminography, and cinefluorography. Their common feature is that they each use X-rays, a form of electromagnetic radiation with defined wavelengths. The X-rays are directed toward the subject's body and penetrate all structures to varying degrees. The resulting image can be made visible on film or visualized on a fluoroscopic screen and then videotaped or photographed.

Still X-rays most often have been used to visualize speech structures from the lateral view. They appear to be of limited utility in speech research since they yield a static, rather than a dynamic, portrayal of the speech structures. Laminography is similar to still X-ray but offers the advantage of visualizing only the structures within a given plane.

Cinefluorography involves the photographing of the intensified image so that dynamic speech processes, rather than a single position, are monitored. Radiation effects are reduced by synchronizing the X-ray generator and the camera shutter. To analyze movement of the articulatory structures, sequences of individual cine-fluorographic frames are traced, and measurements are made from the tracings utilizing radiopaque beads, skeletal structures, and/or articulators covered with a radiopaque substance as referents.

There are a number of problems associated with the use of radiographic techniques that have been reviewed by Bzoch (1970). Danger from radiation exposure requires strict limitations on the speech sample, and the actual acquisition of the data must be under the supervision of a radiologist. The requirement that the body be stabilized limits observations of articulators to a single body position while the same function may differ in other postures due to changes in antigravity muscles.

There are also data-reduction problems. Variations in radiopacity from individual to individual result in reduced reliability of the data measurements. Straight-line emission characteristics of X-rays cause relative enlargement of the periphery, which necessitates the use of correction factors in measurement. Subject instability errors may arise from small movements of the subject's head that alter the positional relationships between reference skeletal structures and articulators. Errors may also occur in the measuring of frames because anatomical structures that have no functional relationship to speech production are used as reference points. Finally, there is the problem of which measurements to make.

In spite of these limitations, cinefluorography offers a view of dynamic activity from a number of articulators at the same time, an important advantage. It is the procedure of choice for investigating structures such as the velopharyngeal mechanism and tongue, which are relatively inaccessible by other techniques.

Ultrasound is useful for observing the dynamic activity of structures without interfering with their activity or exposing the patient to irradiation. Ultrasound is produced by exciting a crystal with an electrical field which changes the crystal's dimensions and produces waves. The ultrasonic waves have the property of being reflected back at the interface (boundary) between two mediums such as the lateral pharyngeal wall and the pharyngeal airspace. The reflected wave is converted into a time-amplitude display since the time between the initiation of the ultrasonic pulses and their return is proportional to the distance from the transmitter to the boundary. This technique has been used to monitor pharyngeal wall (Kelsey, Minifie, and Hixon 1969), tongue (Watkin and Zagzebski 1973), and vocal-fold movement (Minifie, Kelsey, and Hixon 1968). The problems with the technique are that the experimenter is not exactly sure of the point on the structure that she is measuring from, and the transmitter-receiver must be at a 90° angle with the interface. Moreover, in disorders characterized by structural anomalies (cleft palate, partial glossectomee), it may be particularly difficult to identify the point on the structure being monitored.

Strain-gauge transduction theoretically can be used to monitor displacement of any speech structure. In actuality, transducers of this type have been utilized primarily to investigate movements of the jaw (Sussman and Smith 1970a; Abbs and Gilbert 1973; Abbs 1973), velum (Christiansen and Moller 1971), and lips (Sussman and Smith 1970b; Abbs and Gilbert 1973). Strain gauges (Abbs and Watkin 1976) operate on the principle that as a wire is stretched, it is reduced in diameter and increased in length, thus offering greater resistance to the flow of current. Conversely, when these conductors are compressed, there is decreased resistance to current flow. Strain-gauge elements are bonded to a thin metal beam (cantilever) and attached to the structure of interest. Resistance changes proportional to the deformation of the strip occur when the structure is displaced. The resistance changes modulate the current across an amplifier, thereby varying the voltage. The time varying voltage resulting from the structural displacement is graphically displayed.

The advantages of this technique are the ease with which the cantilever beams can be attached to the structures and the absence of subject discomfort. The primary disadvantage is that cantilevers cannot be attached to structures such as the tongue without impeding normal articulatory activity.

We have briefly reviewed only three methods for monitoring structural movement. Descriptions of other techniques, such as high-speed photography, electromagnetic induction, and photoelectric techniques, are available in Abbs and Watkin (1976), Hanley and Peters (1971), Hixon (1972), Harris (1970), and Baken (1987).

AIR PRESSURE—AIR FLOW

Structural movements induce volume changes and produce variations in air pressure and air flow in the speech system. The pressures and flows of interest are displayed in Figure 7–5. The pressures include intraoral, intranasal, subglottic, and

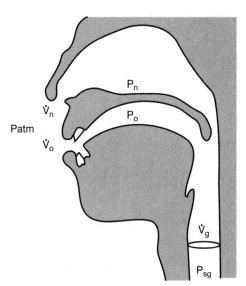

FIGURE 7–5   Speech air pressures and airflows. Air pressures include oral (P_o), nasal (P_n), subglottic (P_{sg}), and atmospheric (P_{atm}). Airflows include glottal (V_g), oral (V_o), and nasal (V_n).

(Adapted from R. Netsell, Speech Physiology. In *Normal Aspects of Speech, Hearing and Language*, eds. F. Minifie, T. Hixon, and F. Williams. Englewood Cliffs, N.J.: Prentice Hall 1973. Used by permission.)

atmospheric. The flows are those across the glottis, the nasal cavity, and the oral cavity. Integration of volume velocity of air flow provides an estimate of volume.

One means of determining lung volume is the *spirometer*. A wet spirometer consists of a bell inverted in a tank of water. Movement of the bell is recorded by a stylus on a slowly revolving drum of paper. The movement of the bell is caused by the subject's breathing through a tube which forces air into the bell. A spirometer can be used to measure lung volumes and capacities. One major drawback of the device is that the magnitude of some measures, such as inspiratory capacity, is highly dependent on the amount of effort expended by the subject. Therefore, multiple trials are usually performed, and the maximum value obtained is considered to be the most valid indicant of performance. A second limitation is that the variables cannot be measured during speech production unless the instrumentation is adapted.

A second means of determining lung volumes is through the use of a *body plethysmograph* (Hixon 1972). It measures air volume as a function of the pressure differential between a chamber in which the subject is placed and the outside atmosphere. The subject is seated in a booth completely enclosed except for the head and neck, which are allowed to project through the top of the chamber. The neck collar provides an airtight seal for the air enclosed in the chamber. During breathing activities, the pressure in the chamber increases and decreases with net inspiratory and expiratory volume changes. With each volume change, gas is displaced through a fine metal screen located in the front wall of the chamber. The flow through the screen is directly proportional to the pressure differential between the chamber and the atmosphere. By integrating the flow sensed by a pressure transducer, a measure of the volume displaced in and out of the chamber is obtained.

The plethysmograph has the advantage of allowing a determination of volume changes during speech production and, therefore, appears to be much more valuable than a wet spirometer. However, it is cumbersome and has not been used extensively in speech research. More recently, a magnatometer system has become the device preferred for measuring movements of the ribcage and abdomen to yield estimates of respiratory apparatus volume changes (Hixon, Mead, and Goldman 1976).

Static measurements of intraoral air pressure may be obtained with a *U-tube water manometer*, which provides an estimate of pressure in centimeters of water displaced, or with a *Hunter Manometer*, which provides a reading in ounces per square inch. The U-tube manometer is constructed of a flexible tube, into which the subject blows, which is connected to a U-shaped glass tube filled with colored water. A scale is marked in centimeters along the side of the tube. A leak tube is used in conjunction with the manometer both to simulate air flow and to prevent valving of the tube with the tongue. Netsell and Hixon (1978) have described a U-tube manometer with a leak tube that simulates pressure and flow values normally associated with phonation. It thereby serves to approximate the glottal resistance of the upper airway. The subject is instructed to blow into a tube for a specified duration while maintaining a prescribed pressure level. Assuming velopharyngeal closure and a tight lip seal around the tube, the method offers an estimate of subglottal pressure. It may be used to differentiate respiratory from laryngeal involvement by estimating the ability of the patient to develop and maintain subglottic pressure under a simulated phonation condition.

The Hunter Manometer works on the same principle as the U-tube. Readings appear on three calibrated dials, and there is a manually operated bleed (leak) valve. Indications of velopharyngeal adequacy are obtained by dividing the reading obtained during a trial with the nares open compared to that obtained with the nares occluded. Theoretically, the ratio should be 1.0. If there is a leak through the velopharyngeal opening with the nares unoccluded, lower ratios are obtained and are an indication of inadequacy. A ratio of 0.89 or less is considered inadequate velopharyngeal closure (Spriestersbach and others 1961).

Dynamic air pressures are monitored by means of a pressure transducer that converts pressure into voltage. This is accomplished by a diaphragm within a transducer. When pressure is exerted on the diaphragm, it is displaced with a resultant change in voltage. The voltage is amplified and displayed on an oscillograph. The intraoral pressure is coupled to the pressure transducer by means of a tube inserted into the oral cavity. The tube is positioned so that its opening is oriented perpendicular to flow to reduce flow artifacts. To obtain bilabial plosive pressure, the tube is entered into the corner of the mouth. To obtain pressures for a large number of consonants, the tube with an oropharyngeal balloon attached to the end is passed through one of the nares to a point below the velopharyngeal space. Another alternative is to place the tube in the dental-gingival sinus so that it enters the oral cavity from behind the last upper molar. Nasal pressure is obtained by sealing the tube to a nasal olive inserted into one of the nares. Subglottic pressure can be obtained by puncturing the trachea between the second and third rings with a hypodermic needle and attaching it to a pressure transducer. These techniques have the advantage of monitoring dynamic pressures during speech production.

Hixon, Hawley, and Wilson (1972) described a simple "homemade" device for measuring respiratory driving pressures using a straw and tall drinking glass filled with water. The water in the glass is calibrated with a ruler. Insertion of the straw to varying depths of the water can be used to determine whether the person tested is capable of generating respiratory driving pressures at levels observed during speech production.

Two systems described by Lubker (1970) are generally used to measure air flow rates occurring during speech. The difference between the systems is in the choice of the sensing device. The sensing element most commonly used to measure airflow is the *pneumotachograph*. This device is based on the principle that as air flows across a resistance the air-pressure drop is proportional to the rate of flow. The pressure drop, or differential, is sensed by a transducer, converted to an electrical signal, amplified, and graphically displayed. This technique for monitoring airflow has the advantage of easy calibration and stability, and it can be used to detect and differentiate between ingressive and egressive flow. The primary disadvantage is that a face mask must be used to trap the flow of air through the device, which places certain restrictions on articulatory movements. Lubker and Moll (1965) have suggested that these restrictions are limited primarily to lip and jaw movements and are highly phoneme-dependent.

The second airflow measuring technique reviewed by Lubker, the *warm-wire anemometer*, uses a heated wire as the airflow sensing element. He noted that

> the basic principle involves the cooling effect of a flow of air on a heated wire through which an electric current is flowing. As the wire is cooled, its resistance to current flow is altered in a systematic manner. The variations in the electrical signal passing through the heated wire, when amplified, recorded, and calibrated, provide a record of flow rate. (p. 209)

The primary advantage of this system is that no face mask is needed to channel the flow of air. Although applications have been made of a single heated wire placed in a tube similar to a pneumotachograph and attached to a mask (Van Hattum and Worth 1967), more recent use has involved the suspension of a series of wires in front of and close to the oral and nasal ports without a mask (Subtelny, Worth, and Sakuda 1966; Subtelny and others 1969). The warm wire or wires may be arranged rather close to the subject's mouth, and their distance must be constant throughout the experiment. Consequently, the subject's head movements need to be restricted, or the apparatus must be attached to the face, or both. The warm-wire system has a number of disadvantages including inability to differentiate between ingressive and egressive flow, poor linearity and frequency response, and difficulties in calibration (Lubker 1970).

These methods allow some means of determining the volume velocity of airflow through the oral cavity and nasal passages. Transglottal airflow can be determined through the use of a plethysmograph (Hixon 1972).

ACOUSTIC ANALYSIS

The *sound spectrograph* is an instrument that visually presents information about the frequency, intensity, and duration of the speech waveform. The speech sample is introduced into the spectrograph via microphone or tape recorder. As the signal is analyzed, a hot-wire stylus records a "picture" of the sound wave on a rotating drum. The spectrogram produced provides a display of frequency on the vertical axis, duration on the horizontal axis, and intensity by the darkness of the trace. Two filter bandwidths may be used for the analysis. A broad band filter provides the best pictorial representation of the waveform for determining formant frequencies, glottal pulse, and segment duration. The narrow band filter is used for determining fundamental frequency, harmonics, and intonational contours. The spectrograph can also be used to obtain line spectra for selected portions of a signal and amplitude and intensity displays. The sound spectrograph has been used extensively in research examining acoustic aspects of both speech production and speech perception. It is an important tool in correlating elements of the acoustic signal with perceived qualities and with acoustic correlates of articulatory gestures. Spectrograms are potentially useful in the diagnosis of voice disorders, where they can be used to supplement other sources of information. Spectrographic data afford physical evidence of perceived vocal abnormalities, such as perturbations of the glottal pulse. The computer-based Speech Laboratory developed by Kay Elemetrics provides numerous acoustical analysis options and to a large extent has replaced the sound spectrograph in clinical practice.

Another device for evaluating the acoustic waveform is the *fundamental frequency indicator* (Hanley and Peters 1971). This instrument is specifically designed to extract the fundamental frequency from the speech waveform. The device may be of value in correlating the maturational development of the larynx and in assessment of voice disorders related to pitch.

The Visi-Pitch developed by Kay Elemetrics is an analog fundamental frequency analyzer that provides an oscillographic display of fundamental frequency and intensity overtime. It was developed specifically for the ease with which it can be used in clinical practice.

A *probe tube microphone assembly* permits the simultaneous recording of oral and nasal acoustic energy in decibels. A probe tube is inserted into the nasal meatus, while the oral signal is recorded by means of a condenser microphone a short distance from the lips. The greater the nasal air flow, the less the difference between the nasal and oral sound pressure levels. This relationship may indicate the degree to which the nasal and oral tracts are coupled during speech and thereby provides an estimate of the adequacy of velopharyngeal closure. A review of this technique is provided by Counihan (1979).

SOME CONSIDERATIONS IN THE SELECTION OF INSTRUMENTATION

We have reviewed only a few of the many instrumental devices available for diagnosis and appraisal of speech disorders. Others run the gamut from the tongue depressor and flashlight to computer analysis of the acoustic signal. A number of factors must be considered before selecting the instrumentation to be used.

1. *The device should be minimally invasive of the patient.* Any instrument that causes the patient discomfort or invades the body should be used with great caution. For example, the implantation of needle or hooked-wire electrodes and the positioning of a nasopharyngeal balloon may be painful and in most cases should be done under the supervision of a physician. This point is doubly important when instruments of this type are used with patients who have chronic debilitating conditions, such as Parkinson's disease.

2. *The procedures should minimally endanger the patient.* This is a postulate of the first point. Some procedures such as cinefluorography produce potentially hazardous radiation and should be used only with qualified personnel available. A basic consideration for all such procedures is that the benefit to be gained must outweigh the risks involved.

3. *The instrumentation should not impede normal speech production.* Some devices may effectively load the structure or structures under study and bring about compensatory articulatory activity. The instrumentation chosen should not alter "typical" or "normal" speech production.

4. *The instrumentation should allow an adequate sampling of connected speech.* Devices such as the oral manometer and wet spirometer cannot be used during connected speech and, therefore, can only be used in a secondary capacity.

5. *If possible, information should be provided about several stages of the speech-production process.* Abbs and Watkin (1976) noted:

   Electromyographic and aerodynamic monitoring represent micro and macro poles in the specification of speech production activity. . . . It would appear worthwhile to observe the mediating variable (viz., structural movement) simultaneously with EMG or air pressures and air flows to facilitate interpretation of these aerodynamic or electromyographic indices of speech system activity.

6. *The speech sample and variables to be measured should be selected with care.* It would seem of little value to measure lower-lip electromyographic activity in a patient with velopharyngeal inadequacy. Likewise, measurement of nasal air flow during production of a bilabial nasal consonant would offer little information about this patient's hypernasality.

Moll (1965) made a similar observation when he emphasized that photographic and radiographic procedures provide information only on structural positions and should be utilized in conjunction with other physiologic research techniques and acoustic and perceptual analyses. The point to be made is that considerable ambiguity may result from attempts to make inferences from only a single stage of the speech-production process.

AN EXAMPLE OF INSTRUMENTATION USED FOR CLINICAL DIAGNOSIS

A review of studies utilizing instrumental approaches to the diagnosis of speech disorders quickly reveals that research, rather than clinical assessment, has been the primary goal of the investigations. In some cases, the two objectives (research and diagnosis) overlap, but the intent is usually to discover characteristics of speech production in a particular disordered group of patients. Our purpose here is to provide an example of data collected for research purposes that contains valuable clinical information and demonstrates the potential of instrumentation.

The example is from Netsell (1969), who recorded intraoral air pressures (using a pressure transducer), rate of nasal airflow (via a pneumotachograph), and the speech signal to determine velopharyngeal competence in cerebral-palsied children. The speech sample included the consonants /t/, /d/, and /n/ to represent voiceless, voiced, and nasal contrasts. The sample was produced under several rate and context conditions.

Speech audio, nasal airflow rate, and intraoral air pressure for a neurologically normal and a dysarthric subject are presented in Figure 7–6. Examination of the figure reveals that except for a slight burst on the initial utterance, no nasal airflow is seen in the production of /ʌtʌdʌ/ by the dysarthric subject. However, during each repetition of /ʌtʌnʌ/, there are two bursts of nasal flow—one for /t/ and one for /n/. It is evident that this patient opened the velopharynx early in anticipation of the /n/ with resultant inappropriate nasal airflow during the /t/. Velopharyngeal closure was achieved during production of /t/ as evidenced by the peaks of intraoral pressure. Since the subject appeared to be able to develop intraoral pressure during production of plosives, the problem is one of timing and not of inability to decrease the area of the velopharyngeal opening during speech production. This finding is important to clinical assessment since remedial procedures vary as a function of the diagnosis. If timing is the problem, as in this example, then a palatal lift may be the optimal form of treatment. If the problem had been due to an inability to adequately close the velopharyngeal port due to a congenitally short palate, then obturation or surgical intervention would be the rehabilitation procedure of choice.

Many other examples of instrumental assessment are available for dysarthria, stuttering, cleft palate, laryngectomy, and voice disorders.

SUMMARY

We have reviewed clinical and instrumental approaches to the evaluation of the speech-production mechanism. Included were a detailed discussion of the structures and functions to be assessed and instrumentation of value in enhancing the observa-

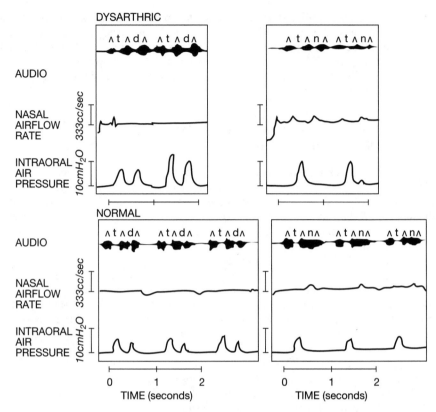

FIGURE 7-6   **Oscillographic recordings of the speech signal (audio), nasal air flow rate, and intraoral air pressure from a dysarthric female and a normal female repeating the utterances /ʌtʌdʌ/ and /ʌtʌnʌ/ (left and right side of the figure, respectively) to illustrate an inappropriate opening of the velopharynx.**

(From R. Netsell, Evaluation of velopharyngeal function in dysarthria. *J. Speech Hearing Res.*, 34, 113–122, 1969. By permission.)

tions made. These procedures are an integral part of the evaluation of patients regardless of the suspected speech and language problems.

REFERENCES

ABBS, J., Some mechanical properties of lower-lip movement during speech production. *Phonetica*, 28, 65–75 (1973).

ABBS, J., AND D. GILBERT, Strain gauge transducer system for lip and jaw motion in two dimensions. *J. Speech Hearing Res.*, 16, 248–256 (1973).

ABBS, J., AND K. WATKIN, Instrumentation for the study of speech physiology. In *Contemporary Issues in Experimental Phonetics*, ed. N. Lass. New York: Academic Press (1976).

ALPERS, B., AND E. MANCALL, *Essentials of the Neurological Examination*. Philadelphia: F. A. Davis Co. (1971).

BAKEN, R., *Clinical Measurement of Speech and Voice*. Boston: College-Hill Press (1987).

BASMAJIAN, J., *Muscles Alive—Their Functions Revealed by Electromyography*. Baltimore: Williams and Wilkins (1967).

BLOOMER, H., Speech defects associated with dental malocclusions and related abnormalities. In *Handbook of Speech Pathology*, ed. L. Travis. Englewood Cliffs, N.J.: Prentice Hall (1971).

BLOOMQUIST, B., Diadochokinetic movements of nine-, ten-, and eleven-year-old children. *J. Speech Hearing Dis.*, 15, 159–164 (1950).

BOONE, D. R., *The Voice and Voice Disorders*, 2nd ed. Englewood Cliffs, N.J.: Prentice Hall (1977).

BOONE, D. R., *The Boone Voice Program for Children: Screening, Evaluation and Referral.* Tigard, Oreg.: C. C. Publications (1980).

BOONE, D. R., *The Voice and Voice Therapy*, 3rd ed. Englewood Cliffs, N.J.: Prentice Hall (1983).

BRAIN, L., AND J. WALTON, *Brain's Diseases of the Nervous System*. London: Oxford University Press (1969).

BZOCH, K., Assessment: Radiographic techniques. *Proceedings of the Workshop, Speech and the Dentofacial Complex: The State of the Art*. Washington, D.C.: ASHA Reports Number 5 (1970).

CASE, J. *Clinical Management of Voice Disorders*, 2nd ed. Austin, Tex.: Pro-Ed (1991).

CHRISTIANSEN, R., AND K. MOLLER. Instrumentation for recording velar movement. *Amer. J. Orthod.*, 59, 448–455 (1971).

COUNIHAN, D., Oral and nasal sound pressure measures. In *Communicative Disorders Related to Cleft Lip and Palate*, 2nd ed., ed. K. Bzoch. Boston: Little, Brown (1979).

DARLEY, F., A. ARONSON, AND J. BROWN, *Motor Speech Disorders*. Philadelphia: W. B. Saunders (1975).

DAVIS, C., AND T. HARRIS, Teachers' ability to accurately identify disordered voices. *Lang. Speech Hearing Serv. Schools*, 23, 136–140 (1992).

DEJONG, R., *The Neurologic Examination*. New York: Hoeber-Harper (1958).

DWORKIN, J., II, Differential diagnosis of motor speech disorders: The clinical examination of the speech mechanism. *J. National Student Speech Hear. Assoc.*, 6, 37–59 (1978).

DWORKIN, J., AND R. CULATTA, *Dworkin-Culatta Oral Mechanism Examination*. Nicholasville, Ky.: Edgewood Press (1980).

ECKEL, F. C., AND D. R. BOONE. The s/z ratio as an indicator of laryngeal pathology. *J. Speech Hearing Dis.*, 46, 147–149 (1981).

FAIRBANKS, G., *Voice and Articulation Drillbook*. New York: Harper & Row (1940).

FENDLER, M., AND W. M. SHEARER, Reliability of the S/Z ratio in normal children's voices. *Lang. Speech Hearing Serv. Schools,* 19, 2 (1988).

FISHER, H., *Improving Voice and Articulation*. Boston: Houghton Mifflin (1966).

FLETCHER, S., R. CASTEEL, AND D. BRADLEY, Tongue-thrust swallow, speech articulation, and age. *J. Speech Hearing Dis.*, 26, 201–208 (1961).

HANLEY, T., AND R. PETERS, The speech and hearing laboratory. In *Handbook of Speech Pathology and Audiology*, ed. E. Travis. Englewood Cliffs, N.J.: Prentice Hall (1971).

HARDY, J., Air flow and air pressure studies. *Proceedings of the Conference: Communicative Problems in Cleft Palate*. Washington, D.C.: ASHA Reports Number 1 (1965).

HARRIS, K., Physiological measures of speech movements: EMG and fiberoptic studies. *Proceedings of the Workshop. Speech and the Dentofacial Complex: The State of the Art*. Washington, D.C.: ASHA Reports Number 5 (1970).

HIXON, T., Some new techniques for measuring the biomechanical events of speech production: One laboratory's experiences. *Proceedings of the Conference. Orofacial Function: Clinical Research in Dentistry and Speech Pathology*. Washington, D.C.: ASHA Reports Number 7 (1972).

HIXON, T., J. HAWLEY, AND K. J. WILSON, An around-the-house device for the clinical determination of respiratory driving pressure: A note on making simple even simpler. *J. Speech Hearing Dis.*, 47, 413 (1982).

HIXON, T., J. MEAD, AND M. GOLDMAN, Dynamics of the chest wall during speech production: Function of the thorax, rib cage, diaphragm, and abdomen. *J. Speech Hearing Res.*, 19, 297–356 (1976).

IRWIN, J., AND O. BECKLUND, Norms for maximum repetitive rates for certain sounds established with the Sylrater. *J. Speech Hearing Dis.*, 18, 149–160 (1953).

JOHNSON, W., F. DARLEY, AND D. SPRIESTERSBACH, *Diagnostic Methods in Speech Pathology*. New York: Harper & Row (1963).

KELSEY, C., F. MINIFIE, AND T. HIXON, Applications of ultrasound in speech research. *J. Speech Hearing Res.*, 12, 564–575 (1969).

KENT, R., J. KENT, AND J. ROSENBEK, Maximum performance tests of speech production. *J. Speech Hearing Dis.*, 52, 367–387 (1987).

LINDBLOM, B., AND J. SUNDBERG, Neurophysiological representation of speech sounds. Paper represented at the XVth World Congress of Logopedics and Phoniatrics, Buenos Aires, Argentina (1971).

LINDBLOM, B., J. LUBKER, AND T. GAY, Formant frequencies of some fixed-mandible vowels and a model of speech motor programming by predictive simulation. *J. Phon.*, 7, 147–161 (1979).

LUBKER, J., Aerodynamic and ultrasonic assessment techniques in speech-dentofacial research. *Proceedings of the Workshop. Speech and the Dentofacial Complex: The State of the Art.* Washington, D.C.: ASHA Reports Number 5 (1970).

LUBKER, J., AND K. MOLL, Simultaneous oral-nasal airflow measurements and cinefluorographic observations during speech production. *Cleft Pal. J.*, 2, 257–272 (1965).

LUNDEEN, D., The relationship of diadochokinesis to various speech sounds. *J. Speech Hearing Dis.*, 15, 54–59 (1950).

MASON, R., Improving the efficiency of the intraoral examination. *J. Tenn. Speech Hearing Assoc.*, 14, 4–10 (1969).

MASON, R., AND W. PROFFIT, The tongue-thrust controversy: Background and recommendations. *J. Speech Hearing Dis.*, 39, 115–132 (1974).

MASON, R., AND C. SIMON, An orofacial examination checklist. *Lang. Speech Hearing Serv. Schools*, 8, 155–164 (1977).

MCKELVEY, J., Performance of normal three- and four-year-old children on ten selected oral motor tasks. Unpublished master's thesis, University of Texas, Austin (1976).

MCWILLIAMS, B., R. MUSGRAVE, AND P. CROZIER, The influence of head position upon velopharyngeal closure. *Cleft Pal. J.*, 5, 117–124 (1968).

MINIFIE, F., C. KELSEY, AND T. HIXON, Measurement of vocal-fold motion using an ultrasonic Doppler velocity monitor. *J. Acous. Soc. Amer.*, 43, 1165–1169 (1968).

MOLL, K., Photographic and radiographic procedures in speech research. *Proceedings of the Conference: Communicative Problems in Cleft Palate.* Washington, D.C.: ASHA Reports Number 1 (1965).

MOORE, G., Voice disorders associated with organic abnormalities. In *Handbook of Speech Pathology*, ed. L. Travis, Englewood Cliffs, N.J.: Prentice Hall (1957).

MURPHY, A., *Functional Voice Disorders.* Englewood Cliffs, N.J.: Prentice Hall (1964).

NETSELL, R., Evaluation of velopharyngeal function in dysarthria. *J. Speech Hearing Dis.*, 34, 113–122 (1969).

NETSELL, R., *Kineseology Studies of the Dysarthrias.* Madison: University of Wisconsin (1975).

NETSELL, R., AND T. HIXON, A noninvasive method for clinically estimating subglottal air pressure. *J. Speech Hearing Dis.*, 43, 326–330 (1978).

NETTER, F., The larynx. *Clinical Symposia.* Summit, N.J.: CIBA Pharmaceutical Company (1964).

PTACEK, P., AND E. SANDER, Maximum duration of phonation. *J. Speech Hearing Res.*, 3, 227–244 (1963).

SCHMIDT, P., F. KLINGHOLZ AND F. Martin, Influence of pitch, voice sound pressure, and vowel quality on the maximum phonation time. *J. Voice*, 2, 245–249 (1988).

SORENSON, D., AND P. PARKER, The voiced/voiceless phonation time in children with and without laryngeal pathology. *Lang. Speech Hearing Serv. Schools*, 23, 163–168 (1992).

SPRIESTERSBACH, D. C., K. L. MOLL, AND H. L. MORRIS, Subject classification and articulation of speakers with cleft palates. *J. Speech Hearing Res.*, 4, 362–372 (1961).

STRONG, P., *Biophysical Measurements.* Beaverton, Oreg.: Tektronix, Inc. (1970).

ST. LOUIS, K., AND D. RUSCELLO, *The Oral Mechanism Screening Examination.* Baltimore: University Park Press (1981).

STONE, R. Issues in clinical assessment of laryngeal function: Contraindications for subscribing to maximum phonation time and optimal frequency. In *Vocal Fold Physiology: Contemporary Research and Clinical Issues*, eds. D. M. Bless and J. H. Abbs. San Diego: College-Hill (1983).

SUBTELNY, J. D., G. KHO, R. MCCORMACK, AND J. SUBTELNY, Multidimensional analysis of bilabial stop and nasal consonants—cineradiographic and pressure-flow analysis. *Cleft Pal. J.*, 6, 263–269 (1969).

SUBTELNY, J., J. WORTH, AND M. SAKUDA, Intraoral pressure and rate of flow during speech. *J. Speech Hearing Res.*, 9, 498–518 (1966).

SUSSMAN, H., AND K. SMITH, Transducer for measuring lip movements during speech. *J. Acous. Soc. Amer.*, 48, 858–860 (1970a).

SUSSMAN, H., AND K. SMITH, Transducer for measuring mandibular movements during speech. *J. Acous. Soc. Amer.*, 48, 857–858 (1970b).

TAIT, N., J. MICHEL, AND M. CARPENTER, Maximum duration of sustained /s/ and /z/ in children. *J. Speech Hearing Dis.*, 45, 239–246 (1980).

VAN HATTUM, R., AND J. WORTH, Airflow rates in normal speakers. *Cleft Pal. J.*, 4, 137–147 (1967).

VAN RIPER, C., *Speech Correction: Principles and Methods*, 6th ed. Englewood Cliffs, N.J.: Prentice Hall (1978).

WAKITA, H., Instrumentation for the study of speech acoustics. In *Contemporary Issues in Experimental Phonetics*, ed. N. Lass. New York: Academic Press (1976).

WARREN, D., Aerodynamics of speech production. In *Contemporary Issues in Experimental Phonetics*, ed. N. Lass. New York: Academic Press (1976).

WATKIN, K., AND J. ZAGZEBSKI, On-Line ultrasonic technique for monitoring tongue displacements. *J. Acous. Soc. Amer.*, 54, 544–547 (1973).

WILSON, D., *Voice Problems of Children*, 2nd ed. Baltimore: Williams and Wilkins (1979).

WILSON, D. K., *Voice Problems of Children*, 3rd ed. Baltimore: Williams and Wilkins (1987).

YANAGIHARA, N., AND Y. KOIKE, The regulation of sustained phonation. *Folia Phon.*, 19, 1–18 (1967).

YANAGIHARA, N., Y. KOIKE, AND H. VON LEDEN, Phonation and respiration: Function study in normal subjects. *Folia Phon.*, 18, 323–340 (1966).

ZEMLIN, W., *Speech and Hearing Science*. Englewood Cliffs, N.J.: Prentice Hall (1968).

8

Assessment Formats for Structural Disorders

Structural deviations are not synonymous with functional differences

Disorders such as laryngectomy, cleft palate, glossectomee, and cerebral palsy result from structural and/or neuromuscular abnormalities. Evaluation of communicative functioning will typically be encompassed within a broader assessment by a team of specialists including otolaryngologists, plastic and reconstructive surgeons, audiologists, physical and/or occupational therapists, and/or orthodontists and prosthodontists, among others. The communicative assessment strategies for these disorders have some procedures in common with problem areas previously discussed, but specialized appraisal tools may also be necessary. Cerebral palsy and severe acquired dysarthrias, in particular, necessitate extending the evaluation to detailed sensorimotor performance analyses in addition to evaluation of speech, language, and cognitive functioning, frequently through adaptations of standardized tests, in order to establish which alternative/augmentative systems function optimally to maximize their communication abilities. The assessment formats for these disorders will be considered because they exemplify the eclectic derivation of evaluative instruments and because they demonstrate the wide range of behaviors that must be quantified in order to determine the communicative disorder(s) to be addressed in treatment.

EVALUATION OF LARYNGECTOMY

There is general agreement (Berlin and Virden 1971; Boone 1983; Gardner 1971; Martin and Hoops 1974; Warner 1971) that a diagnostic evaluation of the laryngectomy should include consideration of factors concerning the surgery; the patient's physical condition, auditory functioning, emotional status, vocation, and articulation and language abilities; the familial attitude toward the patient with esophageal speech; and the use of this information for determining a prognosis for esophageal speech development. The information obtained is clearly prognostic in nature. Since some of the information is acquired before surgery, we will consider preoperative as well as postoperative assessment procedures.

Preoperative Assessment.   Preoperative assessment will include a detailed medical, social, and educational history. The medical history will provide information on conditions that may have a significant bearing on the ability to develop esophageal speech. For example, a history of hernia, abdominal surgery, cleft palate or palatal paresis, pulmonary disease, and colostomy are negative prognostic indicators (Diedrich and Youngstrom 1966). Job duties, leisure-time activities, and the emotional status of the patient should be explored. Patients employed in highly communicative positions and with a history of vocational success are more likely to develop functional esophageal speech. Family attitudes are also important. A supportive, encouraging family accepting of esophageal speech development will have a positive effect on rehabilitation efforts.

Surgical removal of the larynx has a marked impact on oral-peripheral structures. Nevertheless, an examination of the speech-production mechanism should be completed preoperatively. Hearing acuity is also assessed because it is prognostically significant. Berlin (1963) found that 40 percent of the laryngectomies who were poor esophageal speakers had a significant hearing loss. Kahane and Irwin (1975) noted that hearing sensitivity is a critical element in esophageal-voice rehabilitation and may have adverse effects on the control of stoma noise, voice quality, and length of rehabilitation. The audiological battery should include speech discrimination, speech reception threshold, and pure-tone testing.

Other preoperative appraisals may be used. Berlin and Virden (1971) suggested that a preoperative recording of a standard speech passage and plosive production in consonant-vowel or vowel-consonant-vowel contexts be recorded and later compared to esophageal speech. Logemann (1975) recommended that articulatory patterns and rate of speech production be evaluated preoperatively. Finally, an attempt may be made to determine the ability of the patient to produce esophageal phonation. This is of limited value, however, since the structural integrity of the esophagus and oral structures is frequently altered by surgery.

Postoperative Assessment.   Following surgery, a careful review of the surgical report is in order. This is important because it will provide information on the integrity of the apparatus that will be used for esophageal speech. Important information includes reports of denervation of muscular structures of the head and neck, postradiation fibrosis, stenosis of the esophagus, and the extension of the surgery, particularly to excision of the pharynx, base of the tongue, and floor of the mouth.

Attention should be paid to examination of labial, palatal, and lingual structures since they are of primary importance to insufflation of the esophagus. The lips, if there is facial weakness, may not be able to effectively seal air within the intraoral cavity. Likewise, partial removal of the tongue or interruption of the neural supply to the tongue or velopharyngeal mechanism will reduce or prevent insufflation. If the patient has dentures, they should be examined because if they do not fit properly, oral structural movements will be impeded during attempts to force air into the esophagus. Finally, hearing should be reassessed since edema or metastasis of the carcinoma to the auditory nerve may produce hearing impairment.

Instruments for appraising esophageal speech are primarily scaling devices that estimate the proficiency of the patient or monitor the acquisition of alaryngeal speech skills. Perhaps the earliest scale was developed by Wepman, MacGahan, Richard, and Shelton (1953). The seven-point rating scale extends from level 7, no esophageal speech production, to level 1, automatic esophageal speech. Wepman and his associates proposed that the scale be used for self-evaluation and for observation since it serves the dual role of monitoring the progression of esophageal-sound production and providing an estimate of speech proficiency.

Berlin and Virden (1971) developed assessment tasks that have at least face validity in relation to adequate esophageal speech. The four skills evaluated include the reliability of phonation on demand, the maintenance of a short latency between insufflation of the esophagus and vocalization, the maintenance of an optimal duration of phonation, and the ability to sustain phonation during articulation. In order to assess these skills, the patient is asked to perform two tasks: to phonate as long as possible on the vowel /a/ over 20 trials and to repeat the syllable /da/ as many times as possible, without consciously reinflating the esophagus, over 10 trials. The ability to phonate on demand is determined by the percentage of successful vocalizations in 20 trials; any vocalization exceeding 0.4 seconds is considered successful. Maintenance of short latency is measured by finding the mean time between insufflation and production of /a/. Optimal duration is determined by the mean duration of /a/ over 20 trials, and sustaining phonation during articulation is evaluated by recording the mean number of syllables articulated with a single overt insufflation. Berlin and Virden indicated that a good esophageal speaker could phonate reliably on demand with a short latency, sustain a vowel for approximately 2 seconds, and produce approximately 10 syllables per insufflation.

Similar appraisal devices were proposed by Weinberg (1975). He suggested that assessment should be divided into two areas: skill building and speech building. Examples of skill building included determining mean latency, mean duration of phonation, and number of syllables produced on one insufflation. Speech-building assessment included evaluating the patient's ability to produce syllables or words, estimating the intelligibility of speech in conversational settings, and determining the rate of speech production in words per minute.

In summary, assessment of the laryngectomized patient is eclectic. Much of the information gained is biographical in nature and used for determining prognosis. Appraisal tools are limited almost entirely to determining the esophageal-speech proficiency of the patient on the basis of clinical judgment, rather than through standardized appraisal tools.

EVALUATION OF GLOSSECTOMEE

Although there are several clinical case reports and small sample studies of patients who have undergone partial or complete removal of the tongue (Goldstein 1940; Herberman 1958; Massengill, Maxwell, and Pickrell 1970), there has been only one major study of glossectomized patients (Skelly 1973; Skelly and others 1971; Skelly and others 1972). Skelly and others studied the articulatory and phonatory deficits of 25 partial and complete glossectomee patients, and their assessment instruments serve as the primary source for appraisal procedures.

Glossectomees are performed as a lifesaving surgical procedure for cancer of the tongue. The amount of tissue removed is dependent on the site of lesion and metastasis of the disease, and the degree of communicative impairment and dysphagia is dependent upon the amount of tissue resected and the degree of interruption of innervation to the musculature of the head and neck. Partial removal, especially of either the right or left half of the tongue, has far less marked an effect on speech production than complete removal. As would be expected, total removal produces marked deficits in the ability to produce lingual consonants, semivowels, and vowels since the egressive airstream cannot be valved by the tongue, and the tongue is no longer available to alter the resonant characteristics of the vocal tract. Due to the critical role of the tongue in deglutition, drooling and dysphagia are concomitant problems.

There are no standardized tests for the glossectomee. Assessment procedures derive almost wholly from the work of Skelly and others and include consideration of case history and phonatory and articulatory functioning. The case history information and medical and surgical reports provide a social context from which to view the patient and a detailed summary of the anatomical and innervation effects of surgery. Responses to biographical questions and the reading of a standard passage (for example, Arthur the Rat) are tape-recorded to establish baseline performance. The patient is then asked to produce five vowels that are judged by the examiner to determine if they are *distinguishable* from one another and not to determine if they are *identifiable*. This procedure is followed by the patient's production of a vowel (one he produces easily) and the voiced and voiceless labiodental fricatives /v/ and /f/, which are maintained for a maximal duration. Skelly noted that normal duration is approximately 18 seconds, and durations of 14 seconds or less are indicative of laryngeal and/or respiratory problems that should be evaluated further by determining mean duration for each of the 3 phonemes over 3 trials.

The next task is for the patient to produce an open vowel at his highest and then at his lowest pitch followed by glides from highest to lowest and lowest to highest pitch. This procedure, when coupled to the patient's productions of a vowel at the highest pitch and lowest pitch with intervening pauses, provides an estimate of pitch range and additional information regarding the integrity of the respiratory-laryngeal mechanism.

Articulatory abilities are appraised by asking the patient to produce syllables, words, and sentences containing glossal and nonglossal consonants. The glossal and nonglossal consonant productions are then compared and serve as an estimate of residual articulatory facility.

The next task is for the patient to produce words without glossal consonants, such as *pave*, under a number of conditions: with greater labial compression, with greater jaw excursion, at faster and slower rates, at a higher pitch, with the jaw "thrust forward," with vowel prolongation, and with increased intensity. It is evident that the purpose of these tasks is to assess the patient's compensatory abilities following major structural changes of the oral cavity.

Skelly (1973) suggests that a speech sample be used to determine what substitutions are used for glossal consonants, to assess the patient's ability to communicate information, and to provide estimates of intelligibility based upon ratings by the patient, the clinician, and naive listeners. She also recommends that the patient be administered a complete audiological battery, a test for short-term auditory memory, and the *Leiter International Performance Scale*.

In the aggregate, the procedures we have reviewed include primarily nonstandardized instruments, the function of which is to evaluate the residual and compensatory abilities of the speech-production apparatus. These procedures appear intuitively to be adequate for the assessment of the glossectomee, but in the absence of validity and reliability statements, their comparative value cannot be determined. In the end, the value of the information obtained will be at least as much determined by the experience and expertise of the examiner as by the procedures used to obtain the information.

With a few rare exceptions (Backus 1940; Peterson 1973), laryngectomies and glossectomees are adults. We now turn to appraisal procedures for two disorders, cleft palate and cerebral palsy, that are most often evaluated in childhood.

ASSESSMENT OF CLEFT PALATE

Articulation and resonance disorders are the primary communicative deficits associated with cleft palate and arise from the congenital structural abnormalities of the speech-production apparatus. There may be associated deficits in language and auditory acuity, but these problems most often are secondary and are typically mild. The evaluation of the cleft palate patient includes a case history; articulation, resonance, and nasal emission testing; audiological assessment; voice evaluation; and determination of linguistic abilities. We earlier provided information on procedures for acquiring case history information and the steps to be followed in completing an oral-peripheral examination of the speech mechanism. Of major importance to the case history is a detailed summary of the course of surgical, prosthodontic, and therapeutic intervention. The oral-peripheral examination should effectively capture clinical observations on the structural/functional integrity of the speech-production apparatus with special emphasis on the adequacy of the velopharyngeal mechanism. We also previously considered articulation testing, language assessment, voice evaluation, and some aspects of testing velopharyngeal functioning and instrumentation useful for evaluating structural disorders. The focus here is on measures developed specifically with cleft palate patients in mind.

Articulation Tests

The effect of velopharyngeal incompetence is to produce compensations at other constrictions in the vocal tract. Consequently, some of the articulatory behaviors of cleft palate children are different from those produced by children with normal velopharyngeal competence. Behaviors that demonstrate compensatory efforts are attempts to constrict the nares to gain or to maintain intraoral pressure and the substitution of pharyngeal and velar fricatives and glottal stops. The production of these articulatory substitutions exemplifies the efforts made by the speaker to constrict the egressive airstream posterior to the insufficient velopharyngeal valve. Fricatives, affricates, and plosives are most frequently in error because they require the highest intraoral pressure for their production. This is not to say that children with cleft palate will not demonstrate phonological disorders as well since many will; rather, it is to point out that some of the errors will be unique and will involve nasal emission, lack of oral pressure, and marked substitution (McWilliams, Morris, and Shelton 1984) because they are conditioned by a structurally inadequate speech-production apparatus. It is also noteworthy that the substitutions used by the cleft palate patient may persist after surgical and/or prosthetic management has restored velopharyngeal competency since they have become habituated.

One articulation measure already reviewed is the *Iowa Pressure Articulation Test* (IPAT) (Morris, Spriestersbach, and Darley 1961). The test is composed of 43 items selected from the *Templin-Darley Tests of Articulation* (Templin and Darley 1960). Included are fricatives, affricates, and plosives that best discriminate between adequate and inadequate velopharyngeal closure. The errors on the test can be compared to norms from the Templin-Darley test. The sounds in error are also stimulated to determine a prognosis for correction and to separate errors due to physiological inadequacy from those due to delayed phonological development. The IPAT has also been found to be of predictive value in determining the need for secondary management of cleft palate patients (Van Denmark and Morris 1977).

Some of the consonants included on the IPAT are not produced correctly by young children. Van Demark and Swickard (1980) developed a screening articulation test of 25 words emphasizing /p/ and /b/. Administration of the test by means of elicited responses, or alternatively by imitation, to 30 children 30 to 50 months of age yielded high rates of correct production. Since /p/ and /b/ are predictive in discriminating adequate from inadequate velopharyngeal competency (Van Demark 1979), they proposed that the test was useful in identifying those children at greatest risk; children who cannot correctly produce on the test would be considered for additional assessment.

Another articulatory measure developed to assess velopharyngeal function is the *Miami Imitative Ability Test* (Jacobs, Phillips, and Harrison 1970). The test evaluates the ability to imitate acoustic production and articulatory placement for consonants. The measure includes 24 consonants presented in consonant-vowel contexts using the neutral vowel /ʌ/. The patient is instructed to watch and listen as the examiner repeats each syllable three times. The patient is then asked to repeat the syllable. Articulatory placement and acoustic production are scored separately. Responses are assigned one point if produced correctly, one-half point if questionable, or no point if incorrect. Both placement and acoustic scores can range from zero to 24 points. For visible sounds, placement is scored by direct observation. If the placement is not readily visible, the examiner must base her judgment on the visual assessment supplemented by the acoustic production. Since acoustic information must be used to determine placement accuracy, the two evaluational procedures are not independent of one another.

Administration of the test to 129 children with cleft palate and 154 children without orofacial anomalies between 30 and 72 months of age revealed that the cleft-palate children were inferior to the normal group on both evaluations. In fact, at 72 months, cleft-palate children did not have the proficiency on the test of 30-month-old normal children.

The *Bzoch Error Pattern Diagnostic Articulation Test* (described by Bzoch 1979) is based on the articulation characteristics of cleft palate and matched normal control subjects from three to six years of age (Bzoch 1956). The test contains 100 elements (67 single consonants and 33 blends). The single consonants are tested in the initial, medial, and final positions of words and are grouped by manner of production (plosives, fricatives, affricatives, aspirates, glides, nasals). Within each manner grouping, the most peripheral articulations are tested first followed by evaluation of anterior to posterior placements.

Sounds are tested first in the initial position followed by medial and then final positions. Cognate pairs are listed together for the plosive and fricative categories, and the testing of an unvoiced consonant precedes testing of its voiced cognate.

Words with the test element correctly produced are scored as correct whether other elements are correct or not. If the consonant element was produced correctly but was distorted by nasal emission alone, it is scored accordingly. If the test element is produced incorrectly, the child is asked to repeat it two more times, and the most severe error is recorded according to an ascending order of error severity: distortion (due to imprecise articulation), simple substitution (use of another phoneme for the target phoneme), gross substitution (use of velar fricative, pharyngeal fricative, or glottal stop), or omission of the phoneme. Blends are considered, for the purposes of recording and scoring, as single elements. If one or more of the elements of the blend are distorted but all are present, it is scored as a distortion; if part of the blend is missing but some of the sounds are used in place of it (e.g., /th/ for /thr/ in *thread*), it is scored as a simple substitution. Any gross substitution of a blend element is recorded as a gross substitution for the entire blend, and an omission is defined as omission of all blend elements.

The Bzoch test is not particularly unusual. It follows the more traditional format of assessing single elements in the initial, medial, and final positions of words and includes items typically found on many of the articulation tests we reviewed earlier. It is clearly different, however, in its scoring system because it provides error categories that are anticipated for patients with inadequate velopharyngeal closure.

Articulation errors of cleft palate speakers may vary between single words and connected speech. Van Demark (1964) constructed 13 test sentences containing 149 consonant sounds: 56 plosives, 33 fricatives, 31 nasal semivowels, and 29 glides. The sentences contain 21 consonant blends in various combinations. The sentences are constructed to approximate the frequency of occurrence of the various consonant sounds found in the English language. Scoring is accomplished by evaluating the correctness of production of the 149 test consonants. If a consonant is produced incorrectly, the response is categorized according to the manner of production (fricative, plosive, glide, nasal semivowel) and the type of error (distortion-oral, distortion-nasal, glottal stop substitution, substitution, and omission). The test sentences, therefore, provide an estimate of consonant-production accuracy in connected speech.

An important point, based on this discussion, is that articulation test results from the cleft palate child serve a dual purpose. They not only provide information on the articulatory patterns and phonological development of the child but also are useful in determining velopharyngeal competence and effects of the structural anomaly. For example, Philips (1986) noted that a pattern in which fricatives only are nasalized suggests greater velopharyngeal competence than if plosives are also nasalized. She also indicated that posterior compensatory articulations such as pharyngeal fricatives may have an effect on the production of /r/ and /l/ because of the altered articulatory positioning for the high-pressure fricatives.

Clinical Methods of Estimating Velopharyngeal Competence

Nasal emission of air and hypernasality are not the same phenomenon. Both typically result from inadequate velopharyngeal closure, but emission is the audible flow of air through the nasal passages during the production of consonants requiring high intraoral pressure while hypernasality is the acoustic end product of an abnormal coupling of the nasal and oral cavities during voiced segments.

Bzoch (1979) has suggested several clinical tests that yield estimates of nasal emission, hypernasality, and hyponasality. Hyponasality is evaluated because it may be characteristic of patients with overly broad pharyngeal flaps or obturators that effectively valve the velopharyngeal port during the production of nasals. Each test is based on the performance of the patient on 10 items. For the hypernasality test, the patient produces 10 words initiated with /b/ and terminated with /t/. Each word is produced by the patient with the nostrils open and with the nares manually closed. A ratio is determined by counting the number of productions of the 10 on which there is a perceived change of tone. Ten words initiated with /m/ and ended with /t/ are produced with the nares open and occluded on the hyponasality test. Here the number of words that sound the same with the nares open and occluded is used to determine the clinical index of abnormal hyponasality. A nasal-emission clinical index is determined, according to Bzoch, by placing a small paddle wheel in front of the nares during production of 10 bisyllabic words containing /p/ and /b/ in initial and medial word positions. The examiner counts the number of productions on which nasal emission occurs out of the 10 words to determine a ratio.

There are no norms for these clinical tests. However, it can be assumed that a patient with high clinical index ratios on the three measures has abnormal velopharyngeal closure while low ratios are indicative of normal or near normal expected performance.

Another means of evaluating cleft palate speakers is by scaling attributes of their speech production. Subtelny, Van Hattum, and Myers (1972) suggested that this be accomplished by assessing separately the nasality, articulation, and intelligibility of speech samples. The attributes may be rated on a seven-point, equal-interval scale or by other preset criteria. The reliability of the estimates will vary significantly depending on the nature of the speech sample and the procedures used to make the ratings. For example, Counihan and Cullinan (1970) found that the reliability of nasality ratings increased and the degree of ambiguity decreased from vowels to syllables to connected speech rated during backward play to connected speech rated during forward play. Hess (1971) noted that articulatory proficiency was significantly affected by the phoneme type and the stress of the consonant-vowel environment. Moore and Sommers (1973) and Lintz and Sherman (1961) noted that context significantly affected ratings of nasality. Ratings may provide information on nasality and other attributes of speech production, but it must be remembered that the interpretation of these data must be cautious in light of contextual and procedural effects that reduce reliability.

We are in agreement with McWilliams et al. (1984) who noted:

> ... a rating scale is a useful device provided reliability is consistently monitored and provided speech is heard in a variety of contexts ranging from a sentence containing neither high-pressure consonants nor nasals through one loaded with sibilants. (p. 267)

McWilliams and Philips (1979) developed a rating scale to bring together the speech information in order to make a judgment about velopharyngeal adequacy. The scale includes ratings of nasal emission (for example, consistent, inconsistent), facial grimace, nasal resonance (e.g., mild hypernasality, hyponasality), phonation (e.g., mild hoarseness, reduced loudness), and articulation (e.g., omission of fricatives or plosives, glottal stops). The total cumulative score is an estimate of velopharyngeal valving with 0 = competent, 1–2 = competent to borderline competent, 3–6 = borderline to borderline incompetent, and 7 + = incompetent. They noted that there is good agreement between scale ratings and ratings from videofluoroscopic records and that for individuals with scale values greater than 7 instrumental assessment should be undertaken. The scale nicely demonstrates the multiple judgments of articulation, resonance, and phonation that are required to effectively estimate velopharyngeal functioning.

Instrumentation

A mainstay in the assessment of velopharyngeal competence is instrumentation. Perhaps for no other disorder has instrumental analysis had such a large role in evaluation. Typically, clinical results from articulation and resonance are combined with results from instrumental analysis and serve as the basis for determining velopharyngeal competence.

The most frequently used clinical device is the oral manometer, which provides an estimate of velopharyngeal competence by allowing a determination of an intraoral pressure ratio. The ratio is computed by comparing the intraoral pressure obtained with the nares occluded and unoccluded (Morris 1966). However, research findings have questioned the reliability of oral manometer ratios. Noll, Hawkins, and Weinberg (1977) obtained readings of maximum, sustained, positive, and negative pressures from 40 normal six- and seven-year-old children. They found that the majority of the subjects had difficulty generating and maintaining stable positive and negative pressures with the nostrils occluded and unoccluded. They decided that the oral manometric ratio may be of questionable value in predicting velopharyngeal adequacy for speech, particularly if ratio data must be interpreted dichotomously.

A number of other instruments we discussed earlier are available for estimating velopharyngeal competence, including ultrasound, cinefluorography, aerodynamics, endoscopy, and acoustic measurements (Baken 1987; Hollein 1976;

McWilliams et al. 1984; Philips 1986). A combination of approaches is used because of shortcomings associated with each technique. For example, cinefluorography provides information on movement, but since views of structural movement are two-dimensional, small leaks may be missed. Aerodynamic measurements provide data on air pressure and flow during speech production, thereby providing an estimate of the size of the velopharyngeal orifice, but do not result in data that can be used to determine the combination of structural movements that accomplished the valving. The logical procedure is to use combinations of clinical behavioral observations and results from instrumental analysis to yield the best estimate of velopharyngeal closure.

Other Tests

Children with cleft palate frequently have hearing disorders (Hayes 1965) and language deficits (Philips 1986; Philips and Harrison 1969; Smith and McWilliams 1968). Tests for assessing language skills and various types of developmental behaviors were discussed earlier. Choose tests that meet your needs in assessing the linguistic skills of these patients.

EVALUATION IN CEREBRAL PALSY

A practical definition of cerebral palsy—a brain damage syndrome comprised of neuromuscular, sensory, psychological, intellectual, and behavioral disorders—quickly points out the large number of behaviors that may need to be assessed with these patients. If these deficits are viewed from a macroscopic vantage point, it would be expected that a large number of professionals—medical, allied health, and educational—all will contribute assessment data at one time or another if a full description of the cerebral-palsied child is to be obtained.

If we take a more restricted view of the appraisal process by delimiting the areas of concern that are the province of the speech-language pathologist, many of the tests we have previously discussed in this text would also be appropriate to determine communication deficits of cerebral-palsied children, depending partly on the severity of the disorder. The lines of demarcation as to which instruments and which areas of assessment are the province of the speech clinician are not entirely clear—nor should they necessarily be restricted in the context of a team evaluation of the patient. In general, the speech-language pathologist's role in the evaluation process will be dictated by the clinical situation in which he works, the neurophysiological rationale that serves as the basis for the process, and the problems of the patient to be addressed. These somewhat different formats and focuses are seen in assessment approaches proposed by several clinicians.

Crickmay (1966) indicated that an assessment in cerebral palsy should entail evaluation of (1) the ability to move body parts associated with the speech mechanism, such as the head, neck, and shoulders; (2) the ability to do vegetative activities such as sucking, swallowing, biting, and chewing; (3) the ability to manipulate the jaws, lips, and tongue; and (4) the ability to vocalize and speak. She notes further:

> In making this speech assessment, it is necessary to find out which of the patient's reactions are normal, which are pathological and which are primitive but normal. . . . with each reaction tested it is necessary to find out which movements the patient is able to do voluntarily, both with and without emotional stimulation, and which he can only do involuntarily, or merely as a reflex movement in response to a stimulus. (p. 77)

Certainly, Crickmay would not view the language, auditory acuity, and other communication-related deficits to be unimportant since they are included in her therapy regime, but clearly the strategy she proposes focuses squarely on neuromuscular deficits as the primary area of concern.

Hardy (1983) focuses on the evaluation of the speech-production apparatus, including respiratory, phonatory, resonatory, and articulatory systems. He noted that the purpose of evaluating these systems is not only to identify specific characteristics of the speech-production problem and the manner in which the speaker uses the system but also to determine how the system can be used to improve speech production. Assessment procedures are similar to those presented in the chapter on the examination of the speech-production mechanism but with special attention paid to the patterns of performance expected from individuals with cerebral palsy.

A more comprehensive view of the areas in need of assessment is provided by Westlake and Rutherford (1961). They suggest that appraisal procedures, in addition to case history, will include consideration of expressive and receptive language, conceptualization, and vegetative and volitional functioning of the speech-production apparatus. There is some correspondence between Westlake and Rutherford and Crickmay as to the areas to be evaluated, that is, the importance of appraising vegetative and voluntary functioning of the speech-production mechanism. There are similarities in the instruments selected (or not selected); neither Westlake and Rutherford nor Crickmay cite standardized instruments to be used as part of the evaluation. Does this mean that they do not see value in using standardized tests and age-referenced norms? Certainly not. Crickmay points out that "In treating him [the cerebral-palsied child] it is essential at all stages to measure his performance against that of the normal child and to follow the normal developmental pattern as closely as possible," and Westlake and Rutherford observe that two important pieces of information sought in the assessment of expressive behavior are "How does the child's level of oral language usage compare with that of other children of the same chronological age?" and "In what ways are his oral language patterns different from those of other children his age?"

McDonald and Chance (1964) provide a format of evaluation in which the same areas as those cited by Westlake and Rutherford are proposed along with a deemphasis on standardized instruments and an emphasis on age-referenced norms. Lencione (1966) and Mecham, Berko, and Berko (1960), on the other hand, see greater value in standardized tests for appraisal, although the areas of concern as to what is to be assessed are the same. The point to be made is that the instruments and procedures used, the areas to be assessed, and the weight and time afforded each of these areas will be determined in part by the problems demonstrated by the child and in part by the theoretical framework and clinical environment in which the clinician is operating.

Assessment Instruments for Cerebral Palsy

The instruments and procedures you choose for evaluating the cerebral-palsied child will typically include measures of articulation and language. Additionally, a case history will be secured, instrumental data may be obtained to enhance description of speech-production adequacy, and examination of the speech-production mechanism will be performed in an expanded format that considers vegetative, nonverbal, and verbal performance tasks. The exact areas of assessment will depend on the problems demonstrated by the child, the focus and rationale of the assessment, and the availability of information from other professionals. Quite obviously, the appraisal process is not complete, in most cases, without appraisal data from the physician, audiologist, psychologist, occupational and physical therapists, and perhaps educational diagnostician.

Depending on the severity of the disorder, standardized tests may have to be adapted to fit the clinical situation. We cannot provide exact guidelines as to when the test procedures have been sufficiently altered to bring into question the validity and reliability of the test findings. This will depend on the tests and the adaptations made. The important thing to remember is that when assessing the child, there is no substitute for careful observation, detailed description, and clinical judgment when the findings are to be interpreted in light of normative data that serve as the reference for making statements about "normal" and "abnormal" performance.

Several measures have been developed for cerebral-palsied children that may serve to enhance descriptions of their communicative functioning. Denhoff and Holden (1951) studied 100 cerebral-palsied children and compared their performance to that of normal children on 10 motor and communication items from the Gesell scales. Results of the study are displayed as histograms that show average, late normal, and abnormal late development based on the Gesell studies data and the mean performance of the cerebral-palsied children. As would be expected, the cerebral-palsied children were later than the ranges provided for the Gesell children. For example, on "walks alone," the average normal Gesell child accomplished this activity no later than 16 months while the average cerebral-palsied child did not accomplish this skill until 34 months. On "speech—single words," the average normal child would be expected, according to the Gesell data, to have reached this developmental milestone by 11 months while the average cerebral-palsied child did not begin using single words until 28 months. This scale may be helpful because it provides, in addition to normal and late performance in normal children, average development for cerebral-palsied children so that the patient can be compared to a normative reference group and to children with the same diagnosis. Unfortunately, no range is included for the cerebral-palsied children on each task. Denhoff and Holden did report, however, that the performances of the cerebral-palsied children were heterogeneous and that there was overlap with the performance of the Gesell children.

We would like to consider two tests that were developed specifically for cerebral-palsied children—one of articulation and the other of auditory discrimination developed by Irwin. O. C. Irwin, in a large number of studies published in the fifties and sixties, evaluated the communicative abilities of cerebral-palsied children in an effort to develop test instruments standardized specifically for these patients. An *Integrated Test for Use with Children with Cerebral Palsy* (Irwin

1961) is composed of five "short" tests that had been individually standardized on 1,155 cerebral-palsied children. Four of the tests were developed to evaluate consonants; the fifth, to evaluate vowels. The Integrated test is a restandardization of the "short" tests on a group of 147 cerebral-palsied children from 3 to 16 years of age.

The test contains 24 consonants tested in initial, medial, and final word positions (where appropriate) and 11 vowels tested in initial and medial positions. Items are administered by imitation, and the entire test need not be administered at one time since it would be expected that the cerebral-palsied child will fatigue quickly. Items are scored as correct, substituted, omitted, distorted, no response, and neutral (defined as a response that bears no resemblance to the stimulus word). The number of errors of each type on each short test are then tabulated. An alternative list of stimulus words is provided for each of the short tests.

Results of the standardization of the Integrated test are reported as means and variances for boys and girls; for initial, medial, and final word positions for consonants and initial and medial positions for vowels; for spastics and athetoids; for extent of involvement (quadriplegia, hemiplegia, and paraplegia); for left and right hemiplegics; for severity (mild, moderate, and severe); and for severity as a function of extent of involvement. Split-half reliability was found to be 0.98; Kuder-Richardson reliability coefficients were from 0.65 to 0.97; and interobserver agreement was estimated at 90 percent. The validity of the test was reportedly demonstrated to be adequate by means of the method of extreme groups using both articulation scores and ratings of intelligibility.

Given the time and effort expended to develop and standardize the five short tests and the integrated test composed thereof, it might be expected that the test would be on the top of the list when appraising the articulatory development of cerebral-palsied children. However, this has not been the case, and the reasons are apparent. First, no data are available for normal children. Consequently, the performance of the cerebral-palsied child cannot be compared to a normative reference to make statements about the adequacy of his articulatory development. Moreover, even though the performance of cerebral-palsied children is reported on the basis of many factors as previously listed, no mean and variance data are provided as a function of age. These weaknesses preclude the use of the test for making direct comparisons with normal or cerebral-palsied children. The test may serve as a descriptive device that provides a means of quantifying the articulatory behaviors of these children, but it appears to be of less value than articulation tests we discussed in an earlier chapter that were standardized on normal children.

Irwin and Jensen (1963a,b) developed two tests of sound discrimination for cerebral-palsied children. Since they are similar in format and design, we will examine only the first. The test is composed of 30 word pairs. Twenty-five of the pairs differ by a single phoneme (pig–big) or by the presence of a blend versus a singleton consonant (brisket–biscuit). Ten are different in the initial position, 10 in the final position, and 5 in the medial position. Five word pairs are identical and serve as foils. The words are monosyllabic (tin–thin), bisyllabic (frisking–whisking), or multisyllabic (convergent–conversant). It should be noted that many of the stimulus words of the test (cytology–psychology; habitat–habitant) are not found in the vocabulary of young children.

The test was standardized on 153 cerebral-palsied children 6 to 16 years of age with a mean of 10.3 years. Means and standard deviations are provided by two-year intervals except for the first level, which includes only six-year-olds; by mental age; by severity of involvement; and by ratings of speech and language ability. Reliability of the test using a Kuder-Richardson formula was reported to be 0.87. Using the method of extreme groups, significant differences were found in discrimination scores for chronological age, mental age, and ratings of speech and language ability, which Irwin and Jensen considered supportive of the validity of the test.

In light of our earlier stated reservations about the use of auditory discrimination tests, we would not expect this test to be administered to the cerebral-palsied child. However, it serves as another example of a test devised specifically for a group of communicatively handicapped patients but which appears to be of no more worth than comparable tests of the same functions standardized on normal subjects.

In summary, the evaluation format for the cerebral-palsied child is similar to that for other communicatively handicapped patients. There may be small differences depending on the theoretical bases from which the examiner is operating, the age of child, and the severity and type of disorder demonstrated, but the task remains the same—observations are made and quantified so that comparisons with normal performance will allow a determination of communicative ability.

AUGMENTATIVE COMMUNICATION

Augmentative communication refers to all communicative behaviors that augment speech. Vanderheiden and Yoder (1986) point out that nonspeech augmentative behaviors are an important part of the communication process for unimpaired speakers. Gestures, facial expression, and intonational patterning convey much of what is important in the speaker's message. When speech production is compromised due to cognitive, motor, and/or sensory disorders (e.g., cerebral palsy, traumatic brain injury, degenerative neuromuscular diseases), there is a greater reliance on augmentative communication behaviors. Seldom, however, is the disorder sufficient to preclude some oral speech production so that an alternative communication system must be considered. Frequently, augmentative communication abilities are impaired in the patient with limited speech production so that the process of determining the most efficient means of communication requires careful analysis of the communication needs of the patient, her residual capabilities, and systems and strategies that will improve the efficiency of communication. In this section, we address assessment procedures involved in developing an effective communication system for the patient. Consideration of augmentative communication is in harmony with assessment procedures for glossectomee, laryngectomy, and cerebral palsy because, when combined with patients with acquired neurological deficits, these are the primary groups of augmentative patients that the speech-language pathologist works with in medical/educational (re)habilitation environments.

The increased emphasis on augmentative communication during the last 15 years has grown out of three primary areas (Vanderheiden and Yoder 1986): work with communication boards, sign and gestural systems for the deaf, and typing and environmental control systems for the severely handicapped. Vanderheiden and Yoder point out that these areas coalesced in the United States with the passage of

P.L. 94–142, which guarantees to all children, regardless of handicap, equal educational access. The interest in augmentative communication is reflected in the large number of publications that have attempted to bring together important components of augmentative communication rationales, strategies, systems, technology, assessments of augmentative communication rationales, strategies, systems, technology, assessment, and intervention (e.g., Beukelman and Yorkston 1982; Blackstone 1986; Cohen and Shane 1982; Fristoe and Lloyd 1979; Harris and Vanderheiden 1980; Kiernan 1977; McCormick and Shane 1984; Shane and Wilbur 1980; Vanderheiden and Grilley 1976; Yoder and Kraat 1983).

Decisions about augmentative communication candidacy and system selection involve a number of disciplines. Typically included are a speech-language pathologist, social worker, occupational therapist, physical therapist, adaptive engineer, psychologist, and, depending on the disorder, a physician. Professionals from other specialties such as education, computer technology, and audiology may be brought to the assessment based on need. It is expected that each of these specialties will provide information that will be useful in determining communication needs, candidacy for augmentation, and the most appropriate system for the patient.

Assessment will typically take place at critical time points. Yorkston and Karlan (1986) note that "Critical decision making points occur when communication needs are unmet, have changed, or will change substantially in the near future" (p. 164). The changes may be in the patient or in his needs. For example, assessment may be in order for the traumatic brain-injured patient who has regained some oral speech function in that a different augmentative system may allow better matching of oral and augmentative communication options. Evaluation would also be necessary if this patient is to return to a work environment to ensure that communication is sufficient for success in the employment setting.

There are a number of augmentative communication assessment models. The model developed by Beukelman, Yorkston, and Dowden (1985) includes a needs assessment and capability assessment that lead to the customization of an augmentative system that is evaluated by means of performance trials. Other models might be viewed as multistaged with a longitudinal focus in which evaluation of communication needs, environmental factors, and patient capabilities are followed by assessment of the appropriateness of symbol systems, response modes, switches, motor responses, and electronic devices followed by procedures to implement and evaluate the effectiveness of the system. A third model (Larson and Woodfin 1988) emphasizes the interaction of the augmentative communication candidate, the system, and the communicative partner in the framework of evaluation (see Table 8–1). Our discussion focuses on determining communicative needs, patient capabilities, and communication system selection.

Determining communication needs is a critical first step in the assessment process. The needs statements reflect the types of communication tasks the patient must be able to perform in order to function in various situations (Yorkston and Karlan 1986). Beukelman, Yorkston, and Dowden (1985) have provided a list of needs statements related to positioning (e.g., while sitting in bed), communication partners (e.g., several people at a time, someone with poor vision), locations (e.g., single room, outdoors), message needs (e.g., call attention, answer yes-no questions), and modality of communication (e.g., prepare printed messages, communicate via an intercom). Quite obviously, needs statements can be expanded or modified based on the patient. Each of the needs is evaluated to determine whether it is currently met, mandatory (immediately needed), desirable (important but not essential), unimportant, or future (important at some point in time). These decisions are based on interview information provided by the patient, family, teachers, or other communication partners.

There are two identifiable strategies for exploring augmentative communication options (Coleman, Cook, and Meyers 1980). The first approach has the patient "try out" a series of systems and then decide on the system that seems to best meet communication needs. Shortcomings of this approach are that it requires a large base of expensive augmentative communication systems on which to assess the patient; the choice of system is restricted to what is available, and the focus is on the systems rather than on the patient in need of augmentative support. A second approach is to evaluate the patient's communication needs and capabilities which are then used to develop a set of functions and requirements of the system. The functions and requirements are matched to the devices available to decide on the system of choice. The disadvantage of this method is the large commitment of time and funds to the assessment. The two approaches described by Coleman et al. (1980) are approximately equivalent to what Beukelman et al. (1985) and Yorkston and Karlan (1986) describe as criteria-based and comprehensive capability profiling. The two methods are not mutually exclusive, and it is apparent that the choice of approach is at least partially dictated by the type and severity of the communication problem and the environment in which the evaluation is completed.

Patient capabilities are assessed in four major areas: motor abilities, perceptual skills, cognitive/academic skills, and speech and language abilities. Standardized tests may need to be adapted because of the limited response modes of the patient. Adaptation of the administration procedures for these tests may bring into question the validity of the results. Many of these tests do not have norms that are useful for interpreting the performance of multiply handicapped children and adults. Therefore, it is important to utilize informal observation and nonstandardized testing to provide the information about patient capabilities. Goossens and Crain (1986) provide a series of scaling devices, checklists, and interview protocols that can be utilized in conjunction with formal and informal tests to gain a comprehensive evaluation of capabilities. Similarly, Montgomery (1980) includes an intake evaluation protocol for organizing augmentative communication assessment information.

Motor status is evaluated because the more intact the motor system, the larger the number and more efficient the augmentative strategies that will be available to the patient (Silverman 1989). With the patient seated in as comfortable and functional a position as possible, motor abilities of the upper extremities, head and neck, and lower extremities are evaluated for range of motion, strength, endurance, midline crossing, speed, accuracy, control, reliability, and ability to repeat a motion (Montgomery 1986). Silverman (1989) provides motor testing procedures from Daniels and Worthingham (1986) for the upper extremities, face and neck, and trunk and lower extremities. Motor functioning data are used to infer whether the patient would be able to employ a movement in the context of a particular system. An alternative approach would be to directly observe the movement in the context of the augmentative system.

Perceptual abilities are assessed because visual, auditory, and tactile/kinesthetic deficits influence the choice of augmentative communication systems. Auditory and visual acuity can be determined from audiological and ophthalmological examination. However, other abilities such as matching, figure—ground, spatial relationships, problem solving, visual pursuit, and position in space may need to be assessed by direct observation of the patient because administration of standardized tests to the child or adult who cannot point or speak is difficult at best.

Tests and assessment procedures for cognition and academic achievement will vary as a function of the age of the child. Areas include behaviors such as learning rate, attention to task, ability to retain newly learned information, academic performance level in reading and spelling, sound symbol association, and intellectual functioning.

Many of the measures reviewed in previous chapters may be appropriate for evaluation of speech and language abilities. At a minimum, an oral-peripheral examination of the speech mechanism, evaluation of expressive and receptive language functioning, and pragmatics (language use) should be included. Coleman et al. (1980) suggest that the language evaluation should include five prelanguage and three language areas, including attention, matching, memory, sequencing, categorization, vocabulary, grammar, and semantics and pragmatics. Several of these areas would be assessed as part of the evaluation of cognition.

One feature of augmentative communication evaluation is the use of decision-making matrices to determine candidacy for augmentation and the modes and symbol systems that will be used. Shane and Bashir (1980) used 10 areas of clinical concern in a binary choice branching decision matrix to decide whether to elect, reject, or delay implementation of an augmentative communication system. Included were cognitive, oral reflex, language, motor, intelligibility, emotional, chronological age, previous therapy, imitative, and environmental categories. Although the decision-making strategy is helpful as a guide to patient and environmental factors that affect candidacy, it should be pointed out that at no point in the matrix is there a factor that deals directly with the success of the patient in the use of a recommended augmentative communication system. Owens and House (1984) developed matrices to assist in assessment decision making and in implementation of an augmentative communication system. The first matrix deals with binary choice decision making about augmentative communication choices as primary or complementary methods of communication. Factors included on this matrix, the primary purpose of which is to decide on candidacy, are presymbolic and early symbolic skills (cognitive, social/communicative, and receptive language correlates), motor speech abilities, and therapy and environmental factors. The second binary choice matrix deals with deciding on the appropriate augmentative mode. On this matrix, motor skill factors are most important in deciding among manual, nonelectronic, and electronic modes. Matrix factors include manual dexterity and expression, environmental support, physical indicating abilities, purpose and/or comprehension, type of display, and ambulation. The third matrix is used to determine the most appropriate symbol system or code based on cognitive and visual discrimination abilities.

Decision-making matrices should be viewed as guides rather than as formulas for selection of augmentative systems. Their value has been empirically rather than experimentally determined, and it is not uncommon to find patients for whom the matrices must be expanded or adapted. They are important to the extent that they identify important criteria for determining candidacy and the appropriateness of the system recommended.

TABLE 8–1   **Augmentative communication assessment model**

Nonspeaker	System	Partner
Background Information		
Identification	Previous Systems	Identification
Statement of Problem	Current System	Language Dominance
Medical History		Family Nucleus
Developmental History		Current Partners
Treatment History		Commitment
Social/Emotional		
Motivational		
Cognitive		
Previous Test Scores	Specific System	Educational/Training Level
Sensorimotor	Requirements	
IQ Level		
Nonverbal		
Verbal		
Attention		
Memory		
Learning Potential		
Speech		
Intelligibility	Speech Output	Not Applicable
Oral/Motor	Yes/No	
Phonology	Speech Type	
Stimulability		
Language		
Comprehension	Representation System	Not Applicable
Utterance Length	Openness	
Vocabulary	Content	
Production	Form	
MLU	Use	
Grammatical Morphemes	Transparency	
Syntax		
Vocabulary		
Semantic Categories		
Interaction	Interaction	Interaction
Functions	Speed	Awareness of
Discourse	Assertability	Communication
Attention Getting	Display Permanence	Differences
Topic Maintenance	Projection	Awareness of Barriers
Backchannel Responses	Correctability	Facilitation Techniques
Repair Strategies	Expandability	Modeling
Other Discourse Strategies		Waiting
		Teaching
		Question Usage
Educational Testing		
Reading	Not Applicable	Literacy
Spelling		
Writing		
Math		
Number Recognition		

(continued)

TABLE 8–1   Augmentative communication assessment model (continued)

Nonspeaker	System	Partner
Hearing	Not Applicable	
Vision	Not Applicable	
Motor Functioning	Not Applicable	Not Applicable
Positioning		
Posture		
Reflex Integration		
Muscle Tone		
Upper Extremity Functioning		
Hand Functioning		
Motor Control		
Visual Perception		
Sensory Function		
System Access/Use		
Control Site	Portability	Financial Responsibility
Input Mode	Position Independence	Acquisition
Speed/Accuracy	Independence of Use	Development
Fatigue Factor	Intelligibility/Obviousness	Maintenance
Placement of Device	Appropriateness	
Adaptations	Durability	
Financial Responsibility	Total Cost/Funding	
Acquisition	Maintenance	
Development		
Maintenance		
Environmental Interface		
Potential Communication	Cosmesis	Potential Partners
Environments	Vocational/Educational	Lexicon Needs
Lexicon	Compatibility	Technique Needs
Partners	Similarity	
Technique	Training	
Position	Future Adaptability	
	Equipment Interface	

From Larson and Woodfin (1988).

Beukelman and Yorkston (1980) point out that determining the communication needs and capabilities of the patient is only the first phase of the evaluation. A second phase, which they termed "performance evaluation," is the evaluation of the system selected in a variety of communication environments. They noted that although some aspects of performance can be determined in the clinical setting, important information about the ability to generalize the system to different communicative settings, the efficiency of the system with a variety of communicative partners, and the frequency of communication attempts and message types and forms need to be explored. Beukelman, Yorkston, and Dowden (1985) proposed that the performance evaluation include an assessment of controlled drills, message preparation tasks, and interaction training to evaluate more fully and to adapt if necessary the augmentative communication system chosen for the patient.

Several protocols have been developed to determine interactional strategies of augmentative communication system users and their communicative partners. The *Interaction Checklist for Augmentative Communication* (INCH) (Bolton and Dashiell 1984), for example, was developed to assess communicative interaction in as unambiguous a manner as possible. The checklist includes strategies for initiating, facilitating, regulating, or terminating a conversation through five linguistic or nonlinguistic (paralinguistic, kinesic, etc.) modes. After transcribing a communicative interaction, the clinician reviews each of the nonspeaker's utterances and behaviors and categorizes each according to the strategy employed. Initiation strategies include gaining attention, asking questions, or initiating a topic. Maintaining optimal physical distance and seeking help when needed are facilitation strategies; regulation and termination strategies include giving feedback when a message is not understood and indicating when a message has been completed. After identifying the appropriate strategy for a behavior, the mode utilized is noted. Strategies not present in the interaction are assessed for their value in improving communication and may be targeted for intervention.

The INCH is limited in the amount of information yielded concerning communication skills, efficiency, and effectiveness. Although it provides important observations on communicative mode versatility, it does not provide a quantification of the frequency of use of communication strategies. For example, one mode may be used only once to initiate communication, while another mode was used numerous times. The INCH does not provide a systematic means of documenting these differences or the success of the communicative initiations.

Other studies have evaluated the use of interactional strategies by augmentative communication users (Calculator and Dollaghan 1982; Calculator and Luchko 1983; Light, Collier, and Parnes 1985). These studies have addressed methodology for assessing initiations, message intent or type, and communication mode employed. However, there has been less attention paid to communication rate and success and the nonspeaker's range of expression with available vocabulary. Additional important concerns are the reliability of the sampling procedures and the validity of interactional samples. Are the observations typical of what the individual does or are they affected by the situation and time of day? Kraat (1986) points out that care must be taken in gaining a sufficient number of behaviors and communication partners and that the activities and contexts be considered carefully to maximize the reliability and validity of interactions.

Augmentative communication assessment brings together a large part of the appraisal procedures we have discussed to this point. Included are descriptions of cognitive, motor, sensory, language, and adaptive abilities and behaviors and the systematic sampling of communicative behaviors in a variety of contexts with varying content and interactional partners. The critical element is that the observations be made systematically to ensure that the diagnostic questions asked can be answered with the data obtained.

SUMMARY

There are no strong strings that bind the diagnostic procedures and disorders presented in this chapter. We have discussed disorders typically associated with childhood and those acquired later in life; we have provided reasonably complete assessment protocols as well as abbreviated descriptions of procedures; and we have examined informed methods of evaluation as well as tests developed for particular groups of patients. The strings that bind, however, are those that emphasize the need to observe carefully, to quantify completely, and to use clinical judgment when statements regarding "abnormal" performance are to be made.

REFERENCES

BACKUS, O., Speech rehabilitation following excision of the tip of the tongue. *Amer. J. Disabled Child,* 60, 368–370 (1940).

BAKEN, R., *Clinical Measurement of Speech and Voice.* Boston: College-Hill Press (1987).

BERLIN, C., Clinical measurement of esophageal speech: I. Methodology and curves of skill acquisition. *J. Speech Hearing Dis.,* 28, 42–51 (1963).

BERLIN, C., AND V. VIRDEN, Diagnostic techniques for determining methods and potential for teaching alaryngeal speech. In *Therapy for the Laryngectomized Patient,* eds. S. Rigrodsky, J. Lerman, and E. Morrison. New York: Teachers College Press (1971).

BEUKELMAN, D., AND K. YORKSTON, Nonvocal communication: Performance evaluation. *Arch. Phys. Med. Rehabil.,* 61, 272–275 (1980).

BEUKELMAN, D., AND K. YORKSTON, Communication interaction of adult communication augmentation system use. *Topics in Language Disorders,* 2, 39–53 (1982).

BEUKELMAN, D., K. YORKSTON, AND R. DOWDEN, Nonvocal communication: Performance evaluation. *Arch. Phys. Med. Rehabil.,* 61, 272–275 (1985).

BLACKSTONE, S. W., Training strategies. In *Augmentative Communication: An Introduction,* ed. S. W. Blackstone. Rockville, Md.: American Speech-Language-Hearing Association (1986).

BOLTON, S., AND S. DASHIELL, *INCH—INteractional CHecklist for Augmentative Communication.* Huntington Beach, Calif.: INCH Associates (1984).

BOONE, D., *The Voice and Voice Therapy,* 3rd ed. Englewood Cliffs, N.J.: Prentice Hall (1983).

BZOCH, K., An investigation of the speech of preschool cleft palate children. Ph.D. dissertation, Northwestern University, Evanston (1956).

BZOCH, K., Measurement and assessment of categorical aspects of cleft palate speech. In *Communicative Disorders Related to Cleft Lip and Palate,* 2nd ed., ed. K. Bzoch. Boston: Little, Brown (1979).

CALCULATOR, S., AND C. DOLLAGHAN, The use of communication boards in a residential setting: An evaluation. *J. Speech Hearing Dis.,* 47, 281–287 (1982).

CALCULATOR S., AND C. LUCHKO, Evaluating the effectiveness of a communication board training program. *J. Speech Hearing Dis.,* 48, 185–191 (1983).

COHEN, C. G., AND H. SHANE, An overview of augmentative communication. In *Speech, Language, and Hearing: Vol. II, Pathologies of Speech and Language,* eds. N. J. Lass, L. V. McReynolds, J. L. Northern, and D. E. Yoder. Philadelphia: W. B. Saunders (1982).

COLEMAN, C., A. COOK, AND L. MEYERS, Assessing nonoral clients for assistive communication devices. *J. Speech Hearing Dis.,* 45, 515–526 (1980).

COUNIHAN, D., AND W. CULLINAN, Reliability and dispersion of nasality ratings. *Cleft Pal. J.,* 7, 261–270 (1970).

CRICKMAY, M., *Speech Therapy and the Bobath Approach to Cerebral Palsy.* Springfield, Ill.: Charles C Thomas (1966).

DANIELS, L., AND C. WORTHINGHAM, *Muscle Testing: Techniques of Manual Examination,* 5th ed. Philadelphia: W. B. Saunders (1986).

DENHOFF, E., AND R. HOLDEN, *The developmental ladder in cerebral palsy.* Reprinted by National Society for Crippled Children and Adults, Inc., Chicago, Illinois (1951).

DIEDRICH, W., AND K. YOUNGSTROM, *Alaryngeal Speech.* Springfield, Ill.: Charles C Thomas (1966).

FRISTOE, M., AND L. LLOYD, Nonspeech communication. In *Handbook of Mental Deficiency, Psychological Theory and Research,* 2nd ed., ed. N. R. Ellis. Hillsdale, N.J.: Lawrence Erlbaum Associates (1979).

GARDNER, W., *Laryngectomee Speech and Rehabilitation.* Springfield, Ill.: Charles C Thomas (1971).

GOLDSTEIN, M., Speech without a tongue. *J. Speech Dis.,* 5, 65–69 (1940).

GOOSENS, C., AND S. CRAIN, *Augmentative Communication Assessment Resource.* Lake Zurich, Ill.: Don Johnson Developmental Equipment, Inc. (1986).

HARDY, J., *Cerebral Palsy*. Englewood Cliffs, N.J.: Prentice Hall (1983).

HARRIS, D., AND G. VANDERHEIDEN, Augmentative communication techniques. In *Nonspeech Language and Communication*, ed. R. L. Schiefelbusch. Baltimore: University Park Press (1980).

HAYES, C., Audiological problems associated with cleft palate. *Proceedings of the Conference: Communicative Problems in Cleft Palate*. Washington, D.C.: ASHA Reports No. 1 (1965).

HERBERMAN, M., Rehabilitation of patients following glossectomy. *Arch. of Otolaryng.*, 67, 182–183 (1958).

HESS, D., Effects of certain variables on speech of cleft palate persons. *Cleft Pal. J.*, 8, 387–398 (1971).

HOLLEIN, H., Status report on instrumentation useful for craniofacial research. *Cleft Pal. J.*, 13, 138–155 (1976).

IRWIN, O., A manual of articulation testing for use with children with cerebral palsy. *Cerebral Pal. Rev.*, 22, May–June, 1–20 (1961).

IRWIN, O., AND P. JENSEN, A test of sound discrimination for use with cerebral-palsied children. *Cerebral Pal. Rev.*, 24, March–April, 5–11 (1963a).

IRWIN, O., AND P. JENSEN, A parallel test of sound discrimination for use with cerebral-palsied children. *Cerebral Pal. Rev.*, 24, September–October, 3–10 (1963b).

JACOBS, R., B. PHILLIPS, AND R. HARRISON, A stimulability test for cleft palate children. *J. Speech Hearing Dis.*, 35, 354–360 (1970).

KAHANE, J., AND J. IRWIN, Comparison of hearing sensitivity, stoma noise and speech ratings and duration in therapy in 90 esophageal speakers. Paper presented at the Convention of the American Speech and Hearing Association, Washington, D.C. (1975).

KIERNAN, C., Alternatives to speech: A review of research on manual and other forms of communication with the mentally handicapped and other noncommunicating populations. *British J. Mental Subnormality*, 23, 6–28 (1977).

KRAAT, A., Developing intervention goals. In *Augmentative Communication: An Introduction*, ed. S. Blackstone. Rockville, Md.: American Speech-Language-Hearing Association (1986).

LARSON, J., AND S. WOODFIN, Personal communication. Austin, Tex. (1988).

LENCIONE, R., Speech and language problems in cerebral palsy. In *Cerebral Palsy: Its Individual and Community Problems*, ed. W. Cruickshank, Syracuse, N.Y.: Syracuse University Press (1966).

LIGHT, J., B. COLLIER, AND P. PARNES, Communicative interaction between young nonspeaking physically disabled children and their primary caregivers: Part I. Discourse patterns. *Aug. Alt. Communication*, 1, 74–83 (1985).

LINTZ, L., AND D. SHERMAN, Phonetic elements and perception of nasality. *J. Speech Hearing Res.*, 4, 381–396 (1961).

LOGEMANN, J., Assessing alaryngeal voice mechanisms. Paper presented at the Fifteenth Annual Meeting of the International Association of Laryngectomees, Chicago Ill. (1975).

MCCORMICK, L., AND H. SHANE, Augmentative communication. In *Early Language Intervention*, eds. L. McCormick and R. L. Schiefelbush. Columbus, Ohio: Chas. E. Merrill (1984).

MCDONALD, E., AND B. CHANCE, *Cerebral Palsy*. Englewood Cliffs, N.J.: Prentice Hall (1964).

MCWILLIAMS, B. J., H. L. MORRIS, AND R. L. SHELTON, *Cleft Palate Speech*. Philadelphia: B. C. Decker (1984).

MCWILLIAMS, B. J., AND B. J. PHILIPS, *Audio Seminars in Speech Pathology, Velopharyngeal Incompetence*. Philadelphia: W. B. Saunders (1979).

MARTIN, D., AND H. HOOPS, The relationships between esophageal speech proficiency and selected measures of auditory function. *J. Speech Hearing Res.*, 17, 30–85 (1974).

MASSENGILL, R., S. MAXWELL, AND K. PICKRELL, An analysis of articulation following partial and total glossectomy. *J. Speech Hearing Dis.*, 35, 170–173 (1970).

MECHAM, M., M. BERKO, AND F. BERKO, *Speech Therapy in Cerebral Palsy*. Springfield, Ill.: Charles C Thomas (1960).

MONTGOMERY, J., *Nonoral Communication*. Exemplary/Incentive Dissemination Project, ESEA, Title IV-C, Fountain Valley School District/West Orange Consortium for Special Education, Plavan School, Fountain Valley, California (1980).

MOORE, W., AND R. SOMMERS, Phonetic contexts: Their effects on perceived nasality in cleft palate speakers. *Cleft Pal. J.*, 10, 72–83 (1973).

MORRIS, H., The oral manometer as a diagnostic tool in clinical speech pathology. *J. Speech Hearing Dis.*, 31, 362–369 (1966).

MORRIS, H., D. SPRIESTERSBACH, AND F. DARLEY, An articulation test for assessing competency of velopharyngeal closure. *J. Speech Hearing Res.*, 4, 48–55 (1961).

NOLL, J., M. HAWKINS, AND B. WEINBERG, Performance of normal six- and seven-year-old males on oral manometer tasks. *Cleft Pal. J.*, 14, 200–205 (1977).

OWENS, R., AND L. HOUSE, Decision-making processes in augmentative communication. *J. Speech Hearing Dis.*, 49, 18–25 (1984).

PETERSON, H. A., A case report of speech and language training for a two year old laryngectomized child. *J. Speech Hearing Dis.* 38, 275–278 (1973).

PHILIPS, B. J., Speech assessment. *Seminars in Speech and Language*, 7, 297–311 (1986).

PHILIPS, B., AND R. HARRISON, Language skills of preschool cleft palate children. *Cleft Pal. J.*, 6, 108–119 (1969).

SHANE, H., AND A. BASHIR, Election criteria for the adoption of an augmentative communication system: Preliminary considerations. *J. Speech Hearing Dis.*, 45, 408–414 (1980).

SHANE, H., AND R. WILBUR, Potential for expressive signing based on motor control. *Sign Language Studies*, 29, 331–348 (1980).

SILVERMAN, F. H., *Communication for the Speechless*, 2nd ed. Englewood Cliffs, N.J.: Prentice Hall (1989).

SKELLY, M., *Glossectomee Speech Rehabilitation*, Springfield, Ill.: Charles C Thomas (1973).

SKELLY, M., AND OTHERS, Compensatory physiologic phonetics for the glossectomee. *J. Speech Hearing Dis.*, 36, 101–114 (1971).

SKELLY, M., AND OTHERS, Changes in phonatory aspects of glossectomee intelligibility through vocal parameter manipulation. *J. Speech Hearing Dis.*, 37, 379–389 (1972).

SMITH, R., AND B. MCWILLIAMS, Psycholinguistic abilities of children with clefts. *Cleft Pal. J.*, 5, 238–249 (1968).

SUBTELNY, J., R. VAN HATTUM, AND B. MYERS, Ratings and measures of cleft palate speech. *Cleft Pal. J.*, 9, 18–27 (1972).

TEMPLIN, M., AND F. DARLEY, *The Templin-Darley Tests of Articulation*. Iowa City: Bureau of Education Research and Service, Extension Division, University of Iowa (1960).

VAN DEMARK, D., Misarticulations and listener judgments of the speech of children with cleft palate. *Cleft Pal. J.*, 1, 232–245 (1964).

VAN DEMARK, D. R., Predictability of velopharyngeal competency. *Cleft Pal. J.*, 16, 429–435 (1979).

VAN DEMARK, D., AND H. MORRIS, A preliminary study of the predictive value of the IPAT. *Cleft Pal. J.*, 14, 125–130 (1977).

VAN DEMARK, D. R., AND M. A. SWICKARD, A preschool articulation test to assess velopharyngeal competency: Normative data. *Cleft Pal. J.*, 17, 175–179 (1980).

VANDERHEIDEN, G. C., AND K. GRILLEY, *Nonvocal Communication Techniques and Aids for the Severely Physically Handicapped*. Baltimore: University Park Press (1976).

VANDERHEIDEN, G. C., AND D. YODER, Overview. In *Augmentative Communication: An Introduction*, ed. S. Blackstone. Rockville, Md.: American Speech-Language-Hearing Association (1986).

WARNER, J., Vocal rehabilitation following total laryngectomy. *J. Laryng. Otol.*, 85, 577–582 (1971).

WEINBERG, B., Assessing esophageal speech. Paper presented at the Fifteenth Annual Meeting of the International Association of Laryngectomees, Chicago, Ill. (1975).

WEPMAN, J., AND OTHERS, The objective measurement of progressive esophageal speech development. *J. Speech Hearing Dis.*, 18, 247–251 (1953).

WESTLAKE, H., AND D. RUTHERFORD, *Speech Therapy for the Cerebral Palsied*. Chicago: National Society for Crippled Children and Adults, Inc. (1961).

YODER, D., AND A. KRAAT, Intervention issues in non-speech communication. In *Contemporary Issues in Language Intervention (ASHA reports No 12.)*, eds. J. Miller, D. Yoder, and R. L. Schiefelbusch. Rockville, Md.: American Speech-Language-Hearing Association (1983).

YORKSTON, K. M., AND G. KARLAN, Assessment procedures. In *Augmentative Communication: An Introduction*, ed. S. Blackstone. Rockville Md.: American Speech-Language-Hearing Association (1986).

9

Evaluation
of Fluency

Nothing in nature is quite so separate as two mounds of expertise.

Marvin Harris
Cows, Pigs, Wars, and Witches: The Riddles of Culture

In many ways, the evaluation of fluency and/or the diagnosis of stuttering may be a more difficult task than most of the speech and language problems we have discussed to this point. Part of the difficulty arises from the lack of objective measures of stuttering and norms to clearly separate "fluent" from "disfluent" speakers. Stuttering and disfluency are not equivalent terms. Fluency norms are not sufficient to designate a problem that the speaker may have or his listeners may perceive. We obviously need more than a description of speech per se. There are many definitions of stuttering, but there is no single agreed-upon definition. There are no tests for stuttering (Wingate 1978); evaluation is entirely a matter of observation, inquiry, and judgment. This does not mean that our task of appraisal is impossible; it means that we must be careful to be descriptive in our observations, and we must

An earlier version of this chapter was coauthored by Dr. Harold L. Luper.

be chary in our assignment of a diagnostic label. Two types of judgmental errors are possible. The labeling of a normally disfluent child as a stutterer is the error that the stuttering literature seems to have been primarily concerned with, but misjudging the beginnings of stuttering as normal fluency would deny the need for therapeutic intervention—and this may also be a serious error (Adams 1977). What this means, in practical terms, is that to reduce the probability of an error in judgment, we must be concerned with more than just the child's speech.

Within an evaluation framework, a great many different aspects of the speaker, her behavior, and her environment may be considered grist for the diagnostician's mill. In no other communication disorder will it be more obvious that diagnostic evaluation and therapeutic intervention overlap in time. During the course of our therapy regime, we will obviously continue to evaluate and chart behavioral responses, but equally obvious is that our preferred theories of causation and maintenance of stuttering will tend to influence the types of judgments we make during the diagnostic evaluation.

The minimum essential information to be obtained in evaluating stuttering would appear to include at least the following: (1) identification of the speech and nonspeech behaviors that are part of or closely related to the individual's stuttering; (2) measures of the frequency of occurrence of the "stuttering behaviors"; and (3) estimates of the severity of the problem. Most clinicians would also include case history information on areas such as general physical and social development and speech and language development. In addition, since one major purpose of the stuttering evaluation is to make decisions concerning the need for and type of therapy, the stuttering evaluation will normally include some assessment of factors that could affect the success of therapy, such as responses to previous therapy and to trial therapies.

Our concern as diagnosticians must include a complete speech and language appraisal as well as a description of stuttering, normal disfluencies, and associated behaviors that may indicate that a communication barrier exists, as well as a utilization of these findings to highlight danger signs by which the clinician may decide that there is a problem—and who has the problem. We need to know whether the problem is properly called stuttering, whether therapy is indicated, with whom therapy is indicated, the severity of the problem if one exists, and the probabilities of accomplishing a positive therapeutic change.

WHEN IS STUTTERING STUTTERING?

Most definitions of stuttering are not restricted to speech alone but also include references to a negative reaction on the part of the speaker and/or his listeners. Van Riper's (1978) definition is quite succinct: "Stuttering occurs when the forward flow of speech is interrupted abnormally by repetitions or prolongations of a sound, a syllable, or articulatory posture, or by avoidance and struggle reactions" (p. 247). Wingate (1964, p. 488) offered a more elaborate definition but one that also placed the primary emphasis on speech and the speaker. The term "stuttering" means

1. (a) Disruption in the fluency of verbal expression, which is (b) characterized by involuntary, audible or silent, repetitions or prolongations in the utterance of short

speech elements, namely: sounds, syllables, and words of one syllable. These disruptions (c) usually occur frequently or are marked in character and (d) are not readily controllable.

2. Sometimes the disruptions are (e) accompanied by accessory activities involving the speech apparatus, related or unrelated body structures, or stereotyped speech utterances. These activities give the appearance of being speech-related struggle.

3. Also, there are not infrequently (f) indications or reports of the presence of an emotional state, ranging from a general condition of "excitement" or "tension" to more specific emotions of a negative nature such as fear, embarrassment, irritation, or the like. (g) The immediate source of stuttering is some incoordination expressed in the peripheral speech mechanism; the ultimate cause is presently unknown and may be complex or compound.

In terms of speech, those two definitions speak of stuttering disfluencies primarily as related to the production of sounds or syllables. A broader definition of "disfluencies" would include at least eight categories—as defined by Johnson and others (1959). The eight categories include

1. interjections of sounds, syllables, or phrases
2. part-word repetitions—primarily syllables and sounds
3. word repetitions, including words of one syllable
4. phrase repetitions—two or more words
5. revisions—where the content of the phrase is modified
6. incomplete phrases—the thought or the content is not completed
7. broken words—the words are not completely pronounced (e.g., g--oing home)
8. prolonged sounds—usually the initial sound in a word.

Table 9–1 displays mean numbers for each of the eight types of disfluencies for stuttering and nonstuttering children. These data are from *The Onset of Stuttering* studies (Johnson and others 1959) conducted over a period of more than 20 years that included 246 children judged by their parents to be stutterers and 246 children judged by their parents to be nonstutterers.

From the data shown in Table 9–1, it is apparent that both children judged as stutterers and those judged to be nonstutterers displayed some degree of disfluency. The most frequently occurring disfluencies for the nonstuttering children were interjections, revisions, and word repetitions, in that order. Those same three categories of disfluencies were also relatively frequent in the speech of children judged to be stutterers, but the greatest differences between groups occurred on part-word repetitions and sound prolongations. The differences between the samples were statistically significant for only part-word and word repetitions and prolongations, for both boys and girls.

It should be noted that these are mean data. Considerable overlap was shown for individual children within the two groups. In fact, ". . . 20 to 30 percent of the children regarded by their parents as normal speakers spoke with more disfluencies than did 20 to 30 percent of the children who had been for an average of 18 months regarded by their parents as stutterers" (Johnson and others, 1963, pp. 247–248). In other words, we cannot consistently identify stuttering on the basis of either frequency or type of disfluency.

TABLE 9–1   **Mean number of disfluencies per 100 words observed in the speech of 89 stuttering and 89 matched nonstuttering children with a mean age of approximately five years**

Category of Disfluency	STUTTERERS		NONSTUTTERERS	
	Male	Female	Male	Female
Interjections	3.62	4.44	3.13	3.45
Part-word repetitions	5.44	3.93	.61	.83
Word repetitions	4.28	3.65	1.07	1.14
Phrase repetitions	1.14	.84	.61	.58
Revisions	1.30	1.30	1.43	1.38
Incomplete phrases	.34	.22	.23	.28
Broken words	.12	.63	.04	.10
Prolonged sounds	1.67	1.24	.16	.14
Total	17.91	16.25	7.28	7.90

Adapted from W. Johnson and associates. *The Onset of Stuttering*, Minneapolis: University of Minnesota Press, 1959. Used by permission.

Bloodstein (1975) put it this way: "Unfortunately, we have no satisfactory *objective* means of differentiating moments of stuttering from other instances of disfluency. Consequently, the identification of moments of stuttering always involves the judgment of a listener" (p. 4). Johnson (1967) suggested that "there are no 'natural' lines of demarcation between 'normal' and 'abnormal' disfluencies" (p. 238). We commented earlier that some types of disfluencies, notably part-word or syllable repetitions or prolonged sounds, were more likely to elicit a judgment of stuttering than some other types of disfluencies. However, according to Bloodstein (1981), this would still not be sufficient to define stuttering:

> The foregoing discussion has served to raise several fundamental questions. How is stuttering to be defined? What are its measurable dimensions? How is it to be differentiated from other kinds of disfluent behavior including that of normal speech? We have seen that, except for the evaluation of a listener that stuttering has occurred, we as yet have no operational definition serving to characterize the stuttering response in a wholly satisfactory way. On the other hand, we can identify certain features of speech, notably sound or syllable repetitions, broken words, prolonged sounds, and signs of unusual effort or tension that are more closely related than others to what most listeners judge to be stuttering. There are thus hints that with further description we may eventually be able to define stuttering more adequately in terms of its observable features. . . . [and] for investigators who are anxious to define carefully what they mean by stuttering the best definition we appear to be able to offer at present is: whatever is perceived as stuttering by a reliable observer who has relatively good agreement with others. (p. 9)

What the "reliable observer" is likely to respond to as part of the objective judgment (Bloodstein 1975, 1981) may include "associated symptoms" of overt muscular activities; vocal abnormalities; evidence of avoidance, postponement, and escape; or release mechanisms' physiological concomitants such as tremors, eye movements, biochemical changes, and other reflex activity that may or may not be a part of the stutter or even of the stuttering. Many of these same bodily changes have been observed to occur in normal speakers under conditions of excitement and tension. Introspective concomitants also may be part of the "associated symptoms," such as feelings of frustration in an effort to speak, feelings of muscular tension, affective reactions such as apprehension, and so forth, but introspections are not operational definitions.

The number of disfluencies or the types of disfluencies are not sufficient to classify a speaker as stuttering rather than normally disfluent. More often the classification of "stuttering" is assigned to a speaker when we, as observers, note a set of concomitant activities with the act of speaking. But these concomitant activities, as well, may be observed in speakers who are ill at ease—especially children. There is likely to be more uncertainty in the mind of the listener if the speaker is a child and if the question is whether the speech heard is indicative of stuttering or normal child disfluency. In the 1977 issue of the Speech Foundation of America series on stuttering, Ainsworth listed eight "danger signs" indicating that the child has moved beyond the type or level of speech interruptions normal for her age and thereby reflecting stuttering. Ainsworth (pp. 12–16) listed

1. The use of multiple repetitions; more importantly, the repetitions are parts of words and sounds or syllables.
2. The schwa replaces the intended vowel sound in part-word repetitions. The child's repetition such as "go-go-going" is likely to be viewed as normal, but "guh-guh-going" is more likely to be classified as stuttering.
3. The use of prolongations.

These first three are considered "danger" signs when they occur too frequently, in too many situations, and when they begin to affect the child's ability to communicate. They may occur occasionally in all children. The last five danger signs include speech attempts in which there are apparent

4. tremors
5. increases in pitch and loudness
6. struggle and tension
7. momentary looks of fear when saying a difficult word
8. avoidances of words or situations in which stuttering is anticipated

The last five may occur together. According to Ainsworth, the eight danger signs differ from normal interruptions in two ways. The first three distort the speech patterns; the next five occur as the child reacts to interruptions in her speech. They represent behaviors that seriously inhibit the speech flow and disturb communication and indicate that the child is trying to do something about her interruptions. The presence of these danger signs does not necessarily mean that the child *is* stuttering but that she *may* develop a stuttering problem unless something is done.

FREQUENCY OF STUTTERING COUNTS

The bulk of the discussion to this point may seem to imply that the identification of stuttered speech is a simpler task than the identification of "stutterer." The identification of "what words are stuttered," however, is also subject to some variation. Williams and Kent (1958) reported that what the listeners were listening for was important. They asked a group of listeners to identify stutterings in tape-recorded samples of speech. A second group marked the normal interruptions in the same samples. A significantly greater number of stuttering instances were marked when the instructions were to note stuttering, and a greater number of normal disfluencies was marked when the listeners were asked to identify normal interruptions. When asked to note both "stuttering interruptions" and "normal interruptions," the listeners commented that they were confused as to what was normal and what was stuttered.

MacDonald and Martin (1973), in contrast, reported that their data showed stuttering and disfluency as two reliable and unambiguous response classes. The two sets of judges used for their study were college students who were not speech pathologists. Stuttering was not defined for them. The apparent assumption was that "anyone could identify stuttering." One set of judges listened to tape-recorded samples of speech, and they were asked to identify stuttering. From 6 to 11 days later, they were asked to listen to the same tapes but this time were asked to identify normal disfluency. The two listening instructions were reversed for the second group of judges. MacDonald and Martin reasoned that if a response were judged only as stuttering or only as disfluency, the judgments would be considered as unambiguous. If a response were judged (by different listeners or at different times) as both stuttering and disfluency, it would be ambiguous. They reported that of all units judged as stuttering, 71 percent were identified unambiguously as stuttering; and of all disfluency judgments, 85 percent were identified unambiguously. However, only 13 percent of the judged instances of stuttering were agreed upon by more than half of the judges, and 65 percent were agreed upon by less than 10 percent of the judges. Seven percent of the disfluencies were agreed upon by more than half of the listeners, and 50 percent were agreed upon by less than 10 percent of these untrained judges. In other words, the lack of ambiguity did not mean that there was agreement among the listeners as to whether a word was stuttered or normally disfluent. A small group of responses was unambiguously identified as stuttering, and a small group was unambiguously identified as nonstuttering disfluency.

Young (1975) reported that a group of college student judges rated tape-recorded samples of speech as containing more severe examples of stuttering when the rating was done before lunch. It would seem that not only are we likely to be affected by instructions as to what we are listening for (whether these instructions are given internally or externally), but we may even be affected by factors quite unrelated to the speaker's speech performance. High agreement among listeners for word-by-word disfluency judgments are unlikely, according to Young (1975).

Despite some of the problems previously mentioned in making frequency counts, measures of the frequency of stuttering remain one of the most widely used measures of stuttering. Costello and Ingham (1984), after noting many of the difficulties in obtaining reliable measures for identifying specific loci of stuttering moments, point out that frequency counts of the total number of stuttering events can be made with quite satisfactory levels of listener agreement and are probably the "most popular and most sensitive measure of stuttering" (pp. 311–312). They also state that this type of data provides useful information about trends in stuttering across time and "will be appropriately sensitive to clinically significant changes in stuttering frequency." Certainly, most stuttering clients and their parents see reductions in the frequency of stuttering as a necessary goal of therapy. And, importantly for judgments of effectiveness of therapy, *intrajudge* reliability is expected to be higher than *interjudge* reliability.

RATING AND PERCEPTUAL SCALES
OF STUTTERING SEVERITY

While a count of the frequency and category or types of disfluencies is obviously important in our description of speech behavior, the accuracy of this count or the number by itself is apparently insufficient for our diagnostic (problem—no problem) decision. The descriptions and data reviewed to this point would seem to agree on two important aspects:

1. a greater than "usual" number of disfluencies, especially syllable repetitions and sound prolongations, and
2. apparent struggle behavior (facial grimaces and the like) in speech activities, especially those that the listener perceives as demonstrating emotionality or concern for speaking on the part of the child. If these are the relative constants in the determination of stuttering, it would follow that the degree of these behaviors may designate the severity of the problem.

Young (1961) used a nine-point scale for judging the stuttering severity of tape-recorded speech samples. His judges were given explicit definitions of the values of each point from "1" as no stuttering to "9" as severe stuttering, with equal intervals of severity for the points between those two extremes. He also assumed that this elaborate scaling technique would not be practical in most clinical settings. The *Iowa Scale of Stuttering Behavior* (Johnson, Darley, and Spriestersbach 1963) is a similar but less precise scale for rating severity based on frequency and duration of stuttered words plus facial movements and general bodily activity. Scale judgments range from "0" for no stuttering, "1" for *very mild* stuttering on "less than 1 percent of words, little tension, simple disfluency patterns and disfluencies generally less than one second in duration, but no apparent associated bodily movements," to "7" for *very severe* stuttering on "more than 25 percent of words, very conspicuous tension, grimaces averaging more than four seconds in duration, distracting sounds, and very conspicuous grimaces and other associated bodily movements."

Wertheim (1972) approached the classification and measurement of stuttering with both quantitative and qualitative measures. She counted the frequency of the child's disfluencies (prolonged sounds, sound-syllable-word repetitions, broken words, and interjections) and "blocks" ("failure to vocalize in spite of efforts to do so") in answering questions put by the examiner and in conversation with his parents on a prearranged consensus task. The quantitative measure was the count of disfluencies and blocks in the talking situation; the qualitative aspect was what Wertheim defined as the situational stability of the stuttering pattern—that is, whether the child's stuttering was more severe, for example, in a school-like (two-person) situation or in a family situation where the child was interacting with his parents. The definition of "stutterogenic" or sensitive areas had to do with the child's self-concept and his perception of his relative role in school or in home situations. The report of this study does not include numerical data but describes the children as "high" (H) or "low" (L) in frequency of disfluencies and blocks in the two talking situations. The consistency of the child's stuttering frequency (F) and block (B) scores for the two-person versus the family situation was the basis for Wertheim's classification of stuttering subjects as being "invariable," "variable," or "semivariable." A child who was scored as "HH" for both two-person and family situations would be described as severe and of the invariable class; and "LL" in both situations would classify him as mild and invariable. If the pattern of stuttering was dependent on the situation, he would be classified as variable.

Riley (1972, 1980) published a *Stuttering Severity Instrument* (SSI) in which he attempted to calibrate severity on the basis of frequency, duration, and physical concomitants. His scale is designed to be applicable to children or adults by tallying frequency of stuttering in either reading and "job-task" descriptions or, for nonreaders, in their description of picture stories. For readers, a value of from "2" to "9" is assigned for the percentage of words stuttered in reading a 125-word passage. Reading material represented third-grade, fifth-grade, or adult reading levels, according to the capability of the reader. The first 25 words are disregarded, and the next 100 are used to determine percentage of stuttered words. In addition to the reading passage, the stutterer is asked to talk about a job task; for school children, the topic might be a school activity. The job task also is valued from "2" to "9" according to frequency of stuttering. For example, 1 percent of the words stuttered on either reading or job task is scored "2"; 29 percent or greater frequency of stuttering on the job task is rated as "9"; and 27 percent or greater frequency on the reading task is scored "9". The reading score and the job-task score are added and treated as the frequency score. For nonreaders (less than third-grade reading ability), frequency of stuttering in their description of picture stories is scored on a range from 4 to 18 points. Where the Iowa scale utilizes an estimate of average duration of stuttered words, the SSI uses an estimate of duration for the three longest blocks in reading or conversation. The score range is from "1" for fleeting to "7" for more than 60-second estimated duration.

Physical concomitants are rated from "0" (none) to "5" (severe and painful looking) for each of four areas: distracting sounds, facial grimaces, head movements, and extremity movements. In other words, a total of 18 points is possible for frequency, 7 points for duration, and 20 points for physical concomitants.

The total test score (range 0–45) is interpreted as a severity index. A percentile rank is also available to correspond to the SSI total score, but it is not clear from the published data whether these percentile rankings, the total score divisions, and the severity assignment (very mild, mild, moderate, and so forth) are arbitrarily applied. Validity is reported in terms of a ranking correlation between the SSI and the *Iowa Scale of Stuttering Behavior*. It is interesting to note that the validity comparison between these measures was slightly higher (0.89) than interexaminer reliability (0.84) for the SSI. For comparison purposes to record the stutterer's progress in therapy, Riley suggested that the total score and/or scores on each of the three parameters (frequency, duration, and physical concomitants) be charted.

What is consistent among the various scales for stuttering is the inclusion of a judgment of "associated symptoms," whether separately identified or not, and approximate frequency counts of stuttered words. One other common feature is that the judgments are made by listeners, rather than by the speaker and, therefore, may incorporate biases of unknown magnitude. For example, the nine-point scale ratings generated by Young (1961) were derived from 48 listeners who were categorized as stutterers, clinicans, and laypeople. The mean rating for all listeners was 3.84, but stutterers were apparently most critical (mean rating 4.01), followed by clinicians (3.88), and laypeople (3.68). What you know about stuttering apparently makes a difference in your judgment.

Two examples of perceptual scales to be completed by the speakers are Woolf's (1967) *Perception of Stuttering Inventory* (PSI) and the *Communication Inventory* developed by Erickson (1969). The PSI is a descriptive scale designed to be administered to the one who stutters. It consists of 60 statements—20 meant to indicate "struggle," 20 to indicate "avoidance," and 20 to indicate "expectancy." With the PSI scale, the rater is asked to mark as many of the statements as she feels are characteristic of her speech (for example, avoiding talking to people in authority, feeling the interruptions in speech will lead to stuttering, having extra and unnecessary facial movements). The examiner can then total the number of struggle, avoidance, and expectancy items checked and, to some extent, agree or disagree with the rater's check marks.

Erickson's communication attitude scale (S-scale) consists of 39 statements to which the respondent answers "true" or "false." An initial pool of 466 items was administered to a population of 100 nonstutterers and a criterion group of 50 stutterers. The 39 items that best discriminated between the two populations make up the S-scale. In contrast to the PSI, which described behaviors (struggle, avoidance, expectancy) that are frequently or commonly related to stuttering, the S-scale statements do not mention stuttering per se but are concerned with a speaker's confidence in talking (e.g., It is easy for me to talk to important people. I have felt self-conscious when reciting in class. I often have to search for the words I want). The S-scale has also been validated by its relationship to clinician and client ratings of severity, self-ratings of improvement, and self-descriptions of reactions to social conversation.

Behavioral checklists are also available for the diagnostician's use in making observations. They may be viewed as having some intermediate evaluative position between observations of speech-sound productions and perceptual judgments of perceived difficulty and confidence in talking. Behavioral checklists for speech and "associated" behaviors (e.g., Darley, Spriestersbach, and others 1978; Johnson, Darley, and Spriestersbach 1963; Luper and Mulder 1964) typically include type and loci of repetitions, associated tension of the respiratory mechanism, inhaling and exhaling irregularly, facial tension, movements of extremities, turning head sideways, use of avoidance and postponement devices, and the like.

DIAGNOSIS: THE PROBLEM OF STUTTERING—
REACTIONS OF IMPORTANT LISTENERS

The bulk of our discussion to this point has been on the assessment of speech and speaking behavior. The intent of this chapter is to sketch an outline of suggested avenues by which the clinician may describe disfluent speech and associated behaviors that may frequently be categorized as stuttering, to separate between normally disfluent and stuttered speech, and to help define the *problem* of stuttering. Murphy (1962) lists six characteristics by which stuttering may be revealed:

1. Facial contortions, blockings, strugglings, prolongations, breaks in rhythm of speech or other signs of breakdown in the forward flow of speech to a degree that sets the speaker off from his associates
2. An understanding between speaker and listener that stuttering actually has taken place—that is, that the speaker is trying to speak without these interferences, but often fails in the attempt
3. Some feelings of frustration and helplessness brought on by the difficulty plus the fear of possible difficulty
4. Some feelings of fearfulness or concern about the ability to speak at all
5. Anxiety concerning uncertainties—not necessarily connected with speaking—that interferes with speaking ability
6. The speaker having a picture of himself as a stutterer, perhaps a troubled awareness that his way of talking is unnatural and is disturbing to the listener

Note that in none of the six listed criteria is speech fluency the primary concern. The first criterion is not concerned with "breaks in the rhythm of speech . . . ," but rather with the degree that such interruptions in the forward flow of speech "set the speaker off from his associates." In other words, they are perceptions of a listener rather than observations or descriptions and are not necessarily subject to refutation or corroboration on the part of the speaker. What is assumed to be basic to the diagnosis of a problem of stuttering is an interaction between speaker and listener. A case history interview is one basic means of determining the interactive relationship. A second means, of course, is our observation of the interaction between the talker and one of his important listeners. In both cases, perceptual judgments and biases may exist to distort the presenting picture. The attitude scales mentioned earlier can be an important contribution to the interactive relationship between speaker and listeners—and some of the expressed attitudes or perceptions are subject to our clinical review.

Case history forms for stuttering are not necessarily different from the general case history interview we discussed in Chapter 2. That is, the forms contain suggested questions for the interview and not necessarily all of the important probes. Some forms are designed to be administered to parents (or guardian or other knowledgeable adult) when the subject of concern is a child. With older children or adults, many of the same questions may be asked of the speaker directly. Suggested interview items may frequently request descriptions of speech, when the speech that is identified as stuttering began, signs of concern or embarrassment on the part of the speaker, judgments of the adequacy of speaking skills, listing of persons to whom the speaker talks easily and those with whom talking is more difficult, any recent change in speaking proficiency, and other similar questions that may alert the examiner to important interactions. One point bears repeating here from our earlier (Chapter 2) discussion regarding case history information. The "facts" gathered are not necessarily real. The information being supplied, with the best and most honest of intentions, will have been filtered through a set of biases. For example, if you ask the child's mother when the stuttering began, her answer can only indicate when she identified her child's speech as stuttering. According to *The Onset of Stuttering* data, both parents would probably not agree as to the age and date when stuttering began and could probably not tell you how the speech was different on the week or day or month before stuttering was said to have begun. If, in the case interview, you ask the parent if the child was late in learning to talk or late in learning to walk, you will get a judgment based on the parent's internal norms. A *judgment* of "late" may well be an important bit of information reflecting a concern with the child's speaking ability, but it may not be "real." Johnson and others (1959, pp. 61–62) reported that more experimental (stuttering) than control (nonstuttering) group mothers rated their children much slower than the average (at the 0.01 level of confidence), but the differences in mean ages for first words and first sentences were not statistically different (at the 0.05 level of confidence):

> There were no statistically significant differences between the two groups of children with regard to the mean ages, as reported by the mothers, at which they met various specified criteria of development, including the ages at which they spoke their first words and sentences. They were essentially alike also in other aspects of speech development and speech behavior.
>
> The experimental group children were, however, rated somewhat less favorably than were the control group children by their respective parents, particularly with reference to social development. That is, there was a tendency for the experimental group parents to make ratings of their children that were somewhat less favorable than relevant objective data appeared to warrant. (p. 224)

In other words, we are seeking the evaluative judgment of the parent and as much description as possible of the speech in order to determine what that judgment was based on. We need to determine how much reeducation and reevaluation our intervention regime must include.

With other children, or persons who have identified themselves as having a stuttering problem, questions about "when stuttering began," "age of onset," or "earliest memory of stuttering" may well be answered with other than firsthand knowledge. The most likely ages and descriptions quoted (e.g., to questions as to what the speech was like at that time) will probably be what someone told them. It is also entirely logical to have a person say that a stuttering problem began in the second grade or seventh grade or some other milestone she remembers while her mother may say she was concerned about stuttering at the age of four or five. Wingate (1978) has reported that most stutterers are children:

> Stuttering is predominantly a disorder of early childhood. Several sources indicate that approximately 85 percent of cases of stuttering begin well before age five, and most of the remainder before age seven. . . . There is substantial evidence that over 40 percent of the youngsters identified as stuttering before five years of age will no longer be stuttering by the time they are about eight years old. [There is also] ample evidence that recovery from stuttering continues to occur long after age eight. (pp. 255–256)

With persons who have identified themselves as stuttering, or with younger children for whom the parents supply the answers, it is pertinent to ask what, in their opinion, causes stuttering and how the stuttering is maintained. What they believe is the cause can be important to the planning of a therapy regime. It is also important to know whether the answer given denoted *the* theory or *a* theory—in other words, how important is that theoretical base to the client in question. In this and other ways, it can be helpful to find out what the person knows about stuttering and what he thinks can be done about it. "Who else do you know who stutters?" can yield quite different interpretations from the same question. If Uncle Harry stuttered, "but he got over it," the evaluative reaction to the child's speech may be much less negative than if Uncle Harry stuttered, "and I sure don't want my child to have to go through that."

Especially with older children or adults, it may be important to know what, if any, previous therapy has accomplished or what has been done about the stuttering. If therapy had been previously scheduled, you might ask how long it was continued, what was done in therapy, and why the therapy was terminated. If previous therapy was judged to be unsuccessful, as the new clinician you must either plan to do something different from what was done before or at least explain it differently, if you wish the patient to predict a different outcome from last time. When interviewing the parent of a young child, the question more likely would be phrased as "Have any special means been taken by you or anyone else to help him change his speech?" or "Have any changes occurred in his speech recently?" and if so "Do you have any idea what those changes may be attributed to?" With either children or adults, it may be pertinent to ask what has been done (by the speaker) to stop the stuttering, what things have helped the most, and what have helped least. The point of these questions, again, is the informational and theoretical base from which the informant or the speaker is operating.

DEVELOPMENTAL STAGES OF STUTTERING

We have discussed definitions of stuttering and types of disfluencies that may help separate between normal disfluency and stuttering disfluency. We have also discussed fluency counts, attitude scales, behavioral checklists, and case history information to help determine the speaker–listener interaction. We want both general and specific information to help plan the intervention regime. The questions of intervention and the type of intervention (if that is the decision) are based not only on the information gathered in the previous methods, but also on the clinician's definition of degree of stuttering and what that entails. Several categories or degrees of stuttering have been proposed. The following discussion will serve as an example.

Earlier divisions (circa 1930–1940) were usually confined to primary and secondary stuttering.[1] Robinson (1964) used three categories or divisions: begin-

[1]The words "primary" and "secondary" were usually paired with "symptom," therefore, *primary symptoms* or *secondary symptoms* of stuttering. Since the word "symptom" denotes some superficial evidence of a basic underlying fault, usually medical or psychological in nature, one of the theoretical differences of opinion was whether "primary stuttering" was basically different from normal childhood disfluency. If it was, children were first primary and then secondary stutterers. If it was not, then children became stutterers from a normal disfluency stage because of the negative evaluative reaction on the part of important listeners—which the speaker internalized.

From a different frame of reference, Wingate (1978) refers to stuttering as a "primary" speech disorder (fluency) in contrast to neurological disorders, such as Parkinsonism or cerebral palsy, in which there may be fluency disorders that are secondary or result from a more basic problem.

ning stuttering, advanced stuttering, and secondary stuttering. Bloodstein (1960a, 1960b, 1961) defined four stages or phases, which Luper and Mulder (1964) named incipient, transitional, confirmed, and advanced. The three terms—"primary," "beginning," and "incipient"—refer approximately to the same group of children. The most common age of onset of stuttering (specifically, Bloodstein's Phase I) is given as preschool age, and it is for this age group that our most important diagnostic interpretation is whether or not a problem exists and whether the problem is the child's fluency or the listener's evaluation. Phase II (transitional) usually begins in early elementary school; Phase III (confirmed) commonly begins in junior high or high school; and Phase IV (advanced) commonly has its onset in high school or older, according to Bloodstein.

The diagnostic determination of phase of development of stuttering is one base for the choice of intervention techniques. For example, Bloodstein's Phase I child's speech may show episodic periods of fluctuating fluency. Repetitions of syllables and monosyllables are the characteristic speech pattern. The child does not react emotionally to herself as a stutterer; stuttered words are frequently the first words in sentences or are conjunctions, prepositions, and pronouns. The child tends to speak freely in all situations with essentially no fear or embarrassment. With many clinicians, the therapy for this phase may be indirect—working more with the important persons in the child's environment than directly with the child on fluency. The distinguishing characteristic of Phase II (transitional) is the appearance of stuttering primarily when the child talks quickly and gets excited. She stutters equally frequently at home, at school, or with friends. She thinks of herself as a stutterer but talks freely in all situations with little or no concern about stuttering except in special cases or moments of unusual difficulty. The outstanding characteristic of Phase III (confirmed) stuttering is that stuttering is fully developed but without avoidance of speech. The stuttering is essentially chronic although the child will distinctly show more difficulty in some situations than in others. The child in this phase will have developed "secondary symptoms" of postponement and starting and releasing tricks or devices. She is likely to become exasperated, annoyed, or disgusted when she stutters severely, but there is generally no tendency to avoid speaking or any outward appearance of fear or deep embarrassment. The Phase IV stutterer (advanced) views herself as having a serious personal problem. Avoidance, postponement, and starting and release devices are highly developed, and she shows a definite emotional reaction to stuttering, complete with the avoidance of some speaking situations and obvious fear and embarrassment.

Fluency—Developmental and Judgmental

This text is not concerned with therapy except incidentally, but it is obvious that a diagnostic evaluation should also supply information relative to an intervention plan. Fluency, like articulation or language skill, is a dimension of speech that is developmental (Gregory 1973; Starkweather 1986). One of the important aspects of an evaluation for a child referred for professional advice because of a concern with fluency is, therefore, a thorough evaluation of his speech and language skill. Just as we need to know about his disfluency patterns, his reactions to his speech, his general health, and his history of speech and language development, we need to know how he copes with his world in general. It has been mentioned previously that a diagnosis of a stuttering problem is not made purely on the basis of what comes out of the child's mouth. The "problem" may be an evaluative reaction or just lack of "normative" information on the part of the parent. It is not enough for you as an examiner merely to determine to your own satisfaction whether or not the child is normally fluent. The important question to ask yourself, when concerned with a young child, is "What are the likely consequences of the diagnostic judgment?" If the parent were seeking reassurance, your decision that the child was displaying normal speech, language, and fluency may be a welcome corroboration. If the parent were seeking help for a problem she was sure existed, your reassurance of "normal" may or may not be sufficient. One of the important implications of Johnson's definition of the *problem* of stuttering—which we discussed with the three continua—is that in our therapeutic intervention we should work with the one who has the problem. It may be helpful to schedule the child with a group of others who have near-normal language skills for the sake of definition and comparison. In response to the Williams and Kent (1958) data, which suggested that their listeners heard more stuttering when asked to identify stuttering and more normal disfluencies when they were asked to mark normal interruptions, one of the objectives in counseling parents who consider their child to be stuttering is to help them reevaluate some of the child's speech interruptions.

DISFLUENCY AS AN INDEX
OF LANGUAGE SKILL

The basic reason for the child's speech disfluency may be inadequately developed language skills. From somewhat different bases, Weiss (1964), Luchsinger and Arnold (1965), Berry (1938), Froeschels (1958), Wyatt (1969), and Luper (1970) postulated interactions between language skills and stuttering. Many reporters have noted a difference in the fluency of young children depending on the linguistic complexity of the utterance. Muma (1971) reported that more disfluencies occurred in the speech of young children in the production of double-based (complex) sentences than in sentences with a single-based structure. That study did not answer whether the greater number of disfluencies was a function of the language the child used or the child who used the language. Daughtry (1976) attempted to find a partial answer to that question. She separated a group of first-grade children on the basis of more or fewer disfluencies of all types in their repetition of sentences. These two groups of children were then asked to perceptually locate clicks embedded in tape-recorded sentences. On the assumption that children with greater linguistic skill would tend to displace the click to a syntactic boundary (e.g., Fodor and Bever 1965; Garrett, Bever, and Fodor 1965; Ladefoged and Broadbent 1960), a difference in linguistic skill should be reflected in the perceptual accuracy of the click placement. Keeping in mind that the validity of this technique has not been unambiguously established (Olson and Clark 1976), the data from this study indicated that the children in the disfluent group tended to place the clicks more veridically and that the more fluent children tended to displace the click toward a syntactic boundary, thus implying greater language skills for the fluent children. That is, the more fluent children perceived the sentences more in terms of phrase units than as separate words.

Gordon, Luper, and Peterson (1986) reported the number of disfluencies in a group of five-year-old children in repetition of simple and complex sentences and the number of disfluencies in the production of "modeled" sentences of the same types. In the modeled sentence-production task, the subjects were shown a picture frame in which two pictorial examples of a syntactic construction were represented. The examiner produced a sentence describing one of the two pictures. The child's task was to produce a sentence of the same type to describe the second picture. Nearly six times as many disfluencies occurred on the modeling task as on the imitation task, and significantly more disfluencies occurred on complex sentence types than on simple sentences.

Two points are to be made from this discussion. Linguistic skill of the children and the "linguistic weight" of the sentence construction are both expected to have an effect on the number of disfluencies. It is also apparent that a sentence-repetition task is likely to yield less diagnostic description than self-formulated sentences. These three studies were not concerned with stuttering per se but with disfluencies. We assumed earlier that stuttering and disfluency are not the same thing, although they may sometimes be difficult to separate in young children. The specific purpose in commenting on these studies is to stress the importance of language testing with young children referred with a question of stuttering or normal disfluency and the frequent logic of therapy to improve language proficiency with these children as a means of improving fluency.

Differentiation Between Normal and Abnormal Disfluencies

The differentiation between stuttering and normal disfluencies is not at all difficult when the disorder is severe or in more advanced stages. The difficulty is greatest when the disorder is very mild or in the earliest stages of development. One of the reasons for this difficulty, it may be assumed, is the relative subjectivity of the judgments we are asked to make. There are, however, some objective comparisons that can be made. In the seventies, there was a considerable interest in acoustic description of stuttered speech and stuttering speakers. Two such measures are voice onset time (VOT) and reaction time (RT). As used here, VOT is the latency between a speaker's assumption of an articulatory gesture and the initiation of voicing, or the transition between unvoiced and voiced phonemes. RT is the latency between a signal, such as a pure tone delivered through earphones, and the speaker's response—for example, in producing a vowel or tapping a key. There is some evidence that more stuttering occurs when the manner of vocalization (voiced or unvoiced) is changed (Wingate 1976) and that less stuttering occurs when voiceless sounds are removed from a specially constructed passage (Adams and Reis 1971, 1974). Starkweather and others (1976), Adams and Hayden (1976), Cross and Luper (1979) and others have shown that stuttering adults and children are generally slower in reaction time than are nonstutterers and that the stuttering subjects are slower in the transition from unvoiced to voiced sound productions.

Stuttering and nonstuttering speakers have also been shown to differ in vowel duration and transition times (Hand 1979; Zimmerman 1980), which may be a function of what Cooper and Allen (1977) define as a "timing control" problem. The differences between groups are slight, usually ranging under 15 msec, and individual speaker variations are reported in most studies having to do with these types of measures. One point bears repeating in our concern with differentiating between normal disfluency and beginning stuttering. The small, but relatively consistent, differences between groups of stutterers and nonstutterers have been with adults and with "confirmed" samples of children who stutter. We implied earlier in this chapter that there was little difficulty in identifying stuttering adults but that the separation between normal disfluency and stuttering in young children was more difficult and may have different consequences. It should also be remembered that these types of acoustic measures may be made from a sound spectrograph but cannot be made reliably without the aid of such instrumentation.

The instrumental measures were mentioned here to give credence to the statement that frequently appears in clinical reporting that the stuttering child's speech is "jerky." For example, Van Riper (1971) defines stuttering behavior as "a word improperly patterned in time" (p. 15) and reports that the differentiation of normal from abnormal disfluency is made partly on the basis of irregularity of syllable repetitions:

> The few syllabic repetitions which normal speakers show not only occur at the same tempos as the rest of their syllables, but they occur evenly, regularly. When we find a person repeating syllables jerkily rather than smoothly, we tend to diagnose abnormality. (p. 23)

And further:

> The airflow in stuttering repetitions is usually interrupted whereas in the normal speakers it usually continues during disfluencies. Moreover the interruption in stuttering repetitions is usually sudden while in contrast, the syllable of normal nonfluency shows a gradual termination before it is repeated. And there is another characteristic that seems to distinguish the abnormal from the normal syllabic repetitions: the pauses between syllables are much shorter in stuttered repetitions. (p. 25)

Lest we appear to have made it too simple or too precise—lest we appear to have suddenly resolved the distinction between a judgment of normal and abnormal disfluency, remember that the Van Riper descriptions listed here are still subjective. Table 9–2 is a set of relative guideline statements in which many of the behaviors are qualified as "may be present," "often apparent," "usually absent," and so forth.

Along the same lines as the Van Riper checklist is the clinical strategy published by Adams (1977). The five behavioral characteristics utilized by Adams for differentiating normal from abnormal disfluencies include

1. The number of disfluencies per 100 words. Stuttering children are expected to average 10 or more disfluencies per 100 words; their normally disfluent peers average 5 to 6 disfluencies per 100 words.
2. The proportion of the disfluencies that are part-word repetitions and sound prolongations differ. Adams reported that "young stutterers evinced more than four times as many part-word repetitions, and 10 times as many sound prolongations, as normal nonfluent control group children."
3. Part-word repetitions will consist of one to five productions of the unit being repeated with probably more than three iterations ("b-b-b-b-ball"). The nonstuttering children's repetitions will range from one to three productions.

TABLE 9–2   Guidelines for differentiating normal from abnormal disfluency

Behavior	Stuttering	Normal Disfluency
Syllable Repetitions		
a. Frequency per word	More than two	Less than two
b. Frequency per 100 words	More than two percent	Less than two percent
c. Tempo	Faster than normal	Normal tempo
d. Regularity	Irregular	Regular
e. Schwa vowel	Often present	Absent or rare
f. Airflow	Often interrupted	Rarely interrupted
g. Vocal tension	Often apparent	Absent
Prolongations		
h. Duration	Longer than one second	Less than one second
i. Frequency	More than one per 100 words	Less than one per 100 words
j. Regularity	Uneven or interrupted	Smooth
k. Tension	Important when present	Absent
l. When voiced (sonant)	May show rise in pitch	No pitch rise
m. When unvoiced (surd)	Interrupted airflow	Airflow present
n. Termination	Sudden	Gradual
Gaps (silent pauses)		
o. Within the word boundary	May be present	Absent
p. Prior to speech attempt	Unusually long	Not marked
q. After the disfluency	May be present	Absent
Phonation		
r. Inflections	Restricted; monotone	Normal
s. Phonatory arrest	May be present	Absent
t. Vocal fry	May be present	Usually absent
Articulating Postures		
u. Appropriateness	May be inappropriate	Appropriate
Reactions to Stress		
v. Type	More broken words	Normal disfluencies
Evidence of Awareness		
w. Phonemic consistency	May be present	Absent
x. Frustration	May be present	Absent
y. Postponements (stallers)	May be present	Absent
z. Eye contact	May waver	Normal

From C. Van Riper, *The Nature of Stuttering,* Englewood Cliffs, N.J.: Prentice-Hall, Inc., 1971. Used by permission.

4. "The part-word repetitions and sound prolongations of young stutterers seem to be marked by the abrupt, abnormal cessation of voice or air flow through the vocal tract."

5. In their part-word repetitions, the stuttering children are likely to substitute the schwa for the vowel expected[2] ("puh-puh-puh-paper").

If all five of the behavioral characteristics appear to fall on one side or the other of the stuttering-normal disfluency choice, the child can be characterized with relative assurance (according to Adams). The observational results may also be equivocal, with three judgments on one side of the coin and two on the other. If that were the case, the interpretation of choice would probably be conservative. If, as the diagnostician, you were unsure whether the behavior presented was normal disfluency or "incipient" stuttering, Adams's advice is to view the child as normally disfluent but to maintain weekly contacts with the parents and monthly contacts with the child. The child's variations in fluency can be monitored in that way until the diagnostic decision can be made with more confidence.

Pindzola (1986) developed a *Protocol for Differentiating the Incipient Stutterer* that provides a rapid means of making judgments relative to this question. The protocol is an attempt "to synthesize available information from the professional literature in a format designed to guide the clinician in selecting behaviors to count or quantify and interpret the data" (Pindzola and White 1986). The protocol summarizes findings in three areas: auditory behaviors (e.g., types of disfluencies, size of unit affected); visual behaviors (e.g., eye blinks, facial grimaces, head and body movements); and historical and psychological indicators (e.g., duration of the problem, reactions to stuttering).

WHETHER CHILD STUTTERING IS CHRONIC

There are a number of reports in the literature concerning children who once stuttered but who no longer stutter—some because of therapy, some probably in spite of therapy, and some who had no exposure to speech therapy. Cooper (1973) summarized these reports with the assumption that two out of every three stutterers whom speech clinicians meet will recover spontaneously. It is possible that at least some of these "recovered stutterers" were misclassified, but it is also possible that there may be predictive variables concerning the chronicity of stuttering. From this review of the literature, Cooper reported that there does not appear to be a consistent relationship between chronic stuttering and family history of stuttering. There is general agreement that, at least to a degree, the more severe the initial stuttering the more likely it will be maintained and require therapeutic intervention. The duration or length of time the stuttering is reported to have existed does not appear to be related to chronicity. There was no apparent sex bias in the literature; both boys and girls were equally likely to maintain stuttering or to spontaneously recover. It also has been reported—and it is an empirically logical statement—that those who incorporated stuttering into their self-concept were much more likely to remain

---

[2]Montgomery and Cooke (1976) question the prevalence of the schwa vowel in stuttered speech. They played CV segments of stuttered speech to a panel of five judges who were asked to transcribe the vowels they heard. Less than 25 percent were perceived as schwas with the vast majority of the schwa confusions occurring when either /ɝ/ or /aɪ/ were intended.

stutterers (Sheehan and Martyn 1966). There is one other general agreement in the literature regarding chronicity—recovery from stuttering is a gradual process.

For our diagnostic purposes, it is important to remember three items from that chronicity list: (1) The more severe the stuttering, the more likely it will be maintained; (2) the more the speaker's self-concept includes an identification of "stutterer," the more likely stuttering will be maintained; and (3) the recovery from stuttering is a gradual process. The severity variable is important because although there may be disagreement among listeners as to the exact frequency of disfluencies in a child's speech, disagreement is much less likely that a problem exists when stuttering is severe. The self-concept statement highlights the importance of background information and perceptual judgments on the part of the speaker and/or her concerned listeners. And the gradual recovery statement is important to remember for all who are concerned with the therapeutic process on both sides of the table. Therapeutic change is a process, and change occurs by degree and not by decree.

One other very important point relative to the diagnosis of stuttering is highlighted in the following quote from Luper and Ford (1980, p. 273):

> The experienced clinician recognizes also that it is wise to avoid jumping to conclusions on the basis of initial evaluation data. The variability of the occurrence of stuttering and of the conditions which appear to set it off is so great that frequent reevaluation is considered highly important.

THE DIAGNOSIS OF STUTTERING

Conture (1990), after reviewing the "state of the art" definition of stuttering, declared that

> (a) There are no known *objective, listener-independent*, criteria for identifying instances of stuttering or classifying children as stutterers versus normally fluent speakers and (b) there is *no consensus* among experienced clinicians and researchers regarding behavioral definitions of stuttering in childhood or classification of children as stutterers. (p. 3, emphasis in original)

He further quotes Bloodstein (1987, p. 4), who wrote that "the identification of moments of stuttering always involves the judgment of a listener."

Young (1984) points out that "Untrained observers make a clear distinction between stuttering and stutterer, using the former classification more frequently than the latter label, and believe that an individual can stutter without also being a stutterer" (p. 27).

That last statement is possibly the distinction we must keep in mind when we are thinking about the assignment of a diagnostic label for the speech pattern the child presents to us. No talker is completely fluent. The question of whether the relative disfluency of the child represents language skill or a fluency problem should likely dictate the direction of the intervention program. On the other hand, the adult may present a different (easier?) problem. Alfonso (1990) suggests that "Until the distinction between fluent, disfluent, and dysfluent[3] speech is better

---

[3]The prefix *dys* is generally interpreted to mean that there is a basic, probably neurological base for the problem. *Dysfluency* is therefore a symptom. *Dis* as a prefix refers to a relative lack of something. *Disfluency* is a behavior.

understood, the adult stutterer's judgment in the classification of him- or herself as a stutterer and in the fluency-disfluency distinction of his or her speech should be encouraged" (p. 16).

Gordon and Luper (1992a), in a tutorial article concerned with the protocols for differentiation of stuttering from normal disfluency, quote Adams and Webster (1989) concerning the risk of not working with a young child's fluency problem if the problem is stuttering rather than normal disfluency. Basically what Adams and Webster advocate is working with the child whenever there is a question rather than risk not working with one for whom disfluency is the problem, and who would really need the intervention. The primary rationale for this strategy, according to Gordon and Luper (p. 43) is that "the validity of the differential, diagnostic approach has not been established."

Gordon and Luper compared a number of available protocols for, among other things, the quantifiability of the items used and noted that only 4 of the 26 descriptions detailed by Van Riper (reported earlier as Table 9–2) were actions that could be counted. In summary, Gordon and Luper conclude that of the protocols reviewed, "no two protocols are identical, differing in one or more important ways [and that] many of the differences would appear to affect each protocol's usefulness to the clinician" (p. 48). In the second of their two tutorial articles, Gordon and Luper (1992b) suggest that criteria for a differential diagnostic protocol will include a standard size sample and more quantification of specific measures that may differentiate "incipient" or beginning stuttering from normal disfluency.

The preceding summary related to the diagnosis of stuttering was not intended to sound negative or as if it were a hopeless task that we were assigned. An answer to the question of "Is this stuttering or normal disfluency?" is not drastically different from any of our other diagnostic tasks in relation to the child's speech and language skills. There our question is "How shall we most effectively intervene to alleviate what appears to be the problem?" Basically the question would appear to be how we might help this individual become more fluent and less hesitant about speaking. Answers to questions such as these require much more than definitions of what constitutes stuttering. To answer questions about the potential efficacy of a therapy program, we need to have more detailed information about how fluent the individual child may be in what circumstances, and about the quality (efficiency and effectiveness) of his conversational and propositional speech. Ingram (1986, p. 103) suggests that

> in the case of children, stuttering therapy should be primarily concerned with altering speech behavior and very much less concerned with nonspeech behavior variables, although it certainly should not ignore them entirely.

A number of examples of detailed evaluation programs for the initial and continuing evaluation of stuttering have appeared in the literature (e.g., Costello and Ingham 1984; Gregory 1973; Guitar and Peters 1980; Ingham 1986; Pindzola and White 1986; Riley 1972; Van Riper 1973). Typically these protocols include criteria for making judgments of stuttering, lists of the types of situations in which speech samples are to be obtained and often suggestions for obtaining estimates of the client's proclivity for various brief, trial therapies. Gordon and Luper compare and discuss six commonly used protocols (1992a) and then present (1992b) some advantages and limitations in the available protocols as well as make suggestions for further precision in the construction and use of such protocols.

Most evaluation programs recommend the collection of considerable data. For example, Costello and Ingham (1984) advise taking periodic measures from videotaped samples in a least two 10-minute situations within the clinic and a minimum of four 10-minute situations outside the clinic. From these examples, Costello and Ingham measure the percent of syllables stuttered, the duration of individual moments of stuttering, the rate of speaking, the length of stutter-free utterances, and ratings of the quality or naturalness of speech. In addition, they recommended collections of speaking-time logs as measures of the client's ability to change his speech as he experiences brief samples of a number of different types of speaking, such as speaking slowly, prolonging phonation between words, and choral speaking. Their purpose in collecting these data is to help in obtaining base rates for later comparison and to assist in predicting the value of various treatments.

Guitar and Peters (1980) place considerable emphasis on the measurement of the client's attitudes and feelings about speech in addition to evaluating this speech. They also provide brief samples of trial therapy. As a final comment, Ingham (1986) noted that

> Whatever else we disagree about, I am certain that we do agree that stuttering is a variable behavior, and that any assessment procedure must take into account that variability. (p. 103)

Gordon and Luper are opting for delineating behaviors that can be most reliably measured. To paraphrase a quote from Darley included in the first chapter of this text concerning the "scientific method": When we can reduce our observations to numbers, then what we know can at least be measured. And it follows that if our observations can be reliably measured, we can measure change—and the variables that effect the change.

SUMMARY

There is a considerable body of literature available on stuttering. Van Riper collected a bibliography (see Sheehan 1970) of nearly 900 entries for the period from 1950 to 1970. Bloodstein (1975) included more than 950 citations on stuttering in a single text. Andrews et al. (1983) summarized findings from approximately 1,500 research articles. Much is known about stuttering, but there are no objective tests of this speech disorder. There is little that the stutterer does that can be conveyed by available descriptions of nonfluent speech behavior that the nonstutterer does not also do to some extent, and in some instances, in equivalent measure. In spite of the divergent views held on stuttering, it is doubtful that there would be any disagreement that the fundamental observable characteristic of stuttering is a disruption in the flow of speech. Almost certainly the task of diagnosing stuttering will begin with a description of the speech behavior. There is general agreement that stuttering most often includes specific types of disfluencies, but the presence, the frequency, or the articulatory effort with which these disfluencies are produced does not consistently separate between normally disfluent and stuttering speakers. Stuttering always involves a perceptual judgment on the part of a listener (who may also be the talker), and an important variable in the problem of stuttering involves the interaction between the talker and her listener (or listeners).

The bulk of our discussion on stuttering has dealt with a description of disfluency indices and the ubiquitous implication that it may be difficult to separate between beginning stuttering and normal disfluency. The distinction has therapeutic as well as theoretical implications. Luper and Mulder (1964) stated that the examiner's task is to collect the information, summarize the findings, draw conclusions, and make recommendations concerning treatment. Planning for therapy begins with the evaluation. It is the clinician's task to arrive at a reasonable understanding of the child so that therapy can be fitted to the child rather than the child fitted to the therapy. Among the questions to be answered is whether therapy intervention will be direct or indirect. "Even if it is found that a child's speech is normal, it is not enough simply to tell his parents or teacher this" (Luper and Mulder 1964, p. 33).

We have made relatively few specific comments about what stuttering is and what it is not and few specifics about separating between early stuttering and normal disfluency. What we have reported is more a set of descriptions on probabilities than on sureties. In that lack of specificity, we are in concert with most of the authorities on stuttering. Bloodstein (1977), in a state-of-the-art comment, wrote

> The principal questions about stuttering 25 to 50 years ago were What is it? What causes it? How should we treat it? Those were the big questions then, and of course they are still unanswered now. . . . A very large amount of information about stuttering has accumulated. But the basic questions remain [as well as]: . . . What relationship, if any, does early stuttering have to normal childhood disfluency? There are at least three possible answers to this question. First, there may be no relationship whatever. If that is the answer, we will not be very fortunate, . . . because it will leave us in the dark. Second, early stuttering may be the child's effort to avoid normal disfluency. This was Johnson's answer. If it is correct we will be moderately lucky. It is an illuminating hypothesis, but it has proved difficult to verify. Third, early stuttering and normal speech repetitions may be merely the same thing in different degrees. If this is the case we will be very fortunate, because it should be relatively easy to verify it by careful comparative studies of early stuttering and normal disfluency. (pp. 148–149)

Much has been written concerning stuttering since that time, but the definitive answers have still not been verified. With or without an apparent agreement among the scientific community as to the distinguishing characteristics between early stuttering and normal disfluency, it is the clinician's obligation to observe carefully, to describe operationally the speech behavior and the associated mannerisms accompanying the act of speech, to interpret carefully reactions and perceptions of the speaker and her important audience (being aware that these are interpretations and not necessarily facts), and to make judgments concerning any necessary intervention. With older children or adults who stutter, the description of the stuttering behavior and a judgment concerning therapy may be a relatively easy task. With younger children, especially preschoolers, the task is complicated because there is more at stake. One of the concerns the clinician must have has to do with the consequences of the judgment to be pronounced. If a parent is seeking advice and reassurance, it may not be sufficient that you describe the speech behaviors observed in terms of what is to be expected of a child in the process of speech and language development. If the parent is really seeking correction of what she perceives as a problem, reassurance may not be adequate. As a diagnostician, you must make a judgment of the consequences for the child being placed in therapy—and the consequences of not being placed in therapy. Is there a problem? What is the problem? What behaviors (speech and nonspeech) are being demonstrated to indicate a potential or an existing problem? What can be done about it?

REFERENCES

ADAMS, M. R., A clinical strategy for differentiating the normally nonfluent child and the incipient stutterer. *J. Fluency Dis.*, 2, 141–148 (1977).

ADAMS, M. R., AND R. REIS, The influence of the onset of phonation on the frequency of stuttering, *J. Speech Hearing Res.*, 14, 639–644 (1971).

ADAMS, M. R., AND R. REIS, The influence of the onset of phonation on the frequency of stuttering: A replication and reevaluation. *J. Speech Hearing Res.*, 17, 752–754 (1974).

ADAMS, M. R., AND P. HAYDEN, The ability of stutterers and nonstutterers to initiate and terminate phonation during production of an isolated vowel. *J. Speech Hearing Res.*, 19, 290–296 (1976).

ADAMS M. R., AND L. M. WEBSTER, Case selection strategies with children "at risk" for stuttering. *J. Fluency Dis.*, 14, 11–16 (1989).

AINSWORTH, S., ED., *If Your Child Stutters: A Guide for Parents.* Memphis, Tenn.: Speech Foundation of America (1977).

ALFONSO, P. J., Subject definition and selection criteria for stuttering research in adult subjects. In J. A. Cooper, ed., *ASHA Reports #18*, 2–14 (1990).

ANDREWS, G., A. CRAIG, A. FEYER, S. HODDINOTT, P. HOWIE, AND M. NEILSON, Stuttering: A review of research findings and theories circa 1982. *J. Speech Hearing Res.*, 48, 226–246 (1983).

BERRY, M. F., The development history of stuttering children. *J. Pediatrics*, 12, 209–217 (1938).

BLOODSTEIN, O., The development of stuttering: I. Changes in nine basic features. *J. Speech Hearing Dis.*, 25, 219–237 (1960a).

BLOODSTEIN, O., The development of stuttering: II. Developmental phases. *J. Speech Hearing Dis.*, 25, 366–376 (1960b).

BLOODSTEIN, O., The development of stuttering: III. Theoretical and clinical implications. *J. Speech Hearing Dis.*, 26, 67–82 (1961).

BLOODSTEIN, O., *A Handbook on Stuttering.* Chicago: National Easter Seal Society for Crippled Children and Adults (1975, 1981).

BLOODSTEIN, O., Stuttering. *J. Speech Hearing Dis.*, 42, 148–151 (1977).

BLOODSTEIN, O., *The Handbook on Stuttering*, 4th ed. Chicago: The National Easter Seal Society (1987).

CONTURE, E. G., Childhood stuttering: What is it and who does it? In J. A. Cooper, ed., *ASHA Reports #18*, 2–14 (1990).

COOPER, E. B., The development of a stuttering chronicity prediction checklist: A preliminary report. *J. Speech Hearing Dis.*, 38, 2, 215–223 (1973).

COOPER, M. H., AND G. D. ALLEN, Timing control accuracy in normal speakers and stutterers. *J. Speech Hearing Res.*, 20, 55–71 (1977).

COSTELLO, J. M., AND R. J. INGHAM, Assessment strategies for stuttering. In *Nature and Treatment of Stuttering: New Directions*, eds. R. F. Curlee and W. H. Perkins. San Diego: College-Hill Press (1984).

CROSS, D. E., AND H. L. LUPER, Voice reaction time of stuttering and nonstuttering children and adults. *J. Fluency Dis.*, 4, 59–77 (1979).

DARLEY, F. L., D. C. SPRIESTERSBACH, AND OTHERS, *Diagnostic Methods in Speech Pathology*, 2nd ed. New York: Harper & Row (1978).

DAUGHTRY, G. H., The performance of fluent and disfluent seven-year-old males in locating clicks superimposed on sentences. Unpublished paper, University of Tennessee, Knoxville (1976).

ERICKSON, R. L., Assessing communication attitudes among stutterers. *J. Speech Hearing Res.*, 12, 711–724 (1969).

FODOR, J., AND T. BEVER, The psychological reality of linguistic segments. *J. Verb. Learn. Verb. Behav.*, 4, 414–420 (1965).

FROESCHELS, E., Summary statement written in 1955. *Stuttering: Significant Theories and Therapies*, ed. E. F. Hahn. Stanford: Stanford University Press (1958).

GARRET, M., T. BEVER, AND J. FODOR, The active use of grammar in speech perception. *Percep. Psychophys.*, 1, 30–32 (1965).

GORDON, P. A., AND H. L. LUPER, The early identification of beginning stuttering: I. Protocols. *Amer. J. Speech-Language Path.*, 1, No. 3, 43–53 (1992a).

GORDON, P. A., AND H. L. LUPER, The early identification of beginning stuttering: II. Problems. *Amer. J. Speech-Language Path.*, 1. No. 4, 49–55 (1992b).

GORDON, P. A., H. L. LUPER, AND H. A. PETERSON, The effects of syntactic complexity on the occurrence of disfluencies in five-year-old nonstutterers. *J. Fluency Dis.*, 11, 151–164 (1986).

GREGORY, H., *Stuttering: Differential Evaluation and Therapy*. Indianapolis: Bobbs-Merrill (1973).

GUITAR, B., AND T. J. PETERS, *Stuttering: An Integration of Contemporary Therapies*. Memphis, Tenn.: Speech Foundation of America (1980).

HAND, R., An acoustical study of fluent speech in stutterers and nonstutterers. Unpublished Ph.D. dissertation, University of Tennessee, Knoxville (1979).

INGHAM, R. J., Toward a therapy assessment procedure for treating stuttering in children. In *Stuttering Therapy: Prevention and Intervention with Children*. Memphis, Tenn.: Speech Foundation of America (1986).

JOHNSON, W., Stuttering. In *Speech Handicapped School Children*, eds. W. Johnson and D. Moeller. New York: Harper & Row (1967).

JOHNSON, W., AND ASSOCIATES, *The Onset of Stuttering*. Minneapolis: University of Minnesota Press (1959).

JOHNSON, W., F. L. DARLEY, AND D. C. SPRIESTERSBACH, *Diagnostic Methods in Speech Pathology*. New York: Harper & Row (1963).

LADEFOGED, P., AND D. BROADBENT, Perception of sequence in auditory events. *Quart. J. Exper. Psych.*, 12, 162–170 (1960).

LUCHSINGER, R., AND G. E. ARNOLD, *Voice-Speech-Language*. Belmont, Calif.: Wadsworth (1965).

LUPER, H. L., Some speculations on the nature of stuttering in children. *Annual Postgraduate Symposium on Hearing and Speech*, University of Kansas Medical School, Kansas City, 23–27 (1970).

LUPER, H. L., AND R. L. MULDER, *Stuttering: Therapy for Children*. Englewood Cliffs, N.J.: Prentice Hall (1964).

LUPER, H. L., AND S. C. FORD, Disorders of fluency. In *Communication Disorders: An Introduction*, ed. R. Van Hattum. New York: Macmillan (1980).

MACDONALD, J. D., AND R. R. MARTIN, Stuttering and disfluency as two reliable and unambiguous response classes. *J. Speech Hearing Res.*, 16, 691–699 (1973).

MONTGOMERY, A. A., AND P. A. COOKE, Perceptual and acoustic analysis of repetitions in stuttered speech. *J. Commun. Dis.*, 9, 317–330 (1976).

MUMA, J., Syntax of preschool fluent and disfluent speech: A transformational analysis. *J. Speech Hearing Res.*, 14, 428–441 (1971).

MURPHY, A., ed., *Stuttering, Its Prevention*. Memphis, Tenn.: Speech Foundation of America (1962).

OLSON, G., AND H. CLARK, Research methods in psycholinguistics. In *Handbook of Perception: Vol. VII Language and Speech*, eds. E. Carterette and M. Friedman. New York: Academic Press (1976).

PINDZOLA, R. H., *Protocol for Differentiating the Incipient Stutterer*. Auburn, Ala.: Auburn University (1986).

PINDZOLA, R. H., AND D. T. WHITE, A protocol for differentiating the incipient stutterer. *Lang. Speech Hearing Serv. Schools*, 17, 2–15 (1986).

RILEY, G. D., A stuttering severity instrument for children and adults. *J. Speech Hearing Dis.*, 37, 314–322 (1972).

RILEY, G. D., *A Stuttering Severity Instrument for Children and Adults*, rev. ed. Tigard, Oreg.: C. C. Publications (1980).

ROBINSON, F. B., *Introduction to Stuttering*, Englewood Cliffs, N.J.: Prentice Hall (1964).

SHEEHAN, J., ed., *Stuttering: Research and Therapy*. New York: Harper & Row (1970).

SHEEHAN, J. G., AND M. M. MARTYN, Spontaneous recovery from stuttering. *J. Speech Hearing Res.*, 9, 121–155 (1966).

STARKWEATHER, C. W., The development of fluency in normal children. In *Stuttering Therapy: Prevention and Intervention with Children*. Memphis, Tenn.: Speech Foundation of America (1986).

STARKWEATHER, C. W., P. HIRSCHMAN, AND R. S. TANNENBAUM, Latency of vocalization: Stutterers vs. nonstutterers. *J. Speech Hearing Res.*, 19, 481–492 (1976).

VAN RIPER, C., *The Nature of Stuttering*. Englewood Cliffs, N.J.: Prentice Hall (1971).

VAN RIPER, C., *The Treatment of Stuttering*. Englewood Cliffs, N.J.: Prentice Hall (1973).

VAN RIPER, C., *Speech Correction: Principles and Methods*, 6th ed. Englewood Cliffs, N.J.: Prentice Hall (1978).

WEISS, D. A., *Cluttering*. Englewood Cliffs, N.J.: Prentice Hall (1964).

WERTHEIM, E. S., A new approach to the classification and measurement of stuttering. *J. Speech Hearing Dis.*, 37, 2, 242–251 (1972).

WILLIAMS, D., Evaluation. In *Therapy for Stutterers*, ed. C. W. Starkweather. Memphis, Tenn.: Speech Foundation of America (1974).

WILLIAMS, D. E., AND L. R. KENT, Listener evaluations of speech interruption. *J. Speech Hearing Res.*, 1, 124–131 (1958).

WILLIAMS, J. G., A study concerning the relationship of disfluencies to selected linguistic skills. Unpublished master's thesis, University of Tennessee, Knoxville (1974).

WINGATE, M. E., A standard definition of stuttering. *J. Speech Hearing Dis.*, 29, 484–489 (1964).

WINGATE, M. E., Stuttering adaptations and learning: I. The relevance of adaptation studies to stuttering as "learned behavior." *J. Speech Hearing Dis.*, 31, 148–156 (1966).

WINGATE, M. E., *Stuttering: Theory and Treatment*. New York: Irvington Publishers (1976).

WINGATE, M. E., Disorders of fluency. In *Speech, Language and Hearing: Normal Processes and Disorders*, eds. P. H. Skinner and P. Shelton. Reading, Mass.: Addison-Wesley (1978).

WOOLF, C., The assessment of stuttering as struggle, avoidance, and expectancy. *British J. Dis. Comm.*, 2, 158–171 (1967).

WYATT, G. L., *Language Learning and Communication Disorders in Children*. New York: Free Press (1969).

YOUNG, M. A., Predicting ratings of severity of stuttering. *J. Speech Hearing Dis.*, Monogr. Sup. 7, 31–54 (1961).

YOUNG, M. A., Observer agreement for making moments of stuttering. *J. Speech Hearing Res.*, 18, 530–540 (1975).

YOUNG, M., Identification of stuttering and stutterers, In *Nature and Treatment of Stuttering: New directions*, eds. R. Curlee and W. Perkins. San Diego, Calif.: College-Hill Press (1984).

ZIMMERMAN, G., Articulatory dynamics of fluent utterances of stutterers and nonstutterers. *J. Speech Hearing Res.*, 23, 95–105 (1980).

10

Evaluation of Adult Neurological Disorders

... if the patient doesn't agree with the book, throw away the book, not the patient. The patient cannot be wrong.

Kurt Goldstein to Aaron Smith

A host of speech and language disorders result from damage to the brain after communicative skills have been acquired. These disorders are termed *acquired* to contrast them with *congenital* deficits that develop from brain damage incurred before the acquisition of communicative skills. Perhaps no other group of disorders, with the possible exception of stuttering, has been as controversial, as rich in history, or as burdened with a confusing nomenclature.

The controversies that have resulted from attempts to model the functional landscape of the brain and to describe syndromes of impairment associated with particular sites of lesion stem from the brain's complex architecture and operation. The brain is characterized by a dense anatomic connectivity and a continuous activity such that no part is isolated functionally from all other parts. Consequently, a lesion does not destroy a particular cortical area and its corresponding function but deforms the normal patterns of interaction of a whole network of activities. This conceptualization of the nervous system by Lenneberg (1975) may serve as a partial explanation for two conundrums he has eloquently described. First, studies of brain lesions and brain stimulation effects do not agree; that is, cognitive and/or motor activities that are lost due to a lesion are not necessarily the activities observed during stimulation of the same area. Second, patients with widespread cortical damage frequently exhibit similar speech-language deficits while patients with very similar cortical damage can often exhibit very different symptoms.

Given that Lenneberg's conceptualization of neural activity is valid, it is not surprising that early attempts to localize specific functions to circumscribed areas of the brain, as if it were a functional mosaic that only needed to be mapped to be understood, and attempts to describe the brain as equipotential in terms of its ability to subserve a multitude of functions, have led to controversy. At the same time, we, as clinicians, must be cognizant of the fact that these early efforts to impose theoretical constructs on a mechanism of great complexity have been the source for our test models and terminology.

The terms that have evolved to serve as abbreviations for constellations of deficits resulting from brain damage are confusing and serve to obstruct, rather than to facilitate, communication. Consequently, for purposes of discussion and clarification, we will define the major categories of communication disorders to be considered.

DEFINITIONS AND DESCRIPTIONS
OF NEUROGENIC DISORDERS

At birth, both hemispheres of the brain are capable of establishing activity patterns that constitute verbal processes, but as the organism matures, there is a genetically predetermined displacement of verbal functions to the left hemisphere and nonverbal functions to the right hemisphere (Gates and Bradshaw 1977; Krashen 1976). The dominance is functional rather than anatomical, although there are some differences between the left and right hemispheres (LeMay and Geschwind 1978). Consequently, almost all right-handed and most left-handed individuals will have left-hemisphere dominance for speech and language representation.

Damage to the dominant hemisphere will produce disturbances on a variety of tasks, usually affecting some more than others, depending on the site and extent of the lesion. *Aphasia* is a multimodality language disorder characterized by reduced ability to encode and decode linguistic elements. Reading, writing, speaking, and comprehension abilities are involved, and the impairment affects semantic, syntactic, phonological, lexical, and pragmatic aspects of language. Considerable difference of opinion exists as to whether aphasia is best viewed as a singular disorder or as a disorder with a number of identifiable syndromes of impairment. Schuell (1964), for example, described aphasia as a disorder that may be complicated by concomitant sensory, motor, and/or cognitive impairments. In contrast, Goodglass and Kaplan (1972) described a group of identifiable syndromes of aphasia based on similar data.

Apraxia is an inability to voluntarily program movements due to damage to the anterior dominant hemisphere. Oral and limb movements may be affected in addition to speech-related activity. The disorder is considered to be independent of

linguistic deficits and neuromuscular impairment, although these disorders frequently co-occur with apraxia (Darley, Aronson, and Brown 1975; Kent and Rose-
bek 1983). This view of apraxia, however, appears to be under reconsideration
since movement level disturbances are observable in aphasia as well (McNeil and
Kent 1990). A number of aphasiologists (e.g., Goodglass and Kaplan 1972) have
included apraxic symptoms within the classification of Broca's aphasia since the
disorder infrequently occurs independently of language deficits. Typical characteristics of apraxia include groping trial-and-error movements during attempts at
approximating articulatory positions, a high frequency of distortion articulatory
errors (Odell et al. 1990), and prosodic disturbances.

Agnosia is a disorder characterized by an inability to recognize stimuli even
though the sensory pathway to the brain is intact. The patient is aware of the presence of the stimulus but cannot match it to a like stimulus or describe its characteristics. We have chosen to define this disorder because it is a primary diagnostic
label on several test batteries. We wish to point out, however, that there seems to be
relatively little support for its use with the exception of relatively infrequent cases
of cortical deafness or cortical blindness. Penfield and Roberts (1959) observed that
"terms such as those of agnosia . . . do nothing but confuse us. There is not a single
case in the literature of . . . agnosia without other defects."

Damage to the nondominant hemisphere for language (typically the right)
produces a group of deficits that do not specifically impair language but may significantly affect communication. These patients demonstrate poor judgment, inability to follow through on a task that requires several steps for its completion, verbosity, difficulty recognizing faces, intonational patterns and rhythms, and poor
locational and directional skills (Brookshire 1978; Joynt and Goldstein 1975;
Myers 1984). No specific term has been developed for this syndrome.

Acute and chronic bihemispheric structural changes or interference with
neural activity produces disorders that have been termed by Darley (1964) as the
"language of confusion" and the "language of generalized intellectual deterioration" respectively. Neither of these terms has gained wide usage, perhaps because
they encompass broad-based disorders involving cognition as well as language. The
language of confusion is due to a heterogeneous group of disorders as diverse as
closed-head injury, metabolic disturbances, and anoxia subsequent to cardiac arrest.
The condition is characterized, according to Darley, by reduced recognition and
understanding of and responsiveness to the environment, faulty short-term memory,
mistaken reasoning, disorientation in time and space, and behavior that is less adaptive and less appropriate than normal. Clearly, this disorder springs from multiple
etiologies and involves cognition as well as language. Holland (1982), for example,
pointed out that communicative breakdown in closed-head injury involves important components of memory and intellect that have a major bearing on pragmatic
aspects of language. Hagen (1984) has reviewed some important characteristics of
communication disorders arising from cognitive disorganization in closed-head
injury, including decreased auditory, visual, and reading comprehension; disordered expressive language; lack of ability to inhibit verbal expressions; inappropriate word ordering; and inability to recall specific words. Speech and language
deficits associated with brain trauma have been reviewed by Marquardt, Stoll, and
Sussman (1990).

The diagnosis of language of generalized intellectual deterioration also has not gained wide acceptance although the deficits associated with dementia have recently developed into a major area of research. According to Darley (1964), the language of generalized intellectual impairment includes a prominent impairment of memory, particularly for recent events; impoverished, concrete thinking, which may lead to difficulty in coping with simple tasks; emotional and personality changes; and word-finding problems. It is pertinent to note that most of these characteristics deal with cognitive deficits and not with speech and language per se. Bayles (1982) found that patients with dementia demonstrated a particular vulnerability of the semantic system but not of the syntax or phonology systems. Appell, Kertesz, and Fisman (1982) investigated performance of patients with dementia on the *Western Aphasia Battery* and noted that as a group they differed from stroke patients in terms of higher fluency and lower comprehension. No phonemic paraphasias were noted, but these patients showed a high incidence of circumlocutions and semantic jargon. Nicholas et al. (1985) and Richardson and Marquardt (1985) have provided descriptions of speech and language functioning in dementia on a number of dimensions.

Dysarthrias are neuromuscular speech disorders. In other words, speech production is compromised due to paralysis, weakness, and/or incoordination of musculature. Dysarthria may affect the entire speech mechanism, including respiratory, phonatory, and articulatory processes, or be limited to more specific musculature, such as in laryngeal paralysis. The type of dysarthria will depend upon the site of the lesion within the motor pathways. For example, ataxic dysarthria characterized by weakness and incoordination is associated with damage to the cerebellum, and hypokinetic dysarthria with resting tremor, rigidity, and hypokinesis results from damage to the basal ganglia.

It is important to note that none of the acquired neurogenic disorders are mutually exclusive. In fact, it is common to find a patient demonstrating more than one of the disorders described. Our consideration of appraisal procedures will include an examination of standardized tests and assessment protocols useful in characterizing and differentiating among the disorders and a short procedural guide for evaluating the patient. We first focus on aphasia. Assessment of patients with right hemisphere lesions, apraxia, dysarthria, and dysphagia (swallowing disorders) then are considered.

TESTS FOR APHASIA

Numerous test batteries have been developed to evaluate communicative disabilities arising from injury to the dominant hemisphere for verbal skills. In general, they include a number of subtests that evaluate specific subskills of the communicative process, rather than a single estimate of a skill such as writing. As described by Brookshire (1978), during testing one or more input modalities are combined in the presentation of a stimulus, and one or more output modalities are utilized for the response. Inferences regarding the integrity of the processing mechanism are then drawn, based on the output responses to stimuli presented through one or more of the input modalities at various complexity levels. For example, the patient may be presented auditorily with the name of a tool and asked to demonstrate its use. This is an example of an auditory input and a gestural response. Alternatively, the patient may be handed a pencil and asked to name it. Here a visual and a tactile input are coupled to a verbal response. Similar examples can be developed for all combinations of input and output.

Brookshire (1978) has developed a list of criteria for determining the adequacy of a test battery for aphasia. Included are criteria related to representativeness, reliability, treatment planning, validity, and so forth. Not all tests meet these criteria. You will have to decide which criteria are the most important for your purposes. A review of some batteries for the evaluation of aphasia and related disorders may help to provide a basis for your judgment.

Aphasia test batteries can be viewed along a number of dimensions—for example, the qualitative nature of the scoring, the number of test items and subtests, the prognostic value of quantified behaviors, and the ease of administration and interpretation. The tack used here will be a historical perspective because it serves as the best means of interlocking theoretical assumptions about neurogenic communication deficits and the tests constructed to assess these disorders.

Examining for Aphasia (Eisenson 1954) was developed on the premise that aphasic disturbances are impairments in the ability of the patient to handle situations involving significant symbolization manifested in internal symbol processes (thinking) and external symbol processes (speaking, reading, writing). The battery contains 16 subtests divided into two main parts: items used to evaluate abilities to deal with simple recognition or evaluation (predominantly receptive) and items used to evaluate expressive verbal and nonverbal skills (predominantly expressive). The approach of the test follows from the work of Weisenburg and McBride (1935) who classified aphasia on the basis of receptive and expressive functioning.

The test has not been standardized in terms of normative data, stimulus presentation, or scoring responses. No scale or percentage scores or other weighting is provided. Rather, an estimate of the patient's degree of deficit relative to each symbol-function area is made and is categorized as complete, severe, moderate, little, or none. Symbol-function areas include subtests used to determine the presence and severity of aphasic, apraxic, and agnosic disturbances.

The *Language Modalities Test for Aphasia* (Wepman and Jones 1961) was constructed on the basis of the performance of over 200 adult aphasic patients. Factor analysis of the data from these subjects (Jones and Wepman 1961) led the authors to posit two roles for language in the central nervous system: transmissive functions producing nonsymbolic language processes, and integrative functions producing symbolic comprehension and formulation processes. They suggested that dysfunction of the transmissive functions results in agnosias and apraxias and that integration dysfunctions produce aphasias.

The test consists of two forms comparable in difficulty which are presented on film strips 120 frames in length. The two forms of the test allow test-retest evaluations as a means of measuring the stability of the performance of the patient. The initial items on each form of the test are identical and constitute a screening section. Five different types of responses are elicited from the patient: oral, graphic, and three types of matching. Dichotomous scoring is utilized for the screening section and the standardized visual and auditory matching items. For the standardized oral and graphic responses and story-telling sections, the response is scored on a six-point scale and identified as normal, syntactic, pragmatic, jargon, and global. The results of testing are summarized, and the subject is classified according to one of the available categories: pragmatic, semantic, syntactic, jargon, or global aphasia, apraxia, and/or agnosia. Interscorer reliability has been reported to range from 0.88 to 0.96. Alternate form reliability and stability of subject performance are also reported to be high.

The *Minnesota Test for the Differential Diagnosis of Aphasia* (Schuell 1965) contains 47 subtests divided into five areas: auditory disturbances, visual and reading disturbances, speech and language disturbances, visuomotor and writing disturbances, and disturbances of numerical relations and arithmetic processes. Dichotomous scoring is used for most subtests. Scores are summarized on the front sheet of the test form by subtest and area. Schuell has suggested that the subtests can be used to assign a patient to one of five major or two minor categories based on the pattern of impairment. The five major groups include simple aphasia, aphasia with visual involvement, aphasia with sensorimotor involvement, aphasia with scattered findings compatible with generalized brain damage, and irreversible aphasic syndrome. The two minor syndromes are aphasia with partial auditory imperception and aphasia with persisting dysarthria. The prognosis for recovery for each of these groups is provided.

Factor analysis of the scores from 157 aphasic subjects and means, standard deviations, median scores, and percentage of subjects making errors are provided for each subtest. However, no standard scores or numerical indices of severity are provided because Schuell rejected them as "meaningless when dealing with aphasic populations which are heterogeneous in age, intelligence, cultural milieu, medical history, locus and extent of brain damage, and severity and duration of aphasia" (p. 7). Additionally, she stated that "the most effective way of interpreting test data is in terms of clinical signs and total test pattern" (p. 8). Test-retest reliability and interscorer agreement for the test have not been determined.

The *Minnesota Test for the Differential Diagnosis of Aphasia* does not arise from clear-cut theoretical notions. Rather, it is clearly premised on the need to be descriptive in clinical testing because description forms the structure for determining both prognosis and treatment in aphasia.

The *Neurosensory Center Comprehensive Examination for Aphasia* (Spreen and Benton 1969) consists of 20 tests of language performance and 4 tests of visual and tactile function. The 20 language tests assess language comprehension and production, retention of verbal information, and reading and writing. The 4 visual and tactile function tests are designed to detect deficits in these skills and are administered whenever the patient's performance on tests such as visual or tactile naming is subnormal.

Eleven of the tests use sets of common objects with the items in each set sequenced in order of increasing difficulty. Four of the tests are presented on recorded tape. Two use materials from the *Token Test* (McNeil and Prescott 1978). One uses block letters. Four require the use of a small box with a drop curtain so that items can be presented out of the view of the patient. Printed cards and unruled paper are required for reading and copying tasks. Dichotomous scoring is used (correct and incorrect). The examiner should also record incorrect and/or mispronounced correct responses and note any unusual features of performance.

This battery is unique in that there is a provision for construction of a profile of directly comparable percentile scores corrected for age and educational level. Two profile sheets have been developed for this purpose. The first profile is based on the performance of normal adults on the battery. The raw scores are computed for each of the 20 language tests, corrected for age and educational level (where appropriate), and transformed into the corresponding percentile rank of a normal population. The developers suggest that patients without language deficits will perform at the 40th percentile or above. Performance from the 30th to 40th percentile suggests minimal difficulty; from the 20th to 30th percentile, mild impairment; and below the 20th percentile, more severe dysfunction. The second profile allows comparison of the patient's performance with a reference group of aphasic patients. This permits the determination of the patient's strengths and weaknesses relative to the "average" performance of this reference group. Validity and reliability indices have not been reported for this battery.

The *Porch Index of Communicative Ability* (Porch 1971) was designed to assess verbal, gestural, and graphic abilities and was based on the premise that two major requirements of an aphasia examination are high reliability and a scoring system that specifies the nature of the patient's response in terms of multiple dimensions. The test contains 18 subtests (4 verbal, 8 gestural, and 6 graphic), each comprised of 10 items. The responses to the 180 items of the test are scored according to a 16-point binary choice system which considers the accuracy, responsiveness, completeness, promptness, and efficiency of the response. A mean score for each subtest, each modality, and the entire battery is computed from the 180 scored responses. The mean subtest scores can be examined on a Modality Response Summary, which plots subtest scores by modality (verbal, gestural, graphic), and on a Ranked Response Summary, which plots the means in order of decreasing subtest difficulty.

The Porch index was standardized on 280 left hemisphere–damaged patients and 100 bilaterally damaged patients. The test manual includes percentiles for the test as a whole, for each modality and for the mean of the 9 high and 9 low subtests. The means of the 9 low and 9 high subtests and the overall mean are used to plot a recovery curve for the patient. The recovery curve is used to make predictions regarding the patient's eventual communicative functioning based on his performance one month post-onset. At six months post-onset, the mean of the patient's 9 high subtests is considered the best estimate of his eventual maximal level of recovery. The test manual also provides some general guidelines for treatment. Five types of profiles are identified based on test results: (1) aphasia without complications, (2) aphasia complicated by verbal formulation or verbal expression problems, (3) aphasia patterns with accompanying illiteracy, (4) bilateral brain damage, and (5) aberrant patterns suggesting that the communicative disorder is not aphasia. Test-retest reliability has been established at 0.98, although interscorer agreement is somewhat lower.

A large database has been developed for the Porch index since its standardization. For example, Duffy and others (1976) provided subtest, modality, and overall test scores for 130 normal, non–brain-injured adults, and Watson and Records (1978) investigated the effectiveness of the test in assessing specific behavior in senile dementia. The test has also been criticized on the basis of its ordinality (McNeil, Prescott, and Chang 1975) and on its lack of specification of the response, neglect of factors related to communication, distortions in modality scoring, inadequacies of the response categories, statistical treatment of scores, and conceptual limits (Martin 1977).

The *Boston Diagnostic Aphasia Examination* (Goodglass and Kaplan 1972) is based on the assumption that the aphasia deficit is determined by "(a) the anatomical organization of language in the brain, (b) the location of the causative lesion, and (c) the functional interactions (e.g., inhibitory, regulatory, selective) of various parts of the language system" (p. 2). Accordingly, the test battery is geared toward determining the type of aphasic syndrome so that inferences can be made regarding localization of the cerebral lesion; measurement of communicative and related skills over a wide range for initial description and for detecting change in performance over time; and comprehensive assessment of abilities and deficits, which may serve as a guide to therapy.

The battery contains 23 subtests and rating scales designed to assess articulation, loss of verbal fluency, word-finding difficulty, repetition, serial speech, loss of grammar, syntax, auditory comprehension, reading, and writing. Scoring includes plus–minus scores, longhand notation, and rating of conversational and expository speech. The test was standardized on 207 aphasic patients. Based on the range, mean, and standard deviation of the patients' performances, Z-scores were computed, allowing each patient's performance on each subtest to be compared with the normative population scores in standard deviation units. The patient may be assigned to one of several diagnostic categories including Broca's aphasia, Wernicke's aphasia, anomic aphasia, conduction aphasia, and transcortical sensory or motor aphasia based on the rating-scale profile of speech characteristics and Z-scores. The battery also contains supplementary language tests to explore both comprehension and expression skills and supplementary nonlanguage tests, such as reproducing three-dimensional block designs, drawing to command, and so forth. Although test-retest data have not been obtained for this instrument, reliability coefficients based on profiles from 34 patients were from 0.68 to 0.98, which suggests good internal consistency with respect to what the items were measuring. This instrument is unique in that results of testing are used to estimate the site of brain damage responsible for the communicative deficits.

The Boston test has recently undergone a minor revision (Goodglass and Kaplan 1983). Some items within subtests have been reordered, the Body-Part Naming subtest has been eliminated, and three body-part items have been included in the Confrontation Naming subtest. The test booklet has been reorganized, and Z-scores have been converted to percentiles. Normative data are provided for a new sample of 242 aphasic patients, and norms for neurologically normal adults have been included.

The *Aphasia Language Performance Scales* (Keenan and Brassel 1975) was developed because the authors believed that existing aphasia tests had several unsatisfactory conditions: They were time consuming, limited by space and environmental restrictions, tended to break down rapport, and gave little help in planning for therapy. This test is composed of four scales (listening, talking, reading, writing), each containing 10 items. The items on each scale are graded in difficulty and range in linguistic complexity from virtual absence of function to near normal function. The four scales are purported to be independent of one another; that is, performance on items of one scale is not affected by deficits tested on items from another scale.

Each item is scored one point if the response is correct or self-corrected, one-half point if the response is correct following a prompt, and zero points for an incorrect response. The score on each scale is computed and plotted on a summary form that can be used to illustrate the patient's pattern of impairment, severity of the deficit in each modality, and rate of improvement. The Talking Scale was administered to 90 patients by eight speech pathologists to determine internal reliability using the Kuder-Richardson Formula 20 (Keenan and Brassel 1974). This procedure yielded a reliability coefficient of 0.90. In a related study, Basili and others (1974) administered the *Aphasia Language Performance Scales* and subtests of the *Porch Index of Communicative Ability* to 50 aphasic patients. Spearman rank-order correlation coefficients for scale scores and comparable Porch subtest scores ranged from 0.84 to 0.93, which suggested adequate concurrent validity.

The *Functional Communication Profile* (Sarno 1969) begins from an entirely different perspective. Sarno suggested that most clinical tests of aphasia do not take into account the fact that many aphasic patients use gestures to communicate, respond accurately but inconsistently, require a longer period of time to respond even when vocabulary and syntax are intact, and have more difficulty with highly specific tasks. Moreover, she indicated that many of the more standard aphasia batteries are relatively insensitive to minimal impairments and may contain many items to which the severely involved patient cannot respond.

The test consists of 45 integrated communicative behaviors divided into five areas: movement, speaking, understanding, reading, and miscellaneous (including writing and calculation). Ratings of each behavior are made on a continuum along a nine-point scale from zero to normal and take into account "speed, accuracy, consistency, voluntary control without benefit of external cues and compensatory function of the behavior." The ratings are made following informal interaction with the patient in conversational situations and, when necessary, are supplemented with other reports of the patient's abilities. The ratings for each of the five sections and for the entire profile are converted to percentages that reflect the percent of premorbid functioning. A patient functioning at the 60th percentile, for example, would be functioning at 60 percent of her premorbid level. Premorbid capacity, consequently, serves as a reference against which the performance of the patient is measured. The profile of the patient can also be used to visually differentiate between types of verbal impairment. For example, if a patient demonstrates severely impaired speaking skill compared to rated performances on the other sections of the test, she might be described as demonstrating verbal apraxia.

Sarno reported that Taylor and Sands (1965) investigated the interrater reliability of the profile. Three observers rated the performance of 20 aphasic adults. Agreement of the raters, when expressed as Spearman rank-order correlations, ranged from 0.87 to 0.95 for the five sections of the profile. A related study by Greenberg (1969), reported by Sarno, indicated further that investigations have demonstrated that the profile has concurrent and predictive validity, the convergence of these findings suggesting construct validity.

Communicative Abilities in Daily Living (Holland 1979, 1980) is a 68-item test instrument that emphasizes a functional approach to assessing the patient's communicative impairment. The primary focus, according to Holland, is not on whether the message was communicated by verbal or nonverbal means but that it was completed, regardless of the means. Consequently, the test is not modality specific. The Communicative Abilities scale has a three-point scoring system. If the patient's response is successful, whether it has been accomplished by verbal, gestural, or graphic means, it is considered correct and scored as 2. If it was failed, it is scored as 0, and if it is not totally correct, but signifies a communicative relationship to the task item, it is scored as 1. Tasks on the test are everyday activities ranging from responding to and giving social greetings, to differentiating nonverbal signs on restroom doors, to understanding metaphors, to recognizing statements which are unexpected in context. The items are encompassed within simulated, real-world activities, including going to the doctor's office, riding in a car, shopping, using the telephone, and being interviewed by a stranger. The total score is simply the cumulative sum of the item scores.

The *Western Aphasia Battery* (Kertesz 1979, 1982) was designed for clinical and research use. Oral language subtests of the battery (spontaneous speech, comprehension, repetition, naming) are used to assess the type and severity of aphasia. Performance on these subtests is used to assign patients to one of eight aphasia categories: global, Broca's, isolation, transcortical motor, Wernicke's, transcortical sensory, conduction, or anomic aphasia based on taxonomy. Scaled scores from the subtests are used to derive an aphasia quotient (AQ), which is an estimate of aphasia severity (Kertesz and Poole 1974). Similarly, a performance quotient (PQ) is obtained by summing the scaled scores from the reading, writing, praxis, drawing, block design, and calculation subtests and the *Raven Progressive Matrices*. The AQ plus PQ yields a cortical quotient (CQ), which serves an as estimate of cognitive functioning.

The WAB has been standardized on neurologically normal, aphasic, and neurologically impaired nonaphasic subjects (Kertesz 1979, 1982; Shewan and Kertesz 1980) and has adequate reliability and validity. Its unique feature is the derivation of quotients as estimates of verbal, performance, and cognitive functioning.

The Boston Assessment of Severe Aphasia (Helm-Estabrooks et al. 1989) is the most recent addition to diagnostic instruments for aphasia. It is designed to identify and quantify residual abilities in patients with severe aphasia and is best viewed as a general assessment of communicative ability. The test is composed of 61 eclectically derived items divided into 15 sections that range from social greetings and simple conversation to comprehension of number symbols; object naming; and recognition of emotional words, phrases, and symbols. Scoring is qualitative and reflects the modality used, communicative quality, perseveration, and presence of affect by selecting features from a 14-option system. Results from clusters of items including auditory comprehension, praxis, oral-gestural expression, reading comprehension, gesture recognition, writing and visual-spatial tasks and the total score are used to compare the patient tested to a standardization group of subjects with severe aphasia. The cluster scores are based on responses that were fully communicative in the modality specified, which are then summed to obtain a total raw score. The cluster and total scores can be converted to standard scores with a mean of 10 and a standard deviation of 3. Standard scores then can be used to determine percentile ranks and the standard error of measurement.

One hundred and eleven patients with aphasia and/or head injury were field tested with the instrument. Internal consistency based on the total score for a sample of 47 global aphasics was 0.88, somewhat lower than the coefficient of 0.94 for the entire group of severely aphasic subjects. Test-retest reliability for 34 severely aphasic subjects was 0.74; for a sample of 34 global aphasics, 0.75. The test appears to have adequate content validity. Comparison with scores from the *Boston Diagnostic Aphasia Examination* suggests the measure has adequate concurrent validity as well.

ADDITIONAL CONSIDERATIONS IN THE SELECTION OF APHASIA TESTS

Earlier, we noted criteria for evaluating the adequacy of test batteries. Although these may be important variables in your selection of a test, other considerations may enter into your decision.

First, the administration time of the test may influence your choice. The *Aphasia Language Performance Scales* require less than 30 minutes to administer, and the screening tests of the *Minnesota Test for the Differential Diagnosis of Aphasia, Examining for Aphasia*, and *Language Modalities Test of Aphasia* offer a quick means of determining the primary deficits of the patient. Conversely, if time is not a factor and a comprehensive assessment of abilities is required, then the *Boston Diagnostic Aphasia Examination*, which includes supplementary tests for nonlanguage skills and in-depth exploration of expressive and receptive psycholinguistic skills, or the Minnesota test, which contains more items than any other battery, may be your choice.

Second, if you wish to aid in localizing the site of the lesion, then you may choose the Boston test because the results allow the clinician to determine a syndrome of aphasia symptomatology consistent with a specific area of brain damage. Other aphasia tests do not purport to localize the site of the lesion.

Third, standardization of the test to aid in the interpretation of test results may influence your decision. The *Neurosensory Center Comprehensive Examination of Aphasia*, the Boston test, and the *Porch Index of Communicative Ability* provide for a comparison of the patient's results with scores from normal and/or aphasic patients. No standardization data are available for several other tests we have reviewed such as the *Language Modalities Test of Aphasia* or *Examining for Aphasia*.

Obviously, other criteria may dictate your choice of test, such as the degree of auditory or visual emphasis of the battery and the inclusion or noninclusion of gestural subtests. Ultimately, your decision on a test battery will depend on the weight of many if not all of these factors.

Clinical Example

A clinical example may serve to make the interpretations available for different test batteries more apparent. Ms. ET (for English teacher) suffered an occlusion of the left internal carotid artery with resultant aphasia and right hemiplegia following an automobile accident. Two months after discharge from the hospital, she was seen for a speech and language evaluation. Three tests were administered: the *Boston Diagnostic Aphasia Examination*, the *Minnesota Test for the Differential Diagnosis of Aphasia*, and the *Functional Communication Profile*. The Boston and Minnesota tests would typically not both be administered during the course of an evaluation, but we have done so for purposes of comparison. On the Boston test, the Rating Scale Profile of Speech Characteristics was most consistent with a classification of Broca's aphasia. Minnesota test results were as follows: 9 percent errors on the Auditory Comprehension tests, 19 percent errors on Visual and Reading tests, 34 percent errors on Speech and Language tests, 18 percent errors on Visuomotor and Writing tests, and 13 percent errors on Numerical Relations and Arithmetic Processes tests. On the Functional Communication Profile, ET received a 77 percent rating on Movement, 87 percent on Understanding, 57 percent on Speaking, 81 percent on Reading, and 79 percent on Other (telling time, handling money, calculation ability, and the like). The total rating was 77.2 percent. The results of these tests would be expected to reveal some consistencies, and they are evident: The patient demonstrates speaking skills that are more impaired than other aspects of communication.

The finding of a Boston profile consistent with Broca's aphasia suggests that the primary site of lesion is the foot of the third frontal gyrus and surrounding tissue of the left frontal lobe. Results of the Minnesota test are consistent with a Group III–type patient; that is, aphasia with sensorimotor involvement or aphasia with persisting dysfluency (Jenkins and others 1975). The prognosis for recovery for this type of patient is excellent. Finally, results of the Functional Communication Profile suggest that ET's residual communicative abilities in everyday situations are approximately 77 percent of premorbid functioning. Based on these test findings, the best description of the patient's condition would be mild aphasia with verbal apraxia due to damage to the left frontal lobe. The patient functions adequately in everyday communicative situations, and the prognosis for additional recovery is excellent.

Supplementary Tests for Aphasia Test Batteries

While aphasia batteries serve as reasonably comprehensive assessment instruments for aphasia, and to a more limited extent, apraxia and dysarthria, they are insufficient for differential diagnosis of other neurogenic disorders. Darley (1979) observed that a "curious failure in aphasia test development relates to the general absence of built-in ways of distinguishing aphasic patients from patients with language disorders that might be confused with aphasia" and that "test makers have not demonstrated that aphasia can be differentiated from syndromes of confusion, dementia, or psychosis through the use of their tests" (p. 192). Therefore, other tests must be used to allow the examiner to differentially diagnose disorders that may superficially resemble aphasia but are neurologically different. Moreover, other tests and assessment protocols may be needed to evaluate particular neurogenically based linguistic disorders in more detail. Several tests and test protocols will be reviewed, not to serve as an exhaustive listing, but to provide examples of tools available.

The *Token Test* (DeRenzi and Vignolo 1962) was developed to assess high-level auditory comprehension deficits associated with brain damage. The tokens used are large and small squares and circles—blue, green, red, white, and yellow in color. The patient's task is to manipulate the tokens in response to instructions of increasing length and complexity on the five levels of the test. Identification of the different sizes, colors, and shapes of the tokens is required before administration of the test items. Part I includes items such as "Touch the yellow circle"; Part II requires responses such as "Touch the little green circle"; Part III asks the patient, for example, to "Touch the blue square and the yellow square"; Part IV requires the patient to "Touch the little blue square and the little yellow circle"; and Part V asks the patient, for example, to "Put the green square beside the red circle." The test purports to test auditory comprehension, but it is apparent that it also places a considerable burden on the memory skills of the patient.

The *Revised Token Test* (RTT) (McNeil and Prescott 1978) is the result of a major effort to standardize the original test which had undergone numerous modifications. It was standardized in terms of

> (1) a pretest designed to assess the subject's basic knowledge of colors, shapes, and sizes, as well as balanced representation for each; (2) specific colors (shades), materials, and sizes of the tokens; (3) specific placement of the tokens (designed to reduce the visual search aspect of the subject's performance); (4) a consistent order of presentation for each subtest and commands within subtests; (5) a procedure for scoring each linguistic element, each stimulus, each subtest and an overall test mean; and (6) specific rules for applying each of the 15 categories in the evaluative system. (p. 20)

The RTT contains 10 subtests, and responses are scored by means of a 15-point multidimensional scoring system similar to the one used in the *Porch Index of Communicative Ability*. The test was standardized on 90 neurologically normal, 30 left-brain–damaged, and 30 right-brain–damaged adults. Percentiles for overall, subtest, and linguistic element means are provided for the three subject types of the standardization population. Test-retest reliability has been reported at 0.90, intrascorer reliability at 0.97, and interscorer reliability from 0.97 to 0.98. The test appears to be a sensitive instrument for detecting brain damage, and the severity levels obtained appear efficient at differentiating between auditory performance in normal, right-brain–damaged and left-brain–damaged patients.

Only one test that serves to aid in appraising neurogenic linguistic disorders has been reviewed. There are many others that may be used. For example, the *Peabody Picture Vocabulary Test–Revised* (Dunn and Dunn 1981), *Gates Primary Reading Test* (Gates 1958), *Benton Visual Retention Test* (Benton 1974), *Word Fluency Measure* (Borkowski, Benton, and Spreen 1967) and the *Coloured Progressive Matrices* (Raven 1963). The purpose in selecting these tests for administration is to expand the range of testing for particular deficits when they are insufficiently explored by aphasia batteries or to appraise areas of dysfunction not included on the batteries. The initial statement of this section must be reemphasized: There are no tests specifically constructed to investigate communicative deficits associated with dementia, confusion, or psychoses. Therefore, an array of measures may need to be chosen from existing diagnostic materials created for evaluating aphasia and related disorders.

Assessment of Right-Hemisphere Dysfunction

Right-brain damage produces a syndrome of deficits in visuoperceptual functioning, processing of intonation, facial recognition, body topography, and so on. The *Evaluation of Communication Problems in Right Hemisphere Dysfunction* (Burns, Halper, and Mogil 1985) is not a standardized test battery but rather a protocol for assessing behavioral functioning following nondominant hemisphere brain damage. Evaluation is begun by observing the patient in several environmental settings. Included are one-to-one interviews in quiet and distracting environments (i.e., in the patient's room and a hospital waiting area respectively) and a three-way interview with a family member or with another professional. The interviews are used to probe behavioral functions including attention, eye contact, awareness of illness, orientation to place, time, and person, facial expression, intonation, and topic maintenance. Each of these behaviors is rated on a 1-to-5 scale. For example, on "attention," a rating of 1 is assigned if the patient is not alerted by saying his name and if he does not react to simple commands or to a pointing task. A score of 3 is assigned if the patient reacts to auditory information part of the time but is easily distracted, has difficulty shifting tasks, or responds to stimuli without fully assessing aspects of the situation. A rating of 5 is given to a fully responsive patient. The ratings for each of the nine categories are totaled (maximum score = 45) to provide a severity index for each of the three observational settings. Severity ratings range from 9 to 15 for severe (severe deficits in attention, orientation, and communicative interaction) to 40 to 45 for minimal impairment to normal (patient communicates in various contexts but may show subtle integrative skill deficits).

Recommended audiologic assessments include evaluation of hearing acuity as well as administration of tasks of auditory discrimination, recognition, and memory, which may reflect damage to higher auditory association and processing centers. Visuoperceptual testing is suggested to determine the possible presence of left hemianopia, visual neglect, visuospatial deficits, visuomotor disturbances, spatial orientation, memory problems, and visual scanning and tracking problems. Clinical assessment procedures and recommended standardized tests (for example, *Motor-Free Visual Perception Test*) are included for each aspect of the visuoperceptual testing. Evaluation of visual scanning and tracking is completed using a series of four tasks that assess scanning for widely and closely spaced letters and words. Both the number of errors and the time required to complete each of the four tasks are reported.

It is suggested that each patient receives a complete language assessment utilizing an aphasia battery. Additional testing is carried out to assess more thoroughly individual skills in areas such as reading and writing. A specific writing task has been developed as part of the protocol to elicit the types of problems typical of this population of patients. Included are copying a sentence that includes all letters of the alphabet, spelling 10 words to dictation, and writing a narrative of 100 words. Performance on the tasks is rated on a series of eleven 1-to-5 scales, which address visuospatial disorganization, omission of letters, incomplete sentences, run-on sentences, and so on. For example, on Visuospatial Disorganization (superimposed letters and lines diagonally written), a score of 1 is given if it is always present, 3 if it is present 50 percent of the time, and 5 if it is adequate. Obviously, scores of 2 and 4 would be assigned if it is present 25 percent and 75 percent of the time. The total possible score is 55 (11 ratings on 5-point scale).

A *Scale of Pragmatic Communication Skills* is included in the battery in order to assess pragmatic aspects of oral expression, which frequently are included in the syndrome of deficits associated with right-hemisphere lesions. The scale is divided into four sections with rated measures of nonverbal communication behaviors (intonation, facial expression, eye contact, gestures, and proxemics), conversational skills (initiation, turn-taking, verbosity), use of linguistic context (topic maintenance, presupposition, referencing skills), and organization of a narrative. The ratings are based on a dialogue between the clinician and the patient and on a narrative such as retelling a story. The total score is the sum of the ratings (maximum score = 60).

Also recommended as parts of the assessment are evaluation of memory and integrative skills, and several measures for these behaviors are noted (e.g., *Token Test, Detroit Tests of Learning Aptitude*). The *Metaphorical Language Test* is included as part of the testing of integrative skills. It is composed of 10 idiomatic expressions read aloud to or by the patient and which the patient is asked to explain. The responses are scored as incorrect, literal interpretations, repetition of phrase, personal interpretation, partially correct, perseverative response, or normal abstract interpretation. The total possible score is 10. Finally, evaluation of academic skills is recommended. Inclusion of academic tasks such as mathematics provides additional information about deficits associated with the disorder and may be important in planning treatment.

Simmons (1986) reviewed the Rehabilitation Institute of Chicago Evaluation (RICE) and concluded that it had several important shortcomings, including a lack of standardization, insufficient administration and rating instructions, and a lack of harmony between the test format and the authors' theoretical model. She also noted that it did not contain information on administration time, target population, or interpretation of test results. The *Mini Inventory of Right Brain Injury* (Pimental and Kingsbury 1989) attempts to address some of these issues in a single test instrument. The Mini Inventory is intended to identify adults with deficits secondary to right-hemisphere brain damage, to determine the areas of dysfunction and severity of involvement, and to identify strengths and weaknesses to guide treatment planning.

The Mini Inventory is divided into 10 subsections included within the dimensions of visual processing, language processing, emotion and affective processing, and general behavior and psychic integrity. Included in visual processing are visual scanning, integrity of diagnosis (e.g., finger recognition and identification of objects), integrity of body image (visual neglect language and higher level language skills are assessed in the language-processing section). Affect is evaluated in the emotion and affect-processing section and general behavior is assessed in the final section. Several of the subsections include only one or two items. Instructions for item administration are included in the test booklet. Scoring is either dichotomous or quantitative based on the level of impairment (severe = 0, moderate = 1, etc.). Raw scores are calculated for the subsection, for right–left differentiation computed from performance on 10 selected items from subsections, and for the entire test. The right–left differentiation items were chosen for their ability to distinguish left-brain from right-brain damage. Percentages are determined for each subsection and the entire test by dividing the score in each section or the entire test by the number of items. An overall severity rating can be determined from the total score. The seven-step severity continuum extends from profound (0–7 points) to normal (38–43 points). Scores on the left–right differentiation items below 9 are interpreted as a strong probability of right-hemisphere brain damage.

The Mini Inventory was standardized on 30 subject with right-hemisphere brain damage, 30 matched normal subjects, and 13 subjects with left-brain damage.

Interrater reliability for four subjects appeared fair to good ($r = 0.65$ to 0.87). Content validity appears to be sufficient based on item selection. However, criterion validity has not been established from correlations with similar measures or by the ability to predict future performance.

The Mini Inventory is perhaps best viewed as a screening instrument to estimate the presence and severity of right-hemisphere–based lesion effects. Additional standardization with a large number of subjects is required to more fully validate the measure for assessment purposes and to provide additional information on reliability.

We have reviewed only two instruments for assessing right-hemisphere functioning. Other protocols are available (Adamovich and Brooks, 1981; Ross 1986) that may aid in this process. Assessment instruments for right-hemisphere lesions offer an expanded view of communicative functioning and brain damage because they deal with communication domain processes such as affective language, humor, and absurdities that may be of benefit to the assessment of aphasia as well.

Assessment in Brain Trauma

Analogous protocols and assessment are evolving for brain trauma (e.g. Yivisaker and Szekeres 1986) and for dementia (Bayles and Kaszniak 1987; Bayles et al. 1989). Brain trauma produces cognitive and language disturbances that include deficits in memory, visual- and auditory-processing problems, disordered expressive language, and the inability to recall words. Assessment instruments have been developed to explore cognitive and communication deficits associated with traumatic lesions to the brain. The *Brief Test of Head Injury* (Helm-Estabrooks and Hotz 1990) is a 50-item test modeled after the *Boston Assessment of Severe Aphasia*. It is designed to assess orientation and attention, following commands, linguistic organization, reading comprehension, naming, memory and visual-spatial skills. Items are scored on the basis of the type of response (linguistic, gestural) and communicative quality of the response. Perseverative responses also are noted. Scores are computed for each of the seven areas of assessment by determining the number of fully communicative responses, whether linguistic or gestural. The scores from each cluster then can be summed to provide a total score for the test.

The *Brief Test of Head Injury* is in the process of standardization. Preliminary field testing with incomplete or unrevised forms of the test administered to 53 patients with brain trauma revealed adequate internal consistency (0.67 to 0.91) and test-retest reliability (0.52 to 0.81). The test is perhaps best viewed as a general measure of cognitive and language ability in patients with brain trauma. Interpretation of results should be viewed cautiously given the preliminary nature of the standardization.

The *Scales of Cognitive Ability for Traumatic Brain Injury* (SCATBI) (Adamovich and Henderson 1992) is a somewhat more ambitious measure. The test is divided into five scales, including perception and discrimination, orientation, organization, recall, and reasoning. Scores for each scale are summed and can be converted to standard scores or percentiles. Composite scores can be determined from selected combinations of scales as well as for the test in its entirety. The total composite score is the best estimate of overall functioning; the score also can be used to assign the patient's performance to a severity range.

The SCATBI has been standardized on a sample of 244 head-injured patients and 78 non–brain-injured subjects from 15 to 88 years of age. The sample was composed of twice as many males as females. Percentile ranks and standard scores are provided for each of the five scales, lower functioning composite (perception/discrimination, orientation, organization), higher functioning composite (recall, reasoning), and the total score. Test-retest reliability for 33 brain-injured patients retested within eight months ranged from 0.69 (organization) to 0.90 (recall). Concurrent validity is reflected in the agreement of test findings with ratings on the *Rancho Los Amigos Levels of Cognitive Functioning* (Malkmus et al. 1980).

We have briefly reviewed these two measures because they serve to exemplify the expansion of assessment by speech-language pathologists into the domain of cognitive operations in adults with brain trauma. The point to be made is that an understanding of language deficits cannot be obtained or differential diagnosis and treatment planning completed unless there is a firm understanding of the effects of cognitive deficits on language performance.

PROCEDURES FOR ASSESSING NEUROMOTOR DISORDERS

A number of assessment devices have been applied to the evaluation of acquired neuromotor disorders. In general, they are outgrowths of pragmatic clinical procedures frequently included with the neurological examination. We review several of these measures as well as structured test procedures for apraxia, dysarthria, and dysphagia.

Apraxia

DeRenzi, Pieczuro, and Vignolo (1966) developed procedures to evaluate oral and limb apraxia. The test included 10 oral and 10 limb items in which subjects were asked to perform gestures following verbal command and, if necessary, on imitation. Oral gestures included the following: (1) Stick out your tongue, (2) whistle, (3) yawn, (4) try to touch the tip of your nose with your tongue, (5) give a "Bronx cheer" or "raspberry," (6) show how you would kiss someone, (7) show how your teeth chatter when you are cold, (8) click your tongue, imitating the sound of a horse galloping, (9) puff or blow, and (10) clear your throat. Limb gestures included the following: (1) Make the sign of the cross, (2) salute, (3) wave goodbye, (4) threaten somebody with your hand, (5) show that you are hungry, (6) thumb your nose, (7) snap your fingers, (8) make the sign of the horns to designate a cuckold, (9) indicate that someone is crazy, and (10) make the letter O with your fingers. Five categories of response were determined, and each response was scored as 2 (correct), 1 (accurate performance preceded by pause or acceptable performance with defective movement), or 0 (important part of gesture absent, perseveration of preceding item, incorrect oral performance, no response). Determination of the presence and severity of oral and limb apraxia was based on the performance of 40 control subjects, 40 patients with lesions of the right hemisphere, and 134 patients with lesions of the left hemisphere. None of the control or right-brain–damaged subjects received a score of less than 16 on either the oral or the limb tests. Therefore, 16 was used as the cutoff point; that is, patients with scores of 15 or less were classified as apraxic. The cutoff score for separating mild and severe involvement was set at 11.

Darley, Aronson, and Brown (1975) modified the oral apraxia portion of the test by increasing the number of items to 20 and by providing 11 categories for grading the responses. They also presented 18 test words and phrases useful for eliciting verbal apraxic errors, such as "gingerbread," "statistical analysis," "zip-zipper-zippering," and "The shipwreck washed up on the shore." Rosenbek and Wertz (1976) developed a battery of apraxia measures that included verbal, oral, and limb items. The verbal portion requires the patient to prolong vowels, imitate syllable sequences, and produce words and phrases. Responses are transcribed, scored, and analyzed to determine the type and frequency of phonemic and prosodic errors. The oral apraxia section is identical to the 20 items of the Darley and others test, and the limb apraxia test is a modification of the DeRenzi and others test. The oral and limb apraxia responses are graded on an 11-point system similar to that of Darley and others.

DiSimoni (1989) has developed a test instrument, the *Comprehensive Apraxia Test*, that focuses on oral-verbal apractic deficits. Included are subtests that include oral postures and movements, vowels in isolation, alternate motion rates, production of syllables and production of utterances of increasing length, and a nonsense disyllable contextual interference subtest used to assess the effects of context on errors.

We have taken the time to present these procedures for evaluating apraxia to demonstrate the evolution of test batteries to fulfill the need for instruments to measure specific neuromotor deficits associated with left-hemisphere brain damage. With standardization, the batteries may prove to be excellent tools in the differential diagnosis of apractic disorders.

Dysarthria

Individuals with dysarthria require careful examination of the speech production apparatus to determine the extent, type, and severity of neuromuscular impairment. Rosenbek and Wertz (1976) integrated a series of examinations for systematically evaluating cranial nerve function in dysarthria, utilizing speech and nonspeech tasks. Recently, formalized assessment of various aspects of dysarthria have been devised. We review two of these procedures.

The *Frenchay Dysarthria Assessment* (Enderby 1983) was developed as a test to "categorically diagnose dysarthria" (p. 6). The battery contains eight sections with subtests administered according to specific instructions. Sections included are reflex (cough, swallow), respiration, lips, jaw, palate, laryngeal, tongue, and intelligibility (words and sentences). With the exception of the intelligibility tasks, the subtests are not unlike elements of an oral-peripheral examination. For example, Section 3 (Lips) includes five tasks: (1) observing the position of the lips at rest, (2) lip retraction, (3) degree of lip seal that can be attained, (4) alternating lip rounding and retraction, and (5) lip movement during speech. Each task is rated on a five-point (a to e) scale from, for example, "no abnormality" to "severe asymmetry or bilaterally severely affected, little change in position" in observing the lips at rest.

Responses to subtests are recorded on a form with a nine-point bar graph (vertical axis) that lists the individual tasks of each section (horizontal axis). The length of the bar graph filled in is used to reflect the relative degree of difficulty (severity) demonstrated by the patient in completing the task. It should be noted that the clinician is required to translate an a-to-e rating system into the nine-point severity indices. The result is a profile similar to the *Functional Communication Profile*, which shows the pattern of impairment. The test also includes sections for noting factors that may influence overall speech performance (hearing, sight, teeth, language, mood, and posture), for determining speech rate, and for estimating two-point discrimination (sensation) on the upper lip and tongue tip.

The test has been developed for use in categorically diagnosing dysarthria. This interpretation is based on sample profiles provided for five types of dysarthria: (1) upper-motor neuron lesion, (2) mixed upper- and lower-motor neuron lesions, (3) extrapyramidal disorders, (4) cerebellar dysfunction, and (5) lower-motor neuron lesion. The profiles were developed from performance of 85 patients on the assessment. Discriminant function analysis performed on the results found correct assignment in more than 90 percent of the cases tested. There are two major problems with the profiles provided. First, the number of categories is insufficient. For example, extrapyramidal disorders include both hypokinetic and hyperkinetic forms of dysarthria, which have been shown to have distinctive characteristics (Darley, Aronson, and Brown 1969). Second, there are an insufficient number of cases used to develop the profiles. For flaccid dysarthria, we are informed that 10 cases were included; 10 cases are insufficient for establishing a normative reference. The data are further weakened by a lack of subject description. No information is provided about age, and there is only a minimal amount of information concerning etiology.

The validity of the assessment, according to Enderby, is shown by the successful discriminant function analysis and by the successful diagnosis of 22 patients with unspecified neurological lesions from assessment profiles. Interjudge reliability quotients determined from assessments of 113 dysarthric subjects by eight judges varied from 0.79 to 0.92.

The *Frenchay Dysarthria Assessment* is best viewed as an attempt to rate the degree of impairment of the speech-production apparatus as a means of establishing profiles for differential diagnosis. This is certainly a worthwhile endeavor; clinicians consistently use this procedure to make diagnostic decisions about the type of dysarthria demonstrated by the patient. The problem with the *Frenchay Dysarthria Assessment* is the meager database provided to aid the clinician in this process.

Assessment of Intelligibility of Dysarthric Speech

Reduced speech intelligibility is a characteristic of dysarthria regardless of etiology. *Assessment of Intelligibility of Dysarthric Speech* (Yorkston and Beukelman 1981) was developed to measure the intelligibility and speaking rate of individuals with dysarthria. Yorkston and Beukelman note that

> measures of speech intelligibility and speaking rate serve as an index of dysarthric severity, thus enabling the clinician or researcher to (1) rank order different dysarthric speakers; (2) compare performance of a single dysarthric speaker to normal performance; and (3) monitor changing performance over time. (p. 2)

The assessment provides six types of information. Single-word intelligibility can be determined based on the percent of words correctly transcribed or selected by multiple choice from a group of possible options. Sentence intelligibility is based on the percent of words correctly transcribed. Additional sentence-level information includes the speaking rate in words per minute; rate of intelligible speech based on number of intelligible words per minute; and communication efficiency, which is defined as the rate of intelligible speech produced by a dysarthric patient compared to normal speakers.

For the single-word task, the speaker is audio recorded as she produces (preferably by reading) a series of 50 single words generated by randomly selecting one word from a list of 12 similar sounding words for each of 50 items. A listener (not the administrator of the assessment), familiar with the total word pool but not with the 50 words selected for the assessment, judges the sample by choosing the word she thinks has been produced from a list of 12 similar words or by transcribing the word. Responses are scored by the examiner and are reported as percent correct.

Stimuli for the sentence task are two sentences randomly selected at each length from 5 to 15 words (220 words) from a list of 100 sentences provided. The 22 sentences chosen are read by the patient and are audio recorded following presentation by the examiner. The sentences are transcribed by a judge and are then returned to the examiner for scoring. The examiner scores the total number of words correctly transcribed and records the total speaking time. Four types of information may be derived from the data obtained. *Intelligibility*, as with the single-word task, is based on the number of words correctly transcribed divided by the total number of words (on this task words = 220). The total words produced divided by the time required to produce the sentences yields the *speaking rate* in words per minute. *Rate of intelligible speech* is based on the total number of correctly transcribed words divided by the time required to produce the sentences. *Communication efficiency* is defined as the rate of intelligible speech (intelligible words per minute) divided by the mean rate of intelligible speech produced by normal speakers (190 intelligible words per minute).

The number of judges used is dependent on the purposes of testing. If the purpose is to measure change in intelligibility over time, one judge may be sufficient. If the purpose is to determine functional intelligibility level or to compare speakers, more judges are required. Intrajudge and interjudge reliability of word and sentence intelligibility reliability are high and vary from 0.87 to 0.99 (Yorkston and Beukelman 1980).

Several points need to be made about the assessment. The purpose of the test is not to categorize patients by type of dysarthria; rather, results are used to measure changes in intelligibility over time, to compare and to rank dysarthric speakers in severity, and to compare dysarthric speakers to normal speakers on the basis of intelligibility. Determination of intelligibility is one component of the evaluation. Additional protocols are required, for example, to determine which structures are impaired and the effects of these deficits on different aspects of the speech-production process (respiration, phonation, articulation). Strengths of the assessment are the precision and the reliability with which intelligibility can be measured. A negative feature is the need for a judge in addition to the examiner to complete the appraisal process.

Dysphagia

Dysphagia is disordered deglutition or swallowing that results from neurological and neuromuscular diseases, injuries to the head and neck, cancer, and so forth. Approximately 80 percent of the cases are due to neurological disorders (Erlichman 1989). The disorder is not homogeneous and may involve one or more aspects of swallowing, including oral, pharyngeal, and/or esophageal phases of the process.

Within the last 10 years, rehabilitation of dysphagia increasingly has become the role of speech-language pathologists (Asha, 1990). However, evaluational procedures have not been standardized in the assessment and description of patients with swallowing deficits. What has evolved instead is the development of appraisal protocols that group oral-peripheral examination of the patient with results from videofluoroscopic evaluation and ratings of feeding ability.

Perhaps one of the earliest dysphagia assessment protocols was proposed by Larsen (1972). He described an evaluational process for swallowing that included a history (patient complaint, eating habits, food preferred, incidence of choking); examination of the speech mechanism (muscle strength and structural range of motion); evaluation of swallowing (volitional and reflexive); determination of the integrity of taste sensation (sweet, sour, salty); and ability of the patient to masticate and swallow various nutritional substances (liquids, solids, dry, moist). Videofluoroscopy was not a routine evaluational procedure and was not included in the protocol although standardized radiographic procedures are in the process of development (Jones and Donner 1988).

Protocols for deglutition deficits in patients with structural or neurological disorders have been provided by Logemann (1983) and Miller (1984), among others. We review two of these appraisal formats as examples of efforts to capitalize on information from several sets of procedures.

The *BELZ Dysphagia Scale* (Longstreth 1986) takes into consideration a variety of factors that may be used to quantify dysphagia. The Scale is composed of 12 categories on which the patient is rated from 0–3 with 3 reflecting normal performance. The rating categories include a clinical swallowing evaluation, otolaryngology examination, cognition/communication status, physical status, pulmonary function, chest X-ray, videofluoroscopic evaluation of swallowing physiology, tracheostomy tube status, diet consistency, tube feeding, respiratory tract treatments, and gastrointestinal function. Similarly, the *Fleming Index of Dysphagia* (FID) (Fleming and Waver 1987) is a computerized index developed for the purpose of "evaluating the potentially dysphagic patient and for identifying specific deglutition problems needing timely management" (p. 206). The first five items contain demographic information which is coded for patient privacy. Next, 18 items note commonly occurring problems that may result in or be the result of dysphagia. For example, item 7 notes radiographic demonstration of aspiration pneumonia. Each of the items is assigned an impact score and these scores are combined with severity ratings and problem codes to determine the severity of dysphagia, the urgency of need for treatment, and suggestions for patient management. Information from examination, patient interview, and chart review is relied upon for assigning the severity and problem code. Severity is rated on a three-point scale from (1) possible chronic problem or (2) important problem to (3) most critical, needs immediate attention. Multiple problem codes are used, such as (1) problem present, new, and documented and (5) problem not present.

Speech-language pathologists take a leading role in the evaluation of dysphagia. They must rely, however, on multiple sources of appraisal data to determine if a problem exists and the severity of the disorder. Knowledge of normal swallowing and dysphagia and reliance on observation and clinical judgement are critical elements in this process.

CLINICAL PROCEDURES

Differential diagnosis of communicative disorders due to neurological deficits may be difficult due to the overlap of communicative deficits between groups of patients. The acquisition of biographical and medical information in addition to the behavioral testing may be paramount in establishing the diagnosis. A brief procedural guide to the acquisition of the necessary information is provided to facilitate this process.

The History.   In the chapter on case history, we discussed some aspects of information gathering. For patients who have suffered brain damage, a great deal of information can be gleaned from the patient's medical records to supplement information from the standard interview, will provide information on education level, occupation, family history, and so forth. For patients still in the hospital, information from the medical chart will include reports of the medical history, the results of the medical and neurological examination, results of laboratory tests, and nurses' and doctors' notes. The medical history should be reviewed carefully for information regarding earlier incidences of brain damage, periods of confusion or disorientation, and complicating conditions, such as metabolic diseases, cardiac disease, or seizures.

The results of the neurological examination will provide information on the site, size, and nature of the lesion and possible progression of the disorder. Specifically, the neurological examination performed by the physician includes evaluation of mental state, cranial nerves, motor and reflex systems, the cerebellar apparatus, sensory modalities, and the autonomic nervous system. Evaluation of mental state will include assessment of intellectual facility and fund of knowledge; orientation for time, place, and person; memory; attention span; understanding of simple and complex commands; general information; calculation; abstract thinking; and judgment. The cranial nerves are assessed by testing the sensory and motor functions of the areas of the body that they subserve. For example, the integrity of the facial nerve is assessed by evaluating facial movement and the reaction of the face to sensory stimulation such as a pinprick.

Examination of the motor systems will provide information on muscle power, bulk and tone, active and passive movements, involuntary movements, cerebellar functioning, and status of the reflexes. Evaluation of sensory function includes investigation of touch, pain, heat, cold, position, vibration, and a variety of discriminatory senses. An attempt is made to determine what elements of sensation are affected, the degree of involvement, and the areas of sensory impairment or loss. The history may also contain information on past cerebrovascular accidents or disease, associated problems, and medications that may affect behavior. The nurses' notes may offer information on the alertness of the patient; his orientation to time, place, and person; and his adjustment to the problem. The physicians' orders should provide information on the current status of the patient and the treatment program that has been proposed and is being carried out.

Review of all the case history and medical information should provide you with knowledge of the deficits exhibited by the patient, his adjustment to the problem, and the proposed course of treatment and should be reviewed carefully before the patient is seen. The amount and type of information already available may be helpful in your determination of the type of aphasia instrument and related evaluations you wish to make.

Evaluation of the Patient.   Before administering a test battery, it is always helpful to observe the patient in an informal situation. In a hospital, you may visit the patient in his room; in a speech and hearing center, you may visit with him before the formal evaluation begins. This time should be used to assess informally the patient's communicative functioning; to note any significant sensory or motor impairment (visual deficits, hearing loss, hemiplegia); and to determine how closely the patient's condition matches with the available medical information. Determination of sensory and motor problems is crucial because they may suggest ways in which the standard test procedures will need to be modified in the assessment of the patient.

In the formal examination of the patient, the test selected will depend on the type of problems exhibited, the severity of the problems, and complicating conditions, such as sensory or motor impairment. Choose tests and procedures that fulfill your needs (see Table 10–1).

TABLE 10–1   Summary of aphasia test batteries

Test	Description	Norms	Interpretation
Examining for Aphasia (Eisenson 1954)	Subtests dichotomized into primarily receptive and primarily expressive portions. Within each section, subtests divided into those designed to test for subsymbolic or low symbolic function (agnosias, apraxias) and those designed to evaluate high symbolic function (aphasias).	None	Rating of presence and severity of aphasia, apraxia, and agnosia as revealed by subtest performance
Language Modalities Test for Aphasia (Wepman and Jones 1961)	Eleven screening items and two sets of 23 items presented on filmstrips 120 frames in length	Factor analysis of the responses of 168 aphasic patients	Results used to assign patient to categories based upon predominant characteristics of the disorder;

(continued)

TABLE 10–1 Summary of aphasia test batteries (continued)

Test	Description	Norms	Interpretation
	designed to assess auditory compre-hension, verbal expres-sion, reading and writing skills, plus calculation		pragmatic, semantic, syntactic, jargon or global aphasia, and/or apraxia and/or agnosia
Minnesota Test for the Differential Diagnosis of Aphasia (Schuell 1965)	Fifty-seven subtests divided into five major sections: auditory disturbances, visual and reading disturbances, speech and language disturbances, visuo-motor and writing disturbances, disturbances of numerical relations and arithmetic processes. Also includes clinical and severity rating scales and screening version.	Means, standard, deviations, median scores, percentages of 157 subjects making errors on each subtest	Test-score summarization and lists of signs and most discriminating tests used to assign patient to one of five major and two minor prognostic categories based on pattern of impairment
Functional Communi-cation Profile (Sarno 1969)	Forty-five integrated behaviors divided into movement, speaking, understanding, reading, and miscellaneous sections	None. However, sample profiles presented	Ratings converted to percentages for each section and test as a whole. Percentage purported to reflect residual communicative abilities compared to premorbid functioning.
Neurosensory Center Comprehensive Examination of Aphasia (Spreen and Benton 1969)	Twenty tests of lan-guage production and comprehension, reten-tion of verbal informa-tion, reading, writing. Four tests of visual and tactile function	Percentiles for each subtest from perform-ance of neurologically normal and aphasic subjects. Number of subjects unspeci-fied	Some subtests correct-ed for age and educa-tion. Construction of subtest performance profile to compare patient performance to that of normal and aphasic standard-ization populations.
Porch Index of Communicative Ability (Porch 1967, 1971)	Four verbal, 2 auditory, 2 reading, 2 gestural, 2 visual matching subtests, and 6 graphic subtests with 10 items per subtest.	Percentiles for the test as a whole, for each subtest, and for combinations of tests by modality for 280 left-hemisphere brain-damaged and 100 bilaterally brain-damaged subjects.	Overall and gestural, verbal and graphic modality means compared to standard-ization population. Subtest scores plotted as a function of subtest difficulty .Also, recovery curves determined

(continued)

TABLE 10–1   Summary of aphasia test batteries (continued)

Test	Description	Norms	Interpretation
		Also, percentiles for 9 high, 9 low and overall scores. Examples of 5 basic performance patterns provided.	by computation of 9 high, 9 low, and overall test means.
Boston Diagnostic Aphasia Examination (Goodglass and Kaplan 1972, 1983)	Twenty-three subtests used to assess auditory comprehension, oral expression, reading, writing. Ratings of conversational and expository speech on 6 parameters and rating of severity. Also includes 13 language and 14 nonlanguage tests.	Z-score profiles based on the range, mean, and standard deviation of scores from 207 aphasic subjects. Intercorrelation analyses, factor analyses, and reliability coefficients among subtests also provided. Most recent revisions included percentiles.	Overall severity on a 6-point scale, speech characteristics rating on 7 factors, and Z-score profiles used to assign patient to classical aphasic syndromes: Broca's aphasia, Wernicke's aphasia, anomic aphasia, conduction aphasia, transcortical sensory aphasia, transcortical motor aphasia, alexia with a graphia.
Aphasia Language Performance Scales (Keenan and Brassel 1975)	Four scales: listening talking, reading, writing. Each comprised of 10 items.	None	Arbitrary assignments of scores from scales to degree of language impairment
Communicative Abilities in Daily Living (Holland 1980)	Sixty-eight items encompassed within simulated, real-world activities	Means and standard deviations of scores from 130 neurologically normal and 130 aphasic subjects as a function of age, sex, institutionalization, and type of aphasia	Total score is indication of communicative abilities during the course of everyday activities.
Western Aphasia Battery (Kertesz 1982)	Subtests for spontaneous speech, auditory verbal comprehension, repetition, naming, reading, writing, apraxia, and constructional, visuospatial, and calculation tasks plus *Raven Progressive Matrices*	Correlations from 20 subjects on old and new versions of the test for each of the subtests.	Determination of aphasia quotient (AQ) based on performance on oral language subtest performance; cortical quotient (CQ) based on nonverbal subtest scores. Subscore ranges on fluency, comprehension, repetition, and naming subtests used to assign patient to diagnostic

(continued)

TABLE 10–1   Summary of aphasia test batteries (continued)

Test	Description	Norms	Interpretation
			category, including global, Broca's, isolation, transcortical motor, Wernicke's, transcortical sensory, conduction, and anomic classifications.
Boston Assessment of Severe Aphasia (Helm-Estabrooks et al. 1989)	Sixty-one items divided into 15 sections; items range from social greetings and simple conversation to comprehension of numbers, symbols, object naming, and recognition of emotional words, phrases and symbols	Percentile and standard scores based on performance of 111 subjects with severe aphasia (47 with global aphasia)	Item group (cluster) score and total score can be converted to standard scores and percentile ranks

SUMMARY

A large variety of communicative disorders result from damage to the brain after speech and language have been acquired. The problems demonstrated by the patient depend on the site and extent of the brain damage. A number of formal and informal tests to measure these disorders are available, but they vary significantly in the way they view the problem and the means they use to assess deficits. The tests selected for assessing these disorders depend on the type of problem, its severity, and your purposes in testing.

REFERENCES

ADAMOVICH, B., AND R. BROOKS, A diagnostic protocol to assess the communication deficits in patients with right hemisphere damage. In *Clinical Aphasiology Conference Proceedings*, ed. R. H. Brookshire (pp. 244–253). Minneapolis: BRK Publishers (1981).

ADAMOVICH, B., AND J. HENDERSON, *Scales of Cognitive Ability for Traumatic Brain Injury*. Chicago: Riverside Publishing Company (1992).

AMERICAN SPEECH-LANGUAGE-HEARING ASSOCIATION, Skills needed by speech-language pathologists providing services to dysphagic patients/clients. *Asha*, 32 (Suppl. 2), 7–12 (1990).

APPELL, J., A KERTESZ, AND M. FISMAN. A study of language functioning in Alzheimer patients. *Brain Lang.*, 17, 73–91 (1982).

BASILI, A., AND OTHERS, The comparisons between the *Aphasia Language Performance Scales* and two established tests of aphasic impairment. Paper presented at the American Speech and Hearing Association Convention, Las Vegas, Nevada (1974).

BAYLES, K., Language function in senile dementia. *Brain Lang.*, 16, 265–280 (1982).

BAYLES, K., D. BOONE, C. TOMOEDA, AND T. SLAUSON, Differentiating Alzheimer's patients from the normal elderly and stroke patients with aphasia. *J. Speech Hearing Dis.* 54, 74–97 (1989).

BAYLES, K., AND A. KASZNIAK, *Communication and Cognition in Normal Aging and Dementia*. San Diego: College-Hill Press (1987).

BENTON, A., *Benton Revised Visual Retention Test*. New York: Psychological Corporation (1974).

BORKOWSKI, J., A. BENTON, AND O. SPREEN, Word fluency and brain damage. *Neuropsychologia*, 5, 135–140 (1967).

BROOKSHIRE, R. H., *An Introduction to Aphasia*, 2nd ed. Minneapolis: BRK Publishers (1978).

BURNS, M., A. HALPER, AND S. MOGIL, *Clinical Management of Right-Hemisphere Dysfunction*. Rockville, Md.: Aspen Systems Corporation (1985).

DARLEY, F. L., *Diagnosis and Appraisal of Communication Disorders*. Englewood Cliffs, N.J.: Prentice Hall (1964).

DARLEY, F., *Evaluation of Appraisal Techniques in Speech and Language Pathology*. Reading, Mass.: Addison-Wesley (1979).

DARLEY, F., A. ARONSON, AND J. BROWN, Differential diagnostic patterns of dysarthria. *J. Speech Hearing Res.*, 12, 246–269 (1969).

DARLEY, F., A. ARONSON, AND J. BROWN, *Motor Speech Disorders*. Philadelphia: W. B. Saunders (1975).

DeRENZI, E., AND L. VIGNOLO, The Token Test: A sensitive test to detect receptive disturbances in aphasics. *Brain*, 85, 655–678 (1962).

DeRENZI, E., A. PIECZURO, AND L. VIGNOLO, Oral apraxia and aphasia. *Cortex*, 2, 50–73 (1966).

DiSIMONI, F., *Apraxia of Speech: Theoretical and Practical Considerations*. Dalton, Penn.: Praxis House Publishers (1989).

DUFFY, J., AND OTHERS, Performance of normal (nonbrain-injured) adults on the Porch Index of Communicative Ability. In *Clinical Aphasiology: Conference Proceedings 1976*, ed. R. Brookshire. Minneapolis: BRK Publishers (1976).

DUNN, L. M., AND L. M. DUNN, *Peabody Picture Vocabulary Test–Revised*. Circle Pines, Minn.: American Guidance Service (1981).

EISENSON, J., *Examining for Aphasia*. New York: Psychological Corporation (1954).

ENDERBY, P., *Frenchay Dysarthria Assessment*. San Diego: College-Hill Press (1983).

ERLICHMAN, M., Role of speech language pathologists in the management of dysphagia. *Health Technology Assessment Reports (Report No. 1)*. Rockville, Md.: National Center for Health Services Research and Health Care Technology Assessment, U.S. Department of Health and Human Services (1989).

FLEMING, S., AND A. WAVER, Index of dysphagia: A tool for identifying deglutation problems. *Dysphagia*, 1, 206–208 (1987).

GATES, A., *Gates Advanced Primary Reading Test*. New York: Columbia University, Teachers College Press (1958).

GATES A., AND J. BRADSHAW, The role of the cerebral hemispheres in music. *Brain Lang.*, 4, 403–431 (1977).

GOODGLASS, H., AND E. KAPLAN, *The Assessment of Aphasia and Related Disorders*. Philadelphia: Lea & Febiger (1972, 1983).

GREENBERG, F., Measurements of improvement in completed stroke. *Proceedings of Conference on Stroke Predictors*. Chicago, Illinois (1969).

HAGEN, C., Language disorders in head trauma. In *Language Disorders in Adults*, ed. A. Holland. San Diego: College-Hill Press (1984).

HELM-ESTABROOKS, N., AND G. HOTZ, *Brief Test of Head Injury*. San Antonio: Special Press, Inc. (1990).

HELM-ESTABROOKS, N., G. RAMSBERGER, A. MORGAN, AND M. NICHOLAS, *Boston Assessment of Severe Aphasia*. Chicago: Riverside Publishing Company (1989).

HOLLAND, A., Estimates of Aphasic Patients' Communicative Performance in Daily Life. NINCDS 75-05 (NOI-NS-5-2317) (1979).

HOLLAND, A., *Communicative Abilities in Daily Life*. Baltimore: University Park Press (1980).

HOLLAND, A., When is aphasia aphasia? The problem of closed-head injury. In *Clinical Aphasiology Proceedings*, ed. R. Brookshire. Minneapolis: BRK Publishers (1982).

JENKINS, J., AND OTHERS, *Schuell's Aphasia in Adults*. New York: Harper & Row (1975).

JONES, B., AND M. DONNER, Examination of the patient with dysphagia. *Radiology*, 167, 319–326 (1986).

JONES, L., AND J. WEPMAN, Dimensions of language performance in aphasia. *J. Speech Hearing Res.*, 4, 220–232 (1961).

JOYNT, R., AND M. GOLDSTEIN, Minor cerebral hemisphere. In *Advances in Neurology, Vol. 7*, ed. W. Friedlander. New York: Raven Press (1975).

KEENAN, J., AND E. BRASSEL, Development of a scale of aphasic speech impairment. Paper presented at the American Speech and Hearing Association Convention, Las Vegas, Nevada (1974).

KEENAN, J., AND E. BRASSEL, *Aphasia Language Performance Scales*. Murfreesboro, Tenn.: Pinnacle Press (1975).

KENT, R., AND J. ROSENBEK, Acoustic patterns of apraxia of speech. *J. Speech Hearing Res.*, 26, 231–249 (1983).

KERTESZ, A., *Aphasia and Associated Disorders: Taxonomy, Localization, and Recovery*. New York: Grune & Stratton (1979).

KERTESZ, A., *The Western Aphasia Battery*. New York: Grune & Stratton (1982).

KERTESZ, A., AND E. POOLE, The aphasia quotient: The taxonomic approach to the measurement of aphasic disability. *Can. J. Neur. Sciences*, 1, 7–16 (1974).

KRASHEN, S., Cerebral asymmetry. In *Studies in Neurolinguistics, Vol. 2*, eds. H. Whitaker and H. Whitaker. New York: Academic Press (1976).

LARSEN, G., Rehabilitation of dysphagia paralytica. *J. Speech Hearing Dis.*, 37, 187–194 (1972).

LASS, N., AND OTHERS, A normative study of children's performance on the short form of the *Token Test J. Commun. Dis.*, 8, 193–198 (1975).

LeMAY, M., AND N. GESCHWIND, Asymmetries of the human cerebral hemisphere. In *Language Acquisition and Language Breakdown*, eds. A. Caramazza and E. Zurif. Baltimore: Johns Hopkins Press (1978).

LENNEBERG, E., In search of a dynamic theory of aphasia. In *Foundation of Language Development, Vol. 2*, eds., E. Lenneberg and E. Lenneberg. New York: Academic Press (1975).

LOGEMANN, J., *Evaluation and Treatment of Swallowing Disorders*. San Diego: College-Hill Press (1983).

LONGSTRETH, D., The BELZ dysphagia scale. Paper presented at the convention of the American-Speech-Language-Hearing Association, Detroit, Michigan (1986).

MALKMUS, D., B. BOOTH, AND D. KODIMER, *Rehabilitation of the Head-Injured Adult: Comprehensive Adaptive Management*. Downey, Calif.: Professional Staff Association of Rancho Los Amigos Hospital (1980).

MARQUARDT, T., J. STOLL, AND H. SUSSMAN, Disorders of communication in traumatic brain injury. In *Traumatic Brain Injury*, ed. E. Bigler (pp. 181–205). Austin, Tex.: Pro-Ed (1990).

MARTIN, A., Aphasia testing: A second look at the *Porch Index of Communicative Ability*. *J. Speech Hearing Dis.*, 42, 536–546 (1977).

McNEIL, M., AND R. KENT, Motor characteristics of adult aphasic and apraxic speakers. In *Cerebral Control of Speech and Limb Movements*, ed. G. E. Hammond (pp. 349–386) New York: Elsevier Science Publishers (1990).

McNEIL, M., T. PRESCOTT, AND E. CHANG, A measure of PICA ordinality. In *Clinical Aphasiology Conference Proceedings*, ed. R. Brookshire. Minneapolis: BRK Publishers (1975).

McNEIL, M., AND T. PRESCOTT, *Revised Token Test*, Baltimore: University Park Press (1978).

MILLER, R., Evaluation of swallowing disorders. In *Dysphagia Diagnosis and Management*, ed. M. Groher. Boston: Butterworths (1984).

MYERS, P., Right hemisphere impairment. In *Language Disorders in Adults*, ed. A. Holland. San Diego: College-Hill Press (1984).

NICHOLAS, M., L. OBLER, M. ALBERT, AND N. HELM-ESTABROOKS, Empty speech in Alzheimer's disease and fluent aphasia. *J. Speech Hearing Res.*, 28, 405–410 (1985).

ODELL, K., M. McNEIL, J. ROSENBEK, AND L. HUNTER, Perceptual characteristics of consonant production by apraxic speakers. *J. Speech Hearing Dis.*, 55, 345–359 (1990).

PENFIELD, W., AND L. ROBERTS, *Speech and Brain Mechanisms*. Princeton, N.J.: Princeton University Press (1959).

PIMENTAL, P., AND N. KINGSBURY, *Mini Inventory of Right Brain Injury*. Austin, Tex.: Pro-Ed (1989).

PORCH, B., *The Porch Index of Communicative Ability*. Palo Alto, Calif.: Consulting Psychologists Press (1967, 1971).

PRICE, G., C. JONES, R. CHARLTON, AND C. ALLEN, A combined approach to the assessment of neurological dysphagia. *Clin. Otolaryng.*, 12, 197–201 (1987).

RAVEN, J., *Guide to Using the Coloured Progressive Matrices*. London: H. K. Lewis (1963).

RICHARDSON, A., AND T. MARQUARDT, Language skills and communication breakdown in senile dementia. *Aus. J. Human Commun. Dis.*, 13, 75–93 (1985).

ROSENBEK, J., AND R. WERTZ, Veterans Administration Workshop on Motor Speech Disorders, Madison, Wisconsin (1976).

ROSS, D., *Ross Information Processing Assessment*. Austin, Tex.: Pro-Ed (1986).

SARNO, M. T., *The Functional Communication Profile*. New York: New York University Medical Center Rehabilitation Monograph 42 (1969).

SHEWAN, C., AND A. KERTESZ, Reliability and validity characteristics of the Western Aphasia Battery (WAB). *J. Speech Hearing Dis.*, 45, 308–324 (1980).

SCHUELL, H., *Minnesota Test for the Differential Diagnosis of Aphasia*. Minneapolis: University of Minnesota Press (1965).

SIMMONS, N., Review of clinical management of right hemisphere dysfunction, procedure manual, and Rehabilitation Institute of Chicago Examination of Communication Problems in Right Hemisphere Dysfunction (RICE). *Asha*, 28, 72–73 (1986).

SPREEN, O., AND A. BENTON, *Neurosensory Center Comprehensive Examination for Aphasia*. Victoria, B.C.: Neuropsychology Laboratory, University of Victoria (1969).

TAYLOR, M., AND E. SANDS, Reliability measures of the Functional Communication Profile. Paper presented at the American Speech and Hearing Association Convention, Chicago, Illinois (1965).

WATSON, J., AND L. RECORDS, The effectiveness of the Porch Index of Communicative Ability as a diagnostic tool in assessing specific behaviors of senile dementia. In *Clinical Aphasiology: Conference Proceedings 1978*, ed. R. Brookshire. Minneapolis: BRK Publishers (1978).

WEISENBERG, T., AND K. MCBRIDE, *Aphasia*. New York: The Commonwealth Fund (1935).

WEPMAN, J., AND L. JONES, *The Language Modalities Test for Aphasia*. Chicago: Education-Industry Service (1961).

YIVISAKER, M., AND S. SZEKERES, Management of the patient with closed-head injury. In *Language Intervention Strategies in Adult Aphasia*, 2nd ed. R. Chapey. Baltimore: Williams & Wilkins (1986).

YORKSTON, K., AND D. BEUKELMAN, A clinician-judged technique for quantifying dysarthric speech based on single-word intelligibility. *J. Commun. Dis.*, 13, 15–31 (1980).

YORKSTON, K., AND D. BEUKELMAN, *Assessment of Intelligibility of Dysarthric Speech*. Tigard, Oreg.: C. C. Publications (1981).

11

Clinical Reporting and Record Keeping

An expert gives an objective opinion, he gives his own.

Desai

The clinical report in the field of speech pathology and audiology has grown up in this age of accountability. It is no longer adequate or acceptable, if it ever was, for the report of a half-year's therapy contact with a child to be reduced to an informationally empty statement such as: "Johnny is doing well, is more cooperative than at first, and will be continued in therapy." Even if we assume that we know what he is "doing well" at, there are no behavioral descriptions and no measurements on which to base clinical judgments. Accountability implies measurements—measurement as base-line performance and as an increment of progress toward an agreed-upon and stated goal. Accountability demands that the purchaser of services be able to decide whether the benefits to be derived outweigh the investments of time, inconvenience, and money. The documentation of speech and language skill was the concern of the bulk of the preceding chapters. The interpretation and communication of the significance of these performance skills are both the basis and the reason for the clinical report. We discuss three types of clinical reports, according to the purposes for which they are written: the diagnostic or initial evaluation report, the periodic or terminal clinical summary, and the daily contact report. These reports differ in form but not in purpose—each is constructed to communicate necessary clinical information.

WHAT A REPORT IS—AND WHAT IT IS NOT

A report is an answer to a stated or an implied question; therefore, the writer's first task is to determine what question is to be answered and to whom the answer is directed. The question may be whether or not a communication problem exists; or if there is agreement that a problem exists, the question may be what can be done about it. Clinical settings are also an important consideration. As Taylor (1977) has pointed out, not only will form and style differ among similar clinical settings, but specific settings may require specialized types of reporting. For example, a speech consultation in a medical setting is usually brief. The need for clarity and brevity exists in every setting but may be of paramount importance here. The medical speech consultation report does not include the extensive case history information typically found in other parts of the hospital record, and most test details and specifics are not included although they are maintained for your records. Your consultation report for most medical-setting purposes may include only what would have been summary, conclusions, and recommendations of the report you write in another setting. In most medical settings, you are asked to supply a short description of the communication problem presented and what can be done about it.

However, our purpose here is not to outline standards of form for all clinical settings. Purposes as well as local preferences dictate a variety of forms and procedures in report writing. What the variety has in common is that all reports should be designed to communicate the nature of the problem, if one exists, and to outline a plan of care for its remediation. Nation and Aram (1977) outline the diagnostician's task in these words:

> The diagnostician asks himself four interrelated yes/no questions. Can the client change his disordered behavior? Is therapeutic intervention necessary to do so? Are referrals necessary? Is service available? Depending on his answers to these questions, he proceeds to think through the various management alternatives appropriate to the disorder, its causes, and the personal characteristics of the client. He develops a definitive plan of action to offer to the client during the interpretive conference. . . . The information of prime importance to impart is who is going to do what, when, and where. (pp. 332, 328)

A report is not an excuse to pontificate, confabulate, or obfuscate. In other words, one should avoid the unnecessary use of words, such as those contained in the last sentence, because they are less likely to transmit the answer you wish to communicate than if you choose less exotic words. The language used in a report should not be pompous, dogmatic, chatty, or informal, and the information contained should not be confused or obscured by the inclusion of irrelevant statements.

WRITING STYLE

There are a number of publications concerned with writing style in the speech and hearing literature. Notable among them are articles by Jerger (1962), Moore (1969), and Pannbacker (1975). These three have been singled out from the larger number of well-written and informative articles because of the free use of examples of bad writing style they include to help make their points clear. There is general agreement as to what constitutes good writing style (see also Good 1970; Knepflar 1976; Sanders 1972; Wolfle 1967) and few points of disagreement.

Use of Pronouns.   One such point of apparent disagreement is in the use of personal pronouns. Jerger (1962) advocates their use—but not overuse—on the assumption that personal pronouns will make the report sound more natural.

> Nothing livens up dull material like personal references. Use them often. Especially, use personal pronouns like I, me, we, you, she, they, etc. Don't use them to excess— the excessive repetition of anything makes dull reading—but don't be afraid to use them when they are clearly necessary in order to say a thing naturally. (pp. 102–103)

Emerick and Hatten (1974), on the other hand, think that first- and second-person pronouns should be avoided. Johnson and others (1963) stated that the tone of the report should be impersonal and that personal pronouns should be used only to make a statement clearer. English and Lillywhite (1963) advocate the use of personal pronouns only when the writer wishes to emphasize that an opinion or a feeling is being expressed for which she has no immediate objective, supportive evidence. A probable consensus among experienced report writers would be to maintain an impersonal and relatively formal tone in reporting clinical information but not to abrogate personal responsibility, especially in expressing an opinion. In other words, use personal references when necessary. More important than the use of personal pronouns, as such, is the issue of clarity. Jerger (1962) reminds us that in scientific reporting the object is to convey to the reader what you did, why you did it, and what you found.

A comprehensive list of *dos* and *don'ts* specifically applicable to clinical reports would be difficult to write partly because it almost certainly would include many personal preferences and would, therefore, be more biased than stylistic. Moore (1969) liberally quoted from Strunk and White's (1959) *The Elements of Style* in listing a set of rules to be followed in writing clearly and concisely. She listed three primary "symptoms" in determining when writing was defective. According to Moore (1969, p. 535), report writing is defective when it is (1) unintelligible—the report is unclear, (2) conspicuous—the reader pays more attention to how the report is written than to the content, or (3) confusing—if the reader is confused, the writer may well have been confused. Clear thinking cannot be illustrated by fuzzy writing.

Most of Strunk and White's rules are straightforward. For example, "Use definite, specific, concrete language. Prefer the specific to the general, the definite to the vague, the concrete to the abstract" (p. 15). This effectively translates as "say what you mean and mean what you say."

Avoid Jargon.   A number of authors (e.g., Fisher 1969; Knepflar 1976; Taylor 1977; Wolfle 1967) express the admonition to avoid jargon. One of Moore's quoted examples expressed this "conspicuous writing" symptom as

> The patient exhibited apparent partial paralysis of motor units of the superior sinistral fibres of the genioglossus resulting in insufficient lingual approximation of the palatoalveolar region. A condition of insufficient frenulum development was noted, producing not only sigmatic distortion but also obvious ankyloglossia. (p. 536)

Translation: "the patient was tongue-tied and dysarthric." Similarly, a report of "dactyl speech" is not as informative as "finger spelling." Commenting on this same point, Pannbacker (1975) has urged that "only terms in common use by professionals should be used." The difficulty results from the fact that

> [professional workers] all have their jargons; fads abound; authors strain for effects; long words replace short ones, and ignorance, carelessness, a false idea of what constitutes proper style, overuse of the passive voice, and kindred sins all make unnecessary trouble for the readers. (Wolfle 1967, p. 55)

Use of Qualifiers.   One of those kindred sins is the overuse of qualifiers. One Strunk and White rule (quoted by Moore 1969) was to avoid the use of qualifiers; words like "rather," "very," "little," "pretty" "are leeches that infest the pond of prose, sucking the blood of words" (Strunk and White 1959, p. 59). An earlier rule we quoted was to use definite, concrete, specific language. Qualifiers insert a lack of precision and an indefinite tone to otherwise acceptable descriptions. Less experienced report writers are especially prone to hide behind nebulous descriptions—"a little restless," "somewhat delayed," "seems to be," "appears to have"— as if they could abrogate the responsibility of their professional judgment by being less precise. A report *is* a professional opinion and only that. As we discussed at the beginning of this text, there is no ethical requirement that the clinician always be right—only that he makes his best professional judgment based on appropriate tests and observations.

A valid point can be made that not all of our observations and test results can be precisely calibrated or determined. There is a place for "in my opinion" or "it appears to me" statements. Therefore, the suggestion may be made that you go back through and scratch off all the qualifier words after you have finished a report. Then go through again and put back only those that must be included. When we discuss the form or the outline for reports, it will be apparent that sections concerning the history of the problem, the data concerning measurement of the speech and language problem, and your interpretation of the significance of the data and recommendations for amelioration of the problem will contain different types of information.

In the case history report section, some qualifiers such as "Mrs. Jones reported that . . . " or "According to . . . " are appropriate because they remind the reader that the information or judgment is secondhand. When you report performance data gathered from speech-language testing and observations, the report is to be as calibrated and as precise as you can make it, and qualifiers are to be avoided. When you interpret the results, the reader should already be aware that what he is reading is a qualification in that it is not necessarily *the* truth but *your* truth.

One of the more succinct summary sets of report guidelines is that offered by Jerger (1962, p. 104):

1. Write short sentences. Use a new sentence for each new thought.
2. Avoid artificially and pompous embellishment. Write it the way you would say it.
3. Use active verb construction whenever possible. Avoid the passive voice.
4. Use personal pronouns when it is natural to do so.

FORM AND CONTENT OF THE REPORT

A variety of forms are in use as outlines or guidelines for clinical reporting. That is to say that there are many acceptable forms and any form that is functionally adequate to the communicative task is acceptable. For that reason, the example forms for an examination report and for a clinical summary or a progress report included in this chapter are only examples. The form, as such, is of lesser importance than the content to be included, but the use of such an outline form is useful, especially for less experienced report writers, as a reminder of what information should be included. Figure 11–1 is an example format for an initial or diagnostic report outline.

Patient Identification. The identifying information obviously includes the patient's name and address. If the patient is a child, the parents' name is also included. The inclusion of a birth date rather than an age is preferred because it may prevent later confusion in determining the child's specific age.

A file number system is probably in use at every clinical facility. This number system may be a simple numerical sequence or a code (Mueller and Peters 1976) that identifies a patient, the presenting problem, and the clinical setting. The advantages of including a file number on a report are obvious. In the same way as a file number uniquely identifies an individual patient, all reports, tests, and observations *must* be dated. An undated report is useless. In essence, the importance of the detailed heading is that it uniquely identifies a specific set of test results and interpretations for a particular patient at a particular time and place.

One other important feature of the heading is the ICD-9-CM number. In addition to the two sureties of life (death and taxes), add a third. If the Congress legislates a function, a third constant is that the federal government will create an agency. Acronyms are spawned by agencies almost as if they were a requirement. ICD-9-CM is translated as "International Classification of Diseases, 9th Revision, Clinical Modifications," published by the U.S. Department of Health and Human Services. The ICD codes are in three volumes. Volume 1 is a tabular list of diseases; volume 2 is an alphabetic list of diseases; and volume 3 is a tabular and alphabetic list of procedures. A problem such as "Developmental Language Disorder" is a three-digit number—315.31; a procedure such as "Hearing Examination, not otherwise specified" is a two-digit number—95.47. These code numbers are used by Medicare, Medicaid, private insurers, or other third-party payers. "Language Delay" is probably not on the insurance contract list of covered problems, but ICD-9-CM 315.31 may well be.

```
                          EXAM REPORT

                                  (Date report typed)

To: Referring source,
    Address, including zip code
                               Re:  Client's name; File No.
                               Parents:  (if a child)
                                         Address, incl. zip
                               Birthdate:
                               Diagnostic Category:
                               ICD-9-CM #:
                               Date of Evaluation:


HISTORY AND REFERRAL:

  Pertinent birth and early development history; pertinent medical
history; parental description of early speech and language development;
reason for referral--who was concerned for what reason.


SIGNIFICANT FINDINGS:

  Observations and test findings;


RECOMMENDATIONS:

  Disposition--reevaluation, therapy, parental counseling, referral
elsewhere; plus prognosis statement.


                               Reported by:



                               Name, degree, certification
                               Speech Pathologist


                               Assisted by:
                               Student clinician



Copies to: (if any)
```

FIGURE 11–1

There are other lists of codes for these purposes—for example, the CPT numbers (Current Procedural Terminology, published by the American Medical Association). The CPT codes are five-digit numbers (e.g., 92506 "Medical Evaluation of Speech, Language, and/or Hearing Problems"), but these numbers are not appropriate to speech pathology or to audiology services because, by definition, CPT-coded services are under the direction of a physician.

Complaint. If a report is an answer to a question, it helps to know what the question is. The complaint or the reason for the referral should be included in your report as a separate heading or in the history section.

History. The critical guideline for what is to be included in the history section is the word "pertinent." If test findings suggest delayed speech and language, for example, either normal or deviant developmental milestones could be significant. On the other hand, if the patient is an adult who has suffered a stroke, early developmental history would probably not be important, although status before the cerebral damage would be important in terms of expected recovery. The diagnostician in her detective role, as discussed in Chapter 2, is expected to include here the information that could be significant to the problem or problems presented and to the remediation plan proposed.

Examination Results. Knepflar (1976) has suggested separate sections with headings for case history, hearing, speech mechanism, articulation, voice, language, fluency and rate, psychological factors, clinical impressions, and recommendations. Let us agree with Knepflar on the advisability of including all of these observations in the report and suggest that at least the case history, test results and clinical impressions, and summary and recommendations be shown under separate headings. In Chapter 2, we discussed the importance of separating information which was gathered by direct observation (objective) from that which was reported to us (subjective). It is also important to separate test results from interpretation. In contrast, it is less important if you prefer reporting areas of test results by paragraph separation or by separate-heading separation.

There should be no difference of opinion among professionals as to whether a young child's voice and fluency should at least be informally evaluated; the difference of opinion is whether or not "normal" behaviors that were not part of the referral reason bear reporting. Our bias is in favor of this reporting. It takes little time and space to report that "voice quality and fluency were normal" for the child's age, and it at least alerts the reader that we were concerned about the total communication picture.

As we commented earlier, the purpose of the outline for formulation of your report is to cue the reader to the information to be found in different sections. Obviously, it should also remind the writer what is to be included where. The data collected and their significance are a function of the measurement devices used. For example, you may well report that "Henry obtained a vocabulary recognition age-score of 5–7 (chronological age 6–3) on the *Peabody Picture Vocabulary Test–Revised.*" This system immediately does two things. It shows where the data came from, and it provides a comparison by your inclusion of the child's chronological age. In the summary or impressions section, you would report that the vocabulary recognition score was within normal limits for his age. It is important to report how you measured or judged a performance. If you report that the child obtained a language-age score of 6–6 (C.A. 6–6) on the *Utah Test of Language Development* and was, therefore, normal in his expressive language skills, you at least give the knowledgeable reader a chance to disagree. The Utah test is developmental in nature rather than specific to syntax, grammar, and so on. In that sense, you would not have the same theoretical basis for your judgment that expressive language skills were within normal limits that you would have from a structural description obtained from the *Developmental Sentence Scoring* procedure. One more example may help to emphasize the point. If four-year-old Johnny's articulation skill was determined from administration of the *Templin-Darley Screening Test of Articulation*, your report would indicate the number of correct productions.

> Johnny correctly produced 30 of the 50 articulation screening items on the *Templin-Darley Tests of Articulation*. The average performance for a boy of this age is approximately 35 correct, but 23 correct productions is considered adequate. Errors in articulation were primarily on /s/ and /l/ sounds in two- and three-element blends but which Johnny correctly produced in other contexts. Articulation skill is judged as within normal limits for his age, and he is readily intelligible.

If you used a single-phoneme test, as was described in Chapter 3, your judgment of adequate or inadequate would be based on which phonemes were in error and which set of age-of-acquisition norms you chose for comparison.

The point to be emphasized is that your examination data are to be reported as specific to a test, with necessary descriptions or normative comparisons, and that test results are to be separated from the interpretive summary. The examination results are your data. Your interpretation of the significance of the results (in the clinical impressions or summary section) is then your professional judgment. It should be possible for another speech-language pathologist to accept your data and to make a different interpretation of their significance.

Diagnostic Summary (Clinical Impressions).   As the writer of the diagnostic examination report, you are being asked to express your professional opinion. It is appropriate in this section of your report to summarize the pertinent results and to make an interpretation. Earlier, we talked about the use of personal opinions and personal pronouns (English and Lillywhite 1963; Jerger 1962) in making it clear to the reader that what is being expressed as an opinion may go beyond the available data. In other words, this is your truth.

William Rusher (1981), in a book entitled *How to Win Arguments*, described what he termed "expert evidence." He noted that "facts come in various sizes—or perhaps I should say in varying degrees of specific gravity" (p. 78) and that "the best and often the only counter to expert evidence is rival expert evidence" (p. 84). The point to be made is that in a diagnostic report you are reporting the evidence as you see it, and you are the expert. The purpose of your argument (expression of opinion) is that you expect the reader to believe your interpretation.

Recommendations.   Just as the *interpretations* were your professional opinion, so are the *recommendations*. They are your personal judgment as to what you think should be done about the problems you have described. A separate section ensures that you have included this information in your report and that it is readily identifiable. It may also be helpful to the agency or person to whom your report is addressed and whose primary interest may be how you intend to address the problem. The most important statements you write may be those that summarize the problem as you see it and recommend what can be done about it.

The expected outcome, the prognosis, should not be avoided. A prognostic statement is not only required by the ASHA Professional Services Board standards but is required by your professional sense of fair play and logic. If you took your car to the local garage because of an operational problem, you would expect to have some estimate of the time and the cost of repair. Should you do less for the repair (remediation) of the problems you are in charge of fixing? You are expected to provide a prognosis or judgment of what you expect to accomplish with a therapy regime. This is not a guarantee; it is your judgment that the outcome will or will not be favorable and your idea of the duration of the therapy. The ASHA code of Ethics (1992), which enjoins you to "hold paramount the welfare of persons [you] serve professionally" also includes a proscription against misrepresentation: "Misrepresentation also includes the failure to state any information that is material and that ought, in fairness, to be considered."

A further reminder that you are providing your professional judgments—and that you have the responsibility to communicate them—is that

> Individuals shall not provide professional services without exercising independent professional judgment, regardless of referral source or prescription. (Principles of Ethics IV, E)

That statement not only speaks to your training and expertise in specialized and specific areas of the discipline before you attempt the diagnosis and/or intervention, it is also a reminder that you are reporting the test results and observations as *your* professional judgments. You are legally (professionally) and ethically responsible for your judgments. When you work in concert with other professionals—as in many clinical environments such as school systems in which Individualized Educational Plans are established and continued by federal mandates and it is most efficient to have one member of the IEP team do the interpretation to clients/parents—it is still your responsibility, both ethically and legally, to provide considered professional judgments:

> If the speech-language pathologist or audiologist does not communicate findings and recommendations directly to the client, that speech-language pathologist or audiologist remains responsible for ensuring that the findings and recommendations are communicated to the client and relayed correctly and completely by a competent professional. (ASHA 1992, p. 9)

Your legal responsibility includes your obligation to make recommendations, for example, in the school setting what you think is "educationally necessary." Recommendations are not prescriptions—and are not mandates. The agency, the parent, the prospective consumer of your services may choose to ignore your recommendation—or may accept a different recommendation from some other equally trained and certified speech-language professional. That, after all, is what second opinions are about. If one physician recommends that surgery should be considered, a second physician may offer another choice.

Progress Report

A progress report, or therapy summary, by definition, is an answer to a different question. The purpose of the initial or diagnostic evaluation is to provide the database or description of what the problem was like when first identified—at least in your shop. If the initial evaluation was your baseline data, the progress report is a measurement of change as a function of treatment. The progress report outline shown as Figure 11–2 is obviously only an example. Identifying information as previously described is a constant on all reports. In addition, the identification of how long and with what frequency therapy has been scheduled is helpful for a number of comparative and bookkeeping purposes. One obvious example is for the ease of collecting length-of-stay data for audit purposes. That is, how many hours of therapy are usually required in your clinical setting for any particular diagnostic category (an aphasic adult, a cerebral-palsied child, a teenager who stutters, and so on) to reach maximum potential? Of course, not every patient will present the same problems, and not every client responds equally well to the remediation regime, but your range and median hours when compared to those of other clinicians and clinics can tell you something about the relative effectiveness of your therapeutic process. We mentioned the idea of accountability at the beginning of this chapter. It will be discussed more fully in the section concerned with the daily reporting of clinical activities.

Status at Beginning of Period.   By analogy to the examination report, this section of the progress report represents the baseline for the reporting period. Information from the previous description (or descriptions) is briefly abstracted to show the entering baseline performance, the speech-language performance at the beginning of the current period for comparative purposes, and any important considerations that influenced change or lack of change.

Summary of Therapy.   Essentially, a summary of therapy amounts to a statement of what was done or attempted, why and how, and to what effect. Many training programs will require students to write out a specific set of goals and procedures before therapy begins. The difference between the clinician-in-training and the experienced clinician in this respect may be the degree to which the goals and procedures are written out, not the degree to which plans are formulated. For the purposes of the progress report, the critical information is once again a description of current speech and language performance. The more precise your descriptions, the more readily you can determine changes toward the goal originally set, or the modified goal, in your plan-of-care statement. For example, if one of your goals for a child was the inclusion of past-tense morphemes in her speech, your summary may report that "Susan was correct on 80 percent of her regular verb, past-tense endings and 75 percent of the irregular verb endings in structured response situations." This section is a summary or an abstract in the truest sense of the word. All of the details of your day-to-day contact are not included for obvious reasons. It is, however, important to include sufficient description of the *how* and the *why* of your intervention procedure to allow either a continuation of successful procedures or a modification of goals and procedures, if expected progress was not realized. Descriptive statements of this type will allow a comparative audit of procedures at a later time.

```
                              PROGRESS REPORT

Name:                              Clinic No:
Address:                           Diagnostic Category:
                                   ICD-9-CM
                                   Period Covered:   (Quarter, Year)
Phone No:                          Date of Report:   (Date report typed)
School Status:
Birthdate:        Age:

Clinic Schedule:                   Hours Individual (I) Therapy:
  Sessions per week:               Hours Group (G) Therapy:
  Length of session:               Cumulative Hours of I Therapy:
  Number of clinic visits:         Cumulative Hours of G Therapy:


STATUS AT BEGINNING OF PERIOD:

(Short, abstract of information taken from first contact with clinic--
such as diagnostic, reevaluation, hearing report--description of previous
therapy--description of all behaviors (speech, language, attentiveness,
motivation) at the beginning of this reporting period.)


SUMMARY OF THERAPY:

(The summary is to include goals, procedures, results and/or evalua-
tions of the case. Also to be included are description of response to
therapy, impressions of performance, problems in therapy.)


RECOMMENDATIONS

(Be specific so that the reader knows what to expect next and for what
purpose. What is planned in terms of goals and probable methods--and what
is the expected outcome.)




                              _____
                                   (Supervisor will sign here)
                              Supervised by:(Type name, degree)
                                            Speech Pathologist


                              _____
                                            (Sign name)
                              (Type name)    Student Clinician
```

FIGURE 11–2

Recommendations.   The primary requirement in writing recommendations is to be specific. Recommendations are the nearest thing to prescriptions that speech-language clinicians write. Tell the reader what, in your opinion, is to be done as continuation or as modification from what was done in the current therapy period, for what continued or changed purpose, with what frequency, where, by whom, and the expected outcome.

One word has been occurring with some degree of frequency throughout this chapter. That word is "opinion." One chord struck in Chapter 1, and repeated in a number of other places, was the idea of fallibility. The diagnostic instruments and observations we have discussed may not have appraised everything that is important for the formulations of our clinical interaction. If for no other reason than the recognition that this, like other people-oriented professions, is not an exact science, the "in-my-opinion" statement is an acceptable fence-riding hedge. That statement is the basis for the caveat that the report writer must label and separate statements of fact, reports and conjecture, and interpretations. Just as another speech-language pathologist may find it possible to make a different interpretation from your reported data, it may also be possible for him to arrive at a different set of recommendations.

Daily or Therapy Contact Reports

At the beginning of this chapter, we commented on accountability in our evaluation and therapy reporting. Over the last few years, much more attention has been paid to report writing, both as periodic summaries and as daily contact notes. To a large degree, this greater concern and greater precision have been required because of third-party accounting. Medicare, Medicaid, and the federal mandates contained in Public Law 94-142 are examples of this third-party interest. There are two inevitable accompaniments to the occurrence of state and federal support for speech-language and hearing services. One is the proliferation of regulatory guidelines, as mentioned earlier, and the second is the acrostic use of initials to identify what otherwise might have been descriptive phrases. Examples in point for our reporting purposes are PCAs, IEPs, POMR, and SOAP.

PCAs.   PCAs or Patient Care Audits are only peripherally part of our current report writing concern. Patient Care Audits are part of a larger issue identified as quality assurance. An assurance that the services we provide are qualitatively adequate is not only a logical concern, for the provider as well as for the purchaser of services, it is also the implicit reason for all of the recording and reporting of clinical contact. Patient Care Audits are frequently retrospective in the sense that they may be concerned with whether or not we have routinely included in our clinical folders all of the information we have decided is minimal. For example, the members of a clinical group may have decided that all folders for clients seen on an initial speech-language evaluation must include

a. a complete case history form
b. a pure-tone hearing screening
c. a vocabulary assessment
d. an articulation test
e. a measure of receptive and expressive language skill
f. an examination of the oral mechanism

Because we did not specify a number of variables such as age of subjects or degree of cooperation, it would not be logical to assume that 100 percent of the folders to be reviewed for these data will include all of what we decided were minimum requirements. For example, it may be fair to assume that 100 percent of the folders would have a case history interview but that some of the clients were young children on whom we could not get a hearing screening test or a vocabulary test and the like. It would be usual to set our performance criteria at something less than 100 percent but more than 75 percent, if that percentage was considered "minimal."

We may select 90 percent or 85 percent or some other reasonable degree of compliance. Our retrospective review may include all of the cases of this type seen in the previous six months or the last 50 cases of this category or some other representative number. Those folders are pulled from the file and checked to see if they include evidence of the criteria we had chosen. Folders that do not contain all of the listed measures are reviewed by a professional member of the clinic group to see why the noted deficiencies occurred. This information, along with the tally of the percentage of folders that did contain each of the specified measures, is then presented to the entire clinic group for discussion. The identification of deficiencies in the folders or the reports is not to fix blame on individuals but to decide if changes in clinic procedures are necessary to ensure that all the necessary data are collected and reported. It is also possible, as a result of the discussion, that some measures earlier specified as minimal may be deleted from the "minimal" list. The next audit on the same category, at some specified future time, would tell whether the changed procedures had led to the inclusion of the desired data.

Patient Care Audits may be on diagnostic categories, as the previous example; they may be on procedures of therapy or testing and test selection; or they may be outcome audits. An outcome audit is concerned with the effectiveness of the intervention regime. It has to do with total hours of therapy contact and whether the client had reached her maximum potential when dismissed. In the strictest sense, the outcome audit is the real measure of quality of services provided. Drucker (1974), in a text concerned with business management, defines two words that are frequently confused but are pertinent to our discussion of quality of services. The words are "efficiency" and "effectiveness." *Efficiency* is defined as doing well those procedures that we selected; effectiveness is selecting the most appropriate procedures. It is possible to be efficient in procedures that may not be the most effective in outcome. Outcome audits are concerned with the efficiency of effective procedures.

IEPs. Individual Education Plans (IEPs) are mandated by Public Law 94-142. The Education for All Handicapped Children Act of 1975 demanded an appropriate free public education for all handicapped children from 3 to 21 years of age. The Ninety-ninth Congress, in PL 99-457, reauthorized the PL 94-142 legislation and extended the age range downward to include infants. The implementation of this legislation was left to the individual states.[1] The importance of this legislation for our purposes is the reminder of accountability and the importance of communication with the consumer (parent).

The law states that IEPs are to be developed in conjunction with the parent,

[1]The inclusion of children under 5 and over 18 was not required if it was inconsistent with the state law and practice.

the classroom teacher, and a representative of the local educational agency. The PL 99-457 reauthorization is more flexible in organizational mandate than 94-142. For example, classroom teachers will less frequently be involved than early childhood education specialists in educational planning for high-risk infants. To ensure the completeness and appropriateness of the specialized intervention plan, representatives of professional specialties involved in the educational plan may also be included. The IEPs that are developed and periodically reviewed must include

a. a statement of the present levels of educational performance of each such child
b. a statement of annual goals, including short-term instructional objectives
c. a statement of the specific educational services to be provided to each child and the extent to which the child will be able to participate in regular educational programs
d. the projected date of initiation and anticipated duration of such services
e. appropriate objective criteria and evaluation procedures and schedules for determining, at least on an annual basis, whether instructional objectives are achieved

For the purposes of this discussion, our analysis of what the child requires in terms of speech/language/hearing needs is assembled within the framework of his total educational requirements. The items in the IEP obviously require descriptive statements of the problems presented, concise plans for remediation, and goals and objectives that are sufficiently objective to allow measurement. Once again, statements of the problem, descriptive data, interpretations, and recommendations must be separable.

We have been discussing the type of information to be included in a report and the separation of the report into sections for the purpose of easier communication. Watson and Thompson (1983) reported a study in which a group of professionals and a group of parents were asked to make evaluative judgments of the information they received in a postdiagnostic conference. Eighty percent of the professionals and the parents indicated that they gained useful information concerning the child's problem and what to do about it. But more than 10 percent of the parents stated that they failed to understand the findings. As a general rule, the 80 percent "useful" figure is probably high, and the 10 percent "failure to understand" figure may well be low.

POMR—SOAP.   Just as IEPs are usually associated with school programs, POMR and SOAP (Bouchard and Shane 1977) are most often associated with hospital-based programs. POMR stands for Problem Oriented Medical Records. This record-keeping system was not developed specifically for speech-language pathology but like the IEP format can be used effectively by speech-language pathologists. The database is the core of information that is collected for description of the patient. It includes such things as the development of the problem, the present complaint, the life situation insofar as it bears on the problem or the remediation of identified problems, and the results of evaluations from speech pathology and others concerned with the "total" patient. Problems are identified, listed, and numbered on a "problem list" at the front of the patient folder. This list serves as a table of contents and includes the initial plans for patient care as well as a rationale for new testing when appropriate, plans for therapy, and patient education. For example, with a stroke patient, problems identified may include self-help and self-care skills (or activities for daily living), muscle reeducation and locomotion, language and communication, and education of the patient and family as to what to expect in terms of recovery. Problem notes are placed in the daily record and are identified with appropriate problem numbers.

The patient information is placed under four columns in the record, and this is where SOAP comes in. SOAP stands for Subjective, Objective, Assessment, and Plans. The four headings are defined by Bouchard and Shane (1977) as

Subjective	—information supplied by the client and his family including the complaint and the symptoms from their point of view
Objective	—those observations made by the clinician from his viewpoint as well as all objective information received from referral sources
Assessment	—evaluation of the problems presented based on subjective and objective findings—i.e., the measurements
Plans	—plans for further testing, for therapeutic intervention, and for patient education for the numerically identified problems each member of the therapeutic regime is concerned with

This discussion holds no brief for any particular type of daily record keeping. Obviously, some have more relevance for specific settings than others. What is important is the daily, brief, descriptive notation of what happened, when, and to what avail. Daily notes must be recorded in ink and signed by the clinician as part of Medicare regulations. Medicaid is administered by states, so regulations are more variable. One other comment may be appropriate to underline the importance of daily therapy records. They can be considered legal documents and are subject to review and audit, especially for the Special Education Act and Medicare purposes. It probably goes without saying that the certified clinician-in-charge (case manager) writes and signs the daily therapy notes rather than the student-trainee in clinician training programs.

SUMMARY

We have discussed both form and substance of report writing. Listings of dos and don'ts have been provided in a number of published sources for the writing of reports. What they have in common is the insistence on clarity and the requirement that a report communicate information from the writer to the reader. The importance of concise, informative, and descriptive reports cannot be overemphasized. In a legal sense, if the therapeutic contact was not documented and recorded, for all practical purposes it did not occur. A report is a communication that also has relevance beyond the immediate information to be conveyed. Knepflar (1976) expressed it this way:

> The need for effective report writing [is important] to all professionals in our field. How do physicians, dentists, psychologists, social workers, educators, and other professionals judge our capabilities, whether we represent a hospital, a community agency, a public school system, or a college or university? The answer to that question is: through our ability to communicate concisely and effectively, in language that can be easily understood. More often than not, this communication is written rather than oral. (p. xii)

We have discussed three types of clinical reports: initial or diagnostic descriptions, periodic or so-called progress reports of ongoing clinical contact, and special purpose reports including daily record keeping. Outlines for the diagnostic report and for the progress report were included as examples. There is no single acceptable format for writing reports. What is important is that information be included that adequately describes the problem and what will be (or has been) done about it. The interpretation of subjective and objective findings is a professional judgment—and the interpretation of significance and recommendations for what is to be done are statements of the writer's professional opinion. That fact does not make the judgment inherently good, bad, or otherwise. It only means that the writer must be certain that baseline data and interpretations of those data are separable.

REFERENCES

ASHA, Code of Ethics. *ESB Education Standards Board Manual.* Rockville, Md.: American Speech-Language-Hearing Association (1992).

AMERICAN SPEECH-LANGUAGE-HEARING ASSOCIATION, Prescription. *Asha,* 34 (Suppl. 9), 9 (1992).

BOUCHARD, M. M., AND H. C. SHANE, Use of the problem-oriented medical record in the speech and hearing profession (Special Report) *Asha,* 19, 157–159 (1977).

DRUCKER, P. F., *Management: Tasks, Responsibilities, Practices.* New York: Harper & Row (1974).

EMERICK, L., AND J. HATTEN, *Diagnosis and Evaluation in Speech Pathology.* Englewood Cliffs, N.J.: Prentice Hall (1974).

ENGLISH, R., AND H. LILLYWHITE, A semantic approach to clinical reporting in speech pathology. *Asha,* 5, 647–650 (1963).

FISHER, L. I., Reporting: In the schools to the community. In *Clinical Speech in the Schools,* ed. R. J. Van Hattum. Springfield, Ill.: Charles C Thomas (1969).

GOOD, R., The written language of rehabilitation medicine: Meanings and usages. *Arch. Phys. Med. Rehabil.,* 51, 296–336 (1970).

JERGER, J., Scientific writing can be readable. *Asha,* 4, 101–104 (1962).

JOHNSON, W., F. L. DARLEY, AND D. C. SPRIESTERSBACH, *Diagnostic Methods in Speech Pathology.* New York: Harper & Row (1963).

KNEPFLAR, K. J., *Report Writing in the Field of Communication Disorders.* Dansville, Ill.: Interstate Printers and Publishers (1976).

MOORE, M., Pathological writing. *Asha,* 11, 535–538 (1969).

MUELLER, P. B., AND T. J. PETERS, A clinical record-keeping system. *Asha,* 18, 352–353 (1976).

NATION, J. E., AND D. M. ARAM, *Diagnosis of Speech and Language Disorders.* St. Louis, Mo.: C. V. Mosby Co. (1977).

PANNBACKER, M., Diagnostic report writing. *J. Speech Hearing Dis.,* 40, 367–379 (1975).

RUSHER, W. A., *How to Win Arguments.* Garden City, N.Y.: Doubleday & Co. (1981).

SANDERS, L., *Procedure Guides for Evaluation of Speech and Language Disorders in Children.* Danville, Ill.: Interstate Press (1972).

STRUNK, W. JR, AND E. B. WHITE, *The Elements of Style.* New York: Macmillan (1959).

TAYLOR, M. F., Report writing in the medical setting: Some special considerations. *J. Speech Hearing Dis.,* 42, 581–582 (1977).

WATSON, B. U., AND R. W. THOMPSON, Parents' perception of diagnostic reports and conferences. *Lang. Speech Hearing Serv., Schools,* 14, 114–120 (1983).

WOLFLE, D., Bad writing. *Science, N. Y.,* 155, 37 (1967).

Name Index

Subject Index